LIFE AND LEARNING V

PROCEEDINGS OF THE FIFTH UNIVERSITY FACULTY FOR LIFE CONFERENCE

JUNE 1995 AT MARQUETTE UNIVERSITY

edited by
Joseph W. Koterski, S.J.

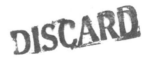

Published by University Faculty for Life
120 New North Building
Georgetown University
Washington, D.C., 20057

Printed in the United States of America

ISBN 1-886387-03-6

Preface

We are pleased to present here all the papers delivered at the fifth annual conference of the University Faculty for Life, held on the Marquette University campus in Milwaukee on June 2-4, 1995.

Special thanks are due to Marquette University and to our local hosts, Professors Al Zanoni and Richard Fehring, for a gracious and well-organized gathering. We would also like to express our gratitude to Mr. E. Lysk Wyckoff, Jr., President of the Homeland Foundation, and to Mrs. Patricia Donahoe, its Program Director, for generous financial support for this conference. And it goes without saying that the success of this meeting and the ongoing work of UFL is due in great part to our President, Fr. Thomas King, S.J., of Georgetown University and to Nora O'Callaghan, UFL's indefatigable office manager.

The wealth of scholarship presented at "Life & Learning V" is here grouped under six general headings, including a category new for these proceedings, "Literary Perspectives" (Koloze, Winderl). The five articles of a political nature (Conley, Liebman, Maloney, Wolfe, and O'Bannon) run the gamut from broadly theoretical issues to questions of nuts-and-bolts community organization. Joined to the remarks of our keynote speaker, Dr. Nigel M. de S. Cameron of Trinity International University, are three other papers from a religious point-of-view (Colliton, Gorman, and Stanford-Rue). We are also pleased to present four articles predominantly legal in focus (Moylan, Collett, Forsythe, and Rue). End-of-life issues are as hotly contested as ever, and two of the conference's papers are studies in this area (Kovach-Wilson-Noonan, Diamond). The pro-life movement itself became the object of study for three of our participants (Beckwith, Cassidy, Crosby). Papers such as these represent precisely the sort of scholarship and research which UFL was founded to promote.

Joseph W. Koterski, S.J.
Fordham University

Acknowledgements

"Shifting the Focus in the Abortion Debate" by Francis J. Beckwith is a revised and expanded version of the article "From Personhood to Autonomy: The Shifting Philosophical and Legal Focus in the Abortion Debate," in *Bioethics and the Future of Medicine*, edited by Nigel Cameron, David Schiedermayer, and John Kilner. Grand Rapids, MI: Eerdmans/Cumbria, UK: The Pasternoster Press, 1995.

The essay by Dr. Nigel M. de S. Cameron is reprinted from *God and Culture: Essays in Honor of Carl F. H. Henry*, edited by D. A. Carson and John D. Woodbridge (Grand Rapids, MI: William B. Eerdmans, 1993), pp. 321-40.

"Effects of Hospice Interventions" by Christine R. Kovach is re-published here with the permission of Nancy Stone Hindlian, Prime National Publishing Corporation, for the *American Journal of Alzheimer's Care and Related Disorders and Research* where it will appear shortly.

The essay by Dr. Christopher Wolfe that appears in this volume is a revised form of "Abortion and Political Compromise" and is printed here with the permission of Rev. Richard John Neuhaus, Editor of *First Things*, where it appeared in Issue #24, June/July 1992.

The article by Dr. Vincent Rue is based upon a previously published work in *Research Bulletin* 9/1 (1995).

Dr. John Crosby's article is an adaptation for UFL of a piece whose definitive text will appear in the summer 1996 issue of *Communio*.

Table of Contents

LEGAL PERSPECTIVES

QUESTIONS AT LIFE'S END

THE PRO-LIFE MOVEMENT

DEMOGRAPHIC POLICY
AND ETHICAL PRINCIPLE

John J. Conley, S.J.

The controversy over the final document approved by the International Conference on Population and Development in Cairo (1994)[1] indicates the bitter political dispute over population policy on the international level. The Cairo battle pivoted around the opposition between two ideological-economical blocs which one might characterize as the coalition of the religious poor and the coalition of the secular affluent. The media often personalized this opposition as a confrontation between Pope John Paul II[2] and President Clinton.[3] Behind the political maneuvers and personal affrontments stands a fundamental controversy concerning the moral principles proper to questions of demographic policy.[4] The negation or, more commonly, the suppression of these principles constitutes the major cause of the growing alliance between international family-planning programs and the ambient culture of death.

In order to excavate the moral controversy at the center of the current political struggle, it is useful to explicitate the ethical principles commonly ignored or distorted by the dominant demographic debate. The first concerns the duty to seek the truth concerning the nature of contemporary demographic shifts, especially in relationship to the earth's environment and economy. The second concerns the violation of human rights masked or even justified by the standard account of population dilemmas. The focus here rests primarily upon the right to life, the right to personal freedom (especially under the rubric of informed consent) and the rights of the family as the fundamental cell of civic society. The political interests served by these moral distortions, as well as the distortions themselves, merit

1

careful scrutiny in the demographic debate.

The first moral principle concerns the duty to seek the truth concerning the nature and social implications of current demographic changes. Obviously, no scientific portrait of the issue is perfectly objective. The frailty of any projection of the future and our incapacity to distance ourselves serenely from statistics fraught with our own destinies render demographic science especially perilous. Even granted these limitations, however, the standard picture of population which has dominated science and popular media in recent decades exhibits little care in the research of demographic trends, little probity in the hypothesization of causes and little sobriety in sketching possible social consequences of these changes. With few exceptions, the scientific-popular literature presents an apocalyptic portrait of a population surge threatening the very survival of humanity and causing a multitude of social evils, ranging from water pollution in Germany to the genocidal conflicts of Rwanda.

Typical of this literature is *The Population Bomb* by biologist Paul Ehrlich.[5] While this tract is an unsophisticated demographic treatise, it remains the most frequently reprinted example of the genre. Indeed, it is the prestigious grandfather of a thousand less forceful pamphlets and op-ed jeremiads.

The Population Bomb develops a grim picture of the population explosion caused by a declining death rate unmatched by a receding birth rate.[6] This demographic imbalance is destroying the finite resources of global nature and human culture. Due to this imbalance, "There is not enough food today... massive famines will occur soon, possibly in the early 1970's, certainly by the 1980's."[7] The population increase is also destroying the natural environment: "The causal chain of deterioration is easily followed to its source. Too many cars, too many factories, too much detergent, too much pesticide..., inadequate sewage treatment plants, too little water, too much carbon dioxide — all can be traced easily to too many people."[8] Population growth becomes the aggravating, if not the principal, cause of social evils such as "starvation, plague and thermonuclear war."

Not surprisingly, Ehrlich conceives vigorous government action as the solution to the impending demographic Armageddon. On the domestic level, he proposes the establishment of a federal Department of Population and Environment to enforce antinatalist policies.[9] Mandatory sex education,[10] luxury taxes for layettes and diapers,[11] and the (now sexist) proposal to find means to produce male first-borns in misogynist societies[12] are features of the government pedagogy. In foreign policy, antinatalist programs would constitute the cornerstone of American assistance to foreign nations.[13]

The Population Bomb's portrait of demographic doom is only a middle-brow example of the framework provided for ethical reflection in demography in recent decades. On a more philosophical level, the works of Garrett Hardin[14] have refined the metaphor of the earth as a swamped "lifeboat" in which we must abandon numerous passengers through a triage of sterilization and abortion.[15] A thousand popular campaigns in the media have reduced Ehrlich's thesis to political slogans. In the pioneering ads of the Campaign to Check the Population Explosion in the 1960's, population growth is touted as the "Threat to peace,"[16] the source of "war and riots,"[17] the cause of soaring crime ("Have you ever been mugged? Well, You may be"),[18] even the source of water pollution ("Warning: the Water you are drinking may be polluted").[19]

Clearly, the apocalyptic anti-population campaigns of the genre of *The Population Bomb* demonstrate scant regard for the facts concerning demography. They ignore obvious trends in the collapse of the birthrate in industrial areas of the North Atlantic community and mask the dramatic lowering of fertility rates in much of the rural South.[20] Their predictions rarely succeed. Condemned as certainly doomed to famine by Paul Ehrlich in 1969,[21] India is now a grain-exporting nation. The efforts to reduce major social evils to the single cause of population growth depend upon the use of correlations which would make a freshman statistics student blush. The contributions of political structure, economic policy and religious tradition to a particular society's balance of benefits and debits are ignored. The numerous counter-examples of densely-populated societies, such as Japan and the Netherlands, are unexamined. The social catastrophes of sparsely-populated nations, such as Somalia, receive inadequate explanation. Even their interpretations of population itself remain limited largely to the question of growth or decline. Other key demographic trends, such as immigration or urbanization, receive scant attention in the efforts to determine the cause of social or environmental disruption.[22]

Such a distortion of demographic science serves several patent interests, if it does not serve the dispassionate truth. The most obvious — and quite explicit — value fostered by such apocalyptic science is the massive intervention of the government into citizens' affective and familial lives. In the alarmist framework, traditional strictures against sterilization and abortion, as well as traditional respect for families to decide their own childbearing, are easily abandoned for the single good of survival. Hardin derides such strictures as antiquated taboos.[23] In this consequentialist ethic, the single end of society is survival of the endangered species and the only reasonable means to the end is vigorous state antinatalist intervention. It is striking that in the philosophical literature concerning demographic policy, the debate tends to pivot around the appropriate degree of state coercion in childbearing[24] rather than around the very justification of such coercion and the verisimilitude of the population crisis which such coercion is alleged to address.

The alarmist distortion of demographic trends not only expands state antinatalist power at the expense of other goods, such as life and personal freedom. It blinds the citizen to other moral duties necessary for the welfare of humanity, especially in the poorer nations. The execution or neglect of these duties often shapes the demographic profile of a particular society. The most obvious neglect concerns the duty to foster economic development. There is little dispute that economic development, especially when accompanied by growing literacy among women, tends to diminish birthrates.   As many critics of the Cairo Conference argued, the novelty of the conference — the link between population and development — received scant treatment in the final document.[25]   To acknowledge this duty, of course, would require the affluent nations to avow the need for sacrifice and technological change. It would require reception of Pope Paul VI's admonition to the United Nations three decades ago: "You must strive to multiply bread so that it suffices for the tables of mankind, and not rather favor an artificial control of birth, which would be irrational, in order to diminish the number of guests at the banquet of life."[26] For contemporary affluent nations, however, the asceticism of sacrifice, technological transfer and trade reform appears too steep. Modest economic aid is increasingly used as a lure for the permanent or temporary sterilization of the poor.[27] For the affluent, campaigns in favor of contraception, sterilization and abortion — promoted through increasingly brutal forms of persuasion — remain preferable to the patient work of economic solidarity, scolarization and political reform of authoritarian regimes.

Perhaps the greatest moral damage operated by survivalist demography is the very loss of the human person as the center of moral concern and civic protection. As the economist Julian Simon remarks in his penetrating critique of Ehrlich's book,[28] Ehrlich only conceives people as a peril. In his preface to *The Population Bomb*, Ehrlich explains that his concern for overpopulation grew out of a trip he made to India. He describes the scene thus: "The streets seemed alive with people. People eating, people washing, people sleeping, people visiting, arguing and screaming..., people defecating and urinating..., people herding animals. People, people, people, people."[29] In this vision, people are simply an invasive threat. There are no scenes of people worshipping or working or singing. Strikingly, there are no individual persons here. There is only a mob to be avoided or reduced as quickly as possible. The racial subtext is hard to avoid. It is a mob of the poor of color, threatening the American professional in his lumbering taxi.

The alarmist version of the demographic issue not only sacrifices the truth. It easily justifies the abolition of fundamental rights of the human person, in particular the right to life and the right to personal integrity.

Alarmist campaigns easily dismiss the right to life of the human fetus and infant as luxuries in an overcrowded boat. Philosophers such as Stephen Mumford[30] justify abortion as a necessary means to the goal of population stabilization and global security. The battle in Cairo pivoted largely around the opposition between those who decried abortion as a means of family planning and those who tacitly urged acceptance of abortion under the rubric of "reproductive health."[31] In his article on demography and the anachronism of traditional rights, Robert McGinn[32] argues that the right to life, like all other rights, has no perduring value. In the rising population, it may be abridged or discarded. The foundation of human rights itself, the inviolate right of the innocent to exist, easily vanishes in the utilitarian framework which claims population reduction as the highest good.

The alarmist account of demographic fact and duty also

weakens the physical and moral integrity of the person, especially the right of the person to determine the size of one's family.   With only nominal criticism by the population lobby, the Chinese government's demographic policies represent the most egregious example of the state's mutilation of this integrity.   The "one child" mandate, enforced by coercive sterilization and abortion, even by torture for the recalcitrant,[33] destroys the right of parents to determine the size and destiny of their family.   The new eugenics edicts, mandating the sterilization of disabled Chinese citizens, radically remove the choice to marry and raise a family.   Such political abberations are not without theoretical warrant from philosophers such as Onora O'Neill,[34] who argues that the putative "right to procreate" is limited to those individuals capable of raising their children according to standards fixed by the state.

Less dramatic, but more widespread, is the sterilization of poor women in conditions which no one would construe as those of "informed consent."   The sudden declines in fertility in Kenya[35] and the Philippines[36] are largely tied to medical programs which systematically sterilized illiterate or semi-literate women rarely apprised of the nature, effects or radicality of the operations performed.   Just as ominous is the increasing use of modest development projects and the popular media to induce poorer citizens to adopt sterilization or contraception in conditions one would rarely describe as those of "knowledge of cause."   The pressure against the poor individual to destroy one's fertility and the right to develop one's family is rooted in the increasing pressure of the affluent nations against poorer nations to reduce fertility through coercive means as a condition of economic aid.

One of the ironies of current demographic programs is that, while the domestic battle uses the rhetoric of "choice" and "reproductive freedom" to justify the abandonment of a comprehensive right to life, the international crusade in favor of population control sacrifices the person's life and autonomy in the name of collective survival. The alarmist account of demographic history and political duty does not simply distort moral values in the discreet domain of family planning. It challenges the right to existence and the right to integrity which constitute the very structure of the person.

In developing an alternative to the alarmist version of demography, the intellectual tasks are multiple. The poor science of the doomsday scenarios must be criticized. The multiple facts concerning human fertility (the problems of financing the welfare state in an aging West, as well of the challenge of large families in certain poor nations) must be equitably presented. The link between economic growth and family stability — and the self-interest of affluent nations who refuse to recognize this link — should be underscored.

The critique of the alarmist account, however, rests primarily upon two moral considerations. It must relentlessly question the means employed by any demographic program and not focus uniquely or primarily upon the utopian end of demographic harmony. In this context, one must scrutinize whether a particular means, such as abortion, kills a human being, rather than simply asking whether widespread abortion relieves population pressure. One must question whether the sterilization programs destroy the integrity and freedom of women, rather than focusing upon whether this program reduces an impoverished population. Second, one must judge demographic programs through the criterion of the perduring goods of the human person. Programs which deliberately destroy the lives, the procreative power and the freedom of individuals fail this personalist test, whatever the putative social benefits may be. When these violations of the person aim especially at the poor on the authority of the apocalyptic lore of the wealthy, the moral disvalues become only greater.

NOTES

1. For a synopsis of the controverted theses in the draft Cairo document, cf. "Excerpts from the Cairo Draft Plan" in *Origins* 24/10 (1994) 187-192.

2. For a presentation of the Vatican position on the conference, cf. John Paul II, "Letter to President Clinton" in *Origins* 23 (1994) 760, and "Population Conference Document Criticized" in *Origins* 23 (1994) 716ff.

3. Cf. Timothy Wirth, "State Department Presentation to Cairo Conference Planning Session" in *Origins* 23 (1994) 757ff.

4. For a theological presentation of such moral principles, cf. Pontifical Council for the Family, "Population Trends: Ethical and Pastoral Dimensions" in *Origins* 24 (1994) 173-186.

5. Cf. Paul Ehrlich, *The Population Bomb* (Binghamton: Ballantine, 1969). For a philosophical critique of Ehrlich's thesis, cf. Craig Waddell, "Perils of a modern Cassandra" in *Social Epistemology* 8/3 (1994) 221-237.

6. Cf. Ehrlich 13-37.

7. Ehrlich 36-37.

8. Ehrlich 57.

9. Cf. Ehrlich 124ff.

10. Cf. Ehrlich 124.

11. Cf. Ehrlich 123.

12. Cf. Ehrlich 124.

13. Cf. Ehrlich 141-154.

14.Cf. Garrett Hardin, *Birth Control* (New York: Pegasus, 1970), *Exploring New Ethics for Survival* (New York: Viking, 1972), *Living Within Limits* (New York: Oxford, 1993).

15. For Hardin's defense of abortion, cf. Garrett Hardin, *Mandatory Motherhood: The True Meaning of "Right to Life"* (Boston: Beacon, 1974).

16. Cf. Lawrence Lader, *Breeding Ourselves to Death* (New York: Ballantine, 1971) 95, 98.

17. Cf. Lader 99.

18. Lader 100.

19. Lader 102.

20. Cf. *The 1990 Revision of the United Nations Global Population Estimates and Projections in Population Studies*, No. 122 (New York: United Nations, 1991).

21. Cf. Ehrlich 143-147.

22. Cf. Pontifical Council for the Family 175-178.

23. Cf. Garrett Hardin, *Living Within Limits: Ecology, Economics and population Taboos* (New York: Oxford, 1993).

24. Cf. Michael Bayles, *Morality and Population Policy* (University of Alabama Press, 1980) for a typical presentation of the public policy dilemma.

25. Cf. John Cardinal O'Connor, "Where's the Development?" in *Catholic New York* (14 April 1994) 5.

26. Cf. Pope Paul VI, "Address to the United Nations General Assembly (Oct. 4, 1965)" in 6 *Acta Apostolica Sedis* 57 (1965) 883.

27. Cf. Christine Vollmer, "Pressure Tactics" in *The Catholic World Report* 4/8 (1994) 40-41.

28. Cf. Julian Simon, *The Ultimate Source* (Princeton: Princeton, 1980) 335-336.

29. Cf. Ehrlich 12.

30. Cf. Stephen Mumford, "Population Growth and Global Security" in *The Humanist* 41/6 (1981) 25-54.

31. On the controversy over this ambiguous phrase, cf. Diarmuid Martin, "Vatican Delegation's presentation to Cairo Conference Planning Session" in *Origins* 23 (1994) 757ff.

32. Cf. Robert E. McGinn, "Demography and the Anachronism of Traditional Rights" in *Applied Philosophy*11/1 (1994) 57-70.

33. Cf. Rene Bel and Adolfo Castaneda,"The Plot Against Life and Family" in *The Catholic World Report* 4/8 (1994) 19-21.

34. Cf. Onora O'Neill, "Begetting, Bearing and Rearing" in *Having Children*, ed. O'Neill (New York: Oxford, 1979) 25-38.

35. Cf. Margaret Ogala, "Case Study: Kenya" in *The Catholic World Report* 4/8 (1994) 26-27.

36. Cf. Mary Pilar Verzosa, "Case Study: Philippines" in *The Catholic World Report* 4/8 (1994) 24-26.

Civilization

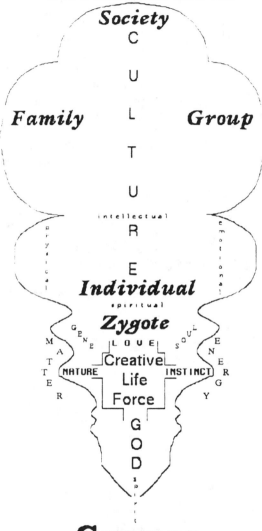

Society

C
U
L
T
U
R
E

Family *Group*

intellectual

physical   emotional

Individual

spiritual

Zygote

GENE   SOUL

LOVE

MATTER   NATURE   Creative   INSTINCT   ENERGY

Life
Force

G
O
D

spirit

Cosmos

DEMOCRACY AND ABORTION

Monte Harris Liebman, M.D.

PART ONE

"...nor shall any State deprive any person of life, liberty or property, without due process of law; nor deny to any person within its jurisdiction the equal protection of the laws." (14th Amendment, U. S. Constitution)

This statement is every individual's assurance that the U.S. Government is bound to protect the right of the individual to "due process" and "equal protection" of the laws even if mob or majority rule should want to do otherwise. This amendment is what upholds the rights of the individual against the might of the majority. It reveals the greatest principle and intent of our nation — to respect the rights of the individual. It matches the strength of the masses with their own government's duty to protect every person under its jurisdiction from injustice, vigilantism and disordered rule. It is the great equalizer that brings balance and order into the democratic system of self rule. Under this rule every person has a right to adjudication before the individual's "life, liberty, or property" can be taken by force.

From July 9, 1868, when this 14th Amendment to the U.S. Constitution was ratified, until January 22, 1973, when the United States Supreme Court ruled the fetus was not a "person," the law protected the right to life of the fetal child. Abortion-on-demand was illegal in most of the United Sates. The *Roe v. Wade* ruling brought down these laws and made abortion legal throughout the entire period of gestation or pregnancy. It allowed the States to prohibit abortion only after viability, the point at which the fetal child can survive outside of the womb.

13

Thus the pre-viable fetal child is now the one exception to the government's mandate to protect the rights of individuals under its jurisdiction. The fetal child is presently denied "due process" and "equal protection of the laws" when it comes to abortion. The fetal child has no effective standing before the law and his or her right to life is not a factor that can impede the mother's right to obtain an abortion. Thus, the fetal child can *lose its life* without adjudication or a hearing in any court in the land and those responsible for the abortion have no accountability to anyone, not even the fetal child's father.

In upholding the right to privacy of the individual, the Supreme Court removed any control over obtaining an abortion. While the court maintains that the unborn is not a "person," it does not take the natural step to determine if it is a human being or when human life begins: "We need not resolve the difficult question or when life begins," stated the Court (*Roe v. Wade*, January 22, 1973).

This disclaimer, however, did not prevent the court from asserting the viewpoint that whatever it is that is growing and developing in the womb is only "potential life": "With regard to the State's important and legitimate interest in potential life, the compelling point is viability" (ibid.). Thus, based on its own beliefs the court concluded the unborn was "potential life" not actual life, and it acted arbitrarily and lifted its 14th amendment protection. It never considered if a life conceived by a woman could ever be non-human! The conclusion from this consideration would not support the court's view that when human life begins is not known or that new life is only "potential life." Not only is the earliest form of the human body scientifically identifiable as human, but it has all of the characteristics of activated actual life.

In its decision, then, the Supreme Court made the one fundamental error that can undermine the entire democratic system. It failed to establish *fact* before moving to the decision. Both the law and majority rule in a democratic system are dependent on fact for relevant governance. Of course, where fact cannot be determined, opinion based on precedent or an innate sense of justice is valid.

But *Roe v. Wade* went against the historical precedent of over 100 years of accepted anti-abortion laws and legislation in the U.S., and it violated that innate sense of justice elaborated in the Declaration of Independence that declared "that all men are created equal, that they are endowed by their Creator with certain unalienable Rights, that among these are Life, Liberty and the pursuit of Happiness." Basing its decision on a formulated protected right to privacy, the court gave women the right to abortion. Because it never decided — by fact or opinion — when human life begins, it never weighed the right to life of new human life against the right to privacy of the mother. Since one of the reasons the anti-abortion laws were established was the medical opinion that the unborn was human and alive, the court should have determined — beyond any reasonable doubt — that the preborn fetal child is not alive or human before it granted the free, indiscriminate and unrestrained right to abortion.

The court's decision in the case of *Roe v. Wade* opened the door to a freedom to kill another human life with impunity. Efforts of the fathers to stop the abortion of their children are thwarted by the system. Efforts to mandate informed consent in which the doctor would have the mother clearly understand that the unborn is alive and human (not merely a clump of undifferentiated biologically unidentifiable cells), the stage of development of her fetal child, the stage of the pregnancy, the abortion procedure, and the possible complications that can occur have been thwarted by the forces seeking to keep abortion on demand legal. Not only is abortion without legal restraints, but responsible, informed consent is not required even though consent would not, in itself, restrain access to abortion or interfere with this presumed right to abortion. Without accountability appropriate information or pertinent laws, freedom is without relevant guidelines; and the freedom to act out without regard for the consequences to another human being is not responsible freedom. It is anarchy, the antithesis of democracy.

It is for this reason that abortion is a contradiction to democracy. It is for this reason that nations and states who love democracy have a legitimate interest in banning abortion as a private right. Like the newly conceived life in the womb, the life of democracy depends on the full disclosure of the facts, relevant accountability and respect for every human life.

PART TWO: THE OATH OF HIPPOCRATES

I swear by Apollo, the physician, and Asclepias and Health and All-Heal and all gods and goddesses that, according to my ability and judgment, I will keep this oath.... I will follow that method of treatment which, according to my ability and judgement, I consider for the benefit of my patients, and abstain from whatever is deleterious or mischievous. I will give no deadly medicine to anyone if asked, nor suggest any such counsel; furthermore, I will not give to a woman an instrument to produce abortion.[1]

In *This Curette for Hire*, Dr. Eugene Diamond states that this legendary oath marked a turning point in human history. He quotes a 1961 personal communication from the anthropologist Margaret Mead revealing the cultural significance of the Oath: "For the first time in our tradition [referring to the Oath] there was a complete separation between killing and curing. Throughout the primitive world the doctor and the sorcerer tended to be the same person."[2] With this oath, the power to kill was forsworn. What a covenant this represented with all of the people physicians henceforth would serve. In a flash this revered and hallowed principle spelled "trust" for the millions of people needing the physician's services and it put the physician on a new ethical plane. Margaret Mead continued: "One profession, the followers of Asclepias, were dedicated completely to life under all circumstances, regardless of rank, age, or intellect--the life of a slave, the life of the Emperor, the life of a foreign man, the life of a defective child."[3] What a principle for governance this is, let alone a principle for care! That any profession would aspire to such an oath of this nature through the tarnished centuries of human chaos and injustice, is most astonishing.

While *Roe v. Wade* discusses in some detail the origins and history of the Oath, the court's text mentions but glosses over the insightful Pythagorean viewpoint, that "the embryo was animate from the moment of conception, and abortion meant destruction of a living being."

Roe cites an authority, Dr. Edelstein, who held that the Hippocratic Oath represented a "Pythagorean manifesto and not the expression of an absolute standard of medical conduct," because the Pythagoreans were not joined by other "Greek thinkers," who "commended abortions." Edelstein further believed that, with the emerging teachings of Christianity, the "Pythagorean ethic" expressed in the Oath became the cornerstone for all medical ethics. Could it be that this small band of Pythagoreans was correct, that the new human life does begin at conception or fertilization? Looking at this astonishing evolution in which an ethic held by a small group of Greeks came to be "a long accepted and revered statement of medical ethics" (*Roe v. Wade*) is a curiosity. How such an early Oath could reflect reality and yet coincide with a new theology is, in itself, an amazing and relevant phenomenon.

THE BEGINNINGS OF THE NEW INDIVIDUAL

There is, and there has been, considerable debate regarding the time that a new individual is formed.

Contrary to the belief and teaching of some, the time and event marking the beginning point is not a matter of opinion. It is a matter of fact. There are a few different ways in which this can be understood and taught. The following presents some ways of verifying the facts of life.

1. *Biological Observations* demonstrate that fertilization normally takes place in the distal part of the oviduct. At this point the egg and the sperm unite, forming a new and unique individual, with its own genetic code, program and processes which are independent of the mother. This new individual is different from both the mother and the father and is a separate individual entity. All of the characteristics of life, namely, growth, reproduction, irritability or response, movement, metabolism and communication appear at that time and as a result of that primordial and essential event — fertilization.

The Pythagoreans were right about the embryo being alive and their Oath fit that reality. Consider the following:

a. "The first scaffolding or rudiment of the body, too, when the brain is nothing more than a limpid fluid, if lightly pricked will move obscurely, will contract and twist itself like a worm or caterpillar, so that it is very evidently possessed with sensation." — William Harvey, father of cardiovascular medicine.[4]

b. "Human development is a continuous process that begins when an ovum from a female is fertilized by a sperm from a male." — Keith L. Moore, *The Developing Human*[5]

c. The frequently cited work of Hertig depicts the earliest stages of human development. The captions in his book read: "Figures 2 and 3 represent the earliest stage of human development thus far observed, the pronuclear ovum."[6]

d. "Roughly 12 hours after the fusion of the chromosomes, the first cell division takes place, and divisions then

continue at intervals of 12 and 15 hours." — Lennart
Nilsson and Lars Hamberger, *A Child is Born*.[7]

e. "The formation, maturation and meeting of a male and
female sex cell are all preliminary to their actual union into
a combined cell, or zygote, which definitely marks the
beginning of a new individual." — Leslie Brainard Arey,
Developmental Anatomy.[8]

f. "It is not my opinion [that a fetus is a human being], but
the teaching of all genetics. It's no doubt a human being
because it's not a chimpanzee.... Now let's take one cell
of a chimpanzee embryo, of a human embryo, of a gorilla
embryo and give it to one of my students in Certificate of
Cytogenetics in Paris, and if he cannot tell you this one is
a human being, this one chimpanzee being, this one is a
gorilla being, he would fail his exam." — Jerome Lejeune,
M.D., Ph.D., Professor of Fundamental Genetics.[9]

2. *Personal Reflection* will reveal that fertilization is the
moment when the self comes into existence. This can be
demonstrated if one asks the question, when one's own life
did begin. Did it begin at fertilization or sometime later,
say 20 minutes later or 20 days later, at birth or 20 years
later? The answer, of course, is at fertilization. One can
also ask if one would be alive if the event of fertilization
had not happened. Again, the answer would prove that any
human's life begins with fertilization, including twins.

3. *Test Tube Fertilization* is now common knowledge and
is an accepted fact. Thus, from this knowledge we can
understand that a new individual is started at the time of
the union of the woman's egg and the man's sperm in the
test tube and then placed in the womb of the mother. The
new individual implanted in the womb was already begun
and in fact was already separate and significantly different
from the mother or father from the instant of his or her
inception at fertilization.[10]

4. *New Generations* begin not when any later stages of development occur, but the next generation or the new generation begins when the new life is generated and created. In the case of the human being, this happens when the first definitive cell that identifies the creation of the new individual — the Zygote — is formed through the union of the mother's egg, and the father's sperm. With the formation of this first cell, the parents have reproduced and the New Generation is begun.

The human family is a genetic, morphologic, individual and social composite. It cannot exist without the presence of any of these factors. That is why we must recognize and protect the primordial cell of every new human life and individual, the *zygote*. Like it or not, and the vanity of some will not, this is everyone's beginning and coming into being. Unseen and unheard, it is *the* most intrinsic part of the human family.

Everything we know today affirms that ancient Pythagorean view quoted in *Roe v. Wade* that "the embryo was animate from the moment of conception, and abortion meant destruction of a living being."

THE FIRST HUMAN RIGHT

"Among other natural rights of the colonists are these: First a right to life. Second, to liberty. Third to property together with the right to support and defend them in the best manner they can. These are the evident branches of, rather than deductions from, the duty of self-preservation, commonly called the first law of nature." — Samuel Adams, Patriot and Member of the Continental Congress[11]

Samuel Adams, one of the few who signed the Declaration of Independence, lists the right to life as the first right of the Colonists, calling this a "natural right," one that is intrinsic to the human condition, one that need not be conferred by authority, one that represents a just claim and entitlement by every living human being. it is a right that one can exercise without consent or restraint, because it is a right without which survival is not possible. It is a right that must be protected and affirmed for those who cannot assert that right for themselves.

Why is this right to life as precious as it is? Why does it demand and deserve priority over all other rights? Both of these questions are answered in the same way. Without the expression of this right, *the existence of life itself*, all other rights are only theories. All rights are predicated on having life. Without life, other rights such as the right to freedom, the right to privacy, the right to property, the right to religious choice, and the right to free speech are all meaningless. The fact of having life is what gives substance and meaning to all other highly esteemed rights. Hence it is the first and most basic right. Abortion, then, through its destruction of the human life in the womb, is the earliest violation of the first most basic of all human rights, the right to life.

REVERSING THE *ROE* PARADOX

It is correct that abortion restricting laws did not become a part of the secular law in the U.S. until the 19th Century.

But it is not correct that it was outlawed solely to protect the health or life of the mother. In fact, the leader of that movement to ban abortions, Dr. Horatio Storer, not only stated that a "child" was involved, but expressed concern for the community as well when he wrote in his prized essay: "Thus it seems that abortion is a crime not merely against the life of the child and health of its mother, and against good morals, but it strikes a blow at the very foundation of society itself." Not only did Dr. Storer's thought extend to the repercussions on the society, but he was concerned with the basis for the abortion choice. He concluded "that sheer ignorance in many honest people, is the spring of the horrible intra-uterine murder which exists among us; why not then, enlighten ignorance."[12]

Why not then? Why not bring the facts of life to the

public? Why not educate people to the details and descriptions of intra-uterine development? Why not let them know there is a difference between an acorn and a human zygote? Why not let everyone know that a zygote, single-celled as it is, has all of the detectable characteristics of life, namely growth, reproduction, irritability or response, movement, metabolism and communication. Why not let everyone know that each stage of life is of equal value (as important as the next) because each stage is dependent on the one before and without origin nothing else is possible for anyone.

Today, we are ruled by an untenable paradox created by the Supreme Court: the legal right to kill without restraint (in most instances), the new human life in any mother's womb. It did this through the development of a presumed right to privacy of women and their doctors.

Like it or not, by legalizing abortion, the Court opened the floodgates to legal abortion and obligated the government to support and protect the exercise of that right. In this way, the government has become complicit to the act of abortion, a condition and situation that is repugnant and reprehensible.

Roe institutionalizes a peculiar form of anarchy, one in which a mother herself can sacrifice the new life she co-created within her body to satisfy her own reasons without regard or concern for the well-being of her child. Yes, people may be free to do as they please but only until their behavior encroaches on another. Then, the behavior must be adjusted so that it does not harm anyone or deprive the other of his or her integrity and rights. Anarchy, being a state of irresponsible self-rule that is free of any governance, disregards the rights and integrity of others. Such is the nature of abortion. It is a form of legalized anarchy!

We must ask the question if anyone has a right to claim entitlements, rights, conditions or privileges which he or she is not willing to grant others. Has anyone the right to deny others the "right to life" he or she has enjoyed? Individuals acting without regard for the similar rights of others threaten society with a personal anarchy and tyranny. Without reciprocal respect of rights, democracy cannot long stand.

The unborn do not create themselves. They are created by others. Their early life is vulnerable to the care and compassion of others. They cannot survive on their own. They require nurturance and protection for survival, growth and development. Since neither their creation, nor their nurturance is under their own control or will, new human beings are dependent on those who create them and can provide for them. The innocence of one's own creation and the helplessness inherent in the unborn create the legitimate and just claim and responsible obligation on their parents to sustain their lives and let them live.

The founding fathers of our nation had an ingenious vision in authoring and establishing our Constitution. Contrary to some beliefs, they did speak to the likes of the preborn: "We the People of the United States, in order to form a more perfect union, establish justice, insure domestic tranquillity, provide for the common defense, promote the general welfare and secure the blessings of Liberty to ourselves and *our posterity*, do ordain and establish this Constitution for the United States of America."[13]

Thus the founding fathers referred to the unborn as "posterity," meaning the generations to come. For those not yet reproducing, "posterity" can only refer to a "potential" life; but to those already reproducing, "posterity" is already present and actualized. Surely, if the genius that created our Constitution saw so far down the road as to provide governance, guidance and order for a remote and potential posterity 200 hundred years hence, that same wisdom must have meant to bestow all of the rights on to all of posterity — even that posterity in its very *beginning* — the *human zygote*.

Understanding that the next generation begins with the first stage of a new human individual's life and not the last or any in between, provides the compelling starting point for reconciliation and reversal of *Roe v. Wade*. For, if the Constitution were meant to be a gift to all, the rights and safeguards granted therein should be *applied* equally to all of our land's "posterity" — inside and outside of the womb. Given this proposition the Supreme Court should reverse *Roe v. Wade* based on this expressed intention in the Preamble of the Constitution and extend to all new human life the first blessing of liberty, the right to live. Witness the words of Thomas Jefferson: "The care of human life and happiness, and not their destruction, is the first and only legitimate object of good government."[14]

These words of Thomas Jefferson and the principle they express are not dead! They are at the heart of the contest for leadership and direction of all civilized governments. They express the core value that unites people, all people, in the drive to ban abortion on demand in the U.S. through all lawful means, including a reversal of *Roe* and the eventual implementation of a Human Life Amendment.

NOTES

1. Cited in *The World Book Encyclopedia*, V.9 (1987).

2. Eugene Diamond, M.D., *This Curette for Hire* (Chicago: ACTA Foundation, 1977) 10.

3. Ibid.

4. William Harvey, *Excitatio de Generatione*, 1651.

5. Keith L. Moore, *The Developing Human* (W.B. Saunders Company — Harcourt Brace Jovanovich, Inc., 1988) 1.

6. Arthur T. Hertig, M.D., *Human Trophoblast* (Springfield: C. C. Thomas, 1968) 19.

7. Lennart Nilsson and Lars Hamberger, *A Child is Born* (New York: Delacorte Press/Seymour Lawrence Bantam Doubleday Dell Publishing Group, Inc., 1990) 57.

8. Leslie Brainard Arey, Ph.D., Sc.D., LL.D., *Developmental Anatomy*, Rev'd. 7th ed. (Philadelphia and London: W.B. Saunders, 1974) 55.

9. Jerome Lejeune, M.D., Ph.D., Professor of Fundamental Genetics and Medicine, Holder of the Kennedy Prize, testimony before the Circuit Court of Blount County, Maryville, Tennessee, Judge Dale Young presiding, August 10, 1989.

10. In 1969 Robert Edwards at the Physiology Laboratory, Cambridge England, successfully fertilized the human egg outside the mother's body. See *Time Table of Technology* (New York: Hearst Books, 1982.

11. Samuel Adams, Patriot and Member of the Continental Congress, "Natural Rights of the Colonists as Men [1773]" cited in *Liberty and Union, Cyclopedia of Patriotism*, ed. Rev. Samuel Fallows, D.D.I. (Chicago and Madison: Midland, 1887) 55.

12. Horatio Storer, *A Proper Bostonian on Sex and Birth Control*, reprint (New York: Arno Press, 1974.

13. The Preamble to the Constitution of the United States of America.

14. Thomas Jefferson, "To the Republican Citizens of Washington County, Maryland, March 31, 1809" in *The Writings of Thomas Jefferson* with explanatory notes by the editor, H. A. Washington (Washington: Taylor and Maury, 1853-54) 8: 165.

YOU SAY YOU WANT A REVOLUTION?
PRO-LIFE PHILOSOPHY AND FEMINISM

Anne M. Maloney

I am a philosophy professor at the College of Saint Catherine — a small, Catholic liberal arts college for women. The focus at St. Catherine's is on its nature as a *women's* college. I am glad that St. Catherine's is a women's college, and very glad to teach there. What continues to frustrate and puzzle me, however, is an all too common notion at St. Kate's that to be pro-woman, one simply must be in favor of abortion rights. I teach Feminist Philosophy, and I am committed irrevocably to the value and importance of women. I see no way to hold the feminist values I do without being at once wholeheartedly pro-life.

I would like to explain my reasons for saying this in the following essay. In the course of my remarks here, I hope to accomplish four things. First, I will outline what I take to be the two major strands in contemporary feminist thinking. I will term one of them "Androgynous Ideal Feminism" and the other "Woman Ideal Feminism." Second, I will show that Androgynous Ideal Feminism is truly a wolf in sheep's clothing, that what many feminists call an *androgynous* worldview is in fact a worldview which posits what is *male* as what is valuable. Third, I will show that Woman Ideal Feminism may be a more honest and accurate mirror of authentic feminist thinking. Fourth, I will outline and briefly analyze the theory of one Woman Ideal thinker, Nel Noddings, in order to show that, despite her own pro-abortion stance, a careful and consistent reading of the principles which she espouses can only give rise to a worldview which embraces the distinctive value of women and a wholeheartedly pro-life point of view.

THE ANDROGYNOUS IDEAL FEMINISTS

What I am here calling the Androgynous Ideal Feminists include those feminists who describe themselves as "Liberal Feminists," some of the "Radical Feminists," and "Social Feminists." In contemporary feminist scholarship, these would be among the most discussed and credible versions of feminism.

Androgynous Idealists maintain that women will never achieve equality in the world until they have all the same rights and privileges which men currently enjoy. For example, Liberal Feminists point out that the ability to reason is the foundation for having rights, and women can reason as well as men can. In fact, say Liberal Feminists, women and men are *different* at all only because of social conditioning; there are no essential differences between men and women. Betty Friedan points out that boys and girls are treated differently from birth, and but for that, there would *be* no significant differences between men and women. Women are *not* intrinsically more intuitive, more emotional, more concrete or relationship-oriented than men.[1] We are simply reared to be that way.

What about the fact that biology dictates that it is women, not men, who conceive, generate, and nourish their young? Liberal Feminists consider such data irrelevant. Just as height and weight are incidental to who I am, so too are my sexual characteristics. In the ideal society which Liberal Feminists envision, there would still be physiological males and females, but physiology would be incidental. To facilitate equal opportunity for all, Liberal Feminists propose free contraception, abortion on demand, and twenty-four hour daycare.

Some Radical and Socialist Feminists take a different approach in their pursuit of the androgynous ideal. These feminists acknowledge readily that the differences between men and women, both physiological and psychological, are significant and do much to determine the status of women.

It is fine for the Liberal Feminists to maintain that women and men are equally rational and posit equal opportunity for all. But equal opportunity does not mean very much if Joe pursues his interests without ever getting pregnant or nursing his children, and Edith must pursue her interests while doing both of these things. This, say many Radical and Socialist Feminists, is not a fair race; men automatically have a head-start. Thus do the Radical Feminists say that gender is the source of all forms of oppression of women: gender structures how men and women dress, eat, work, have sex, and view themselves. If the problem is gender, then gender must be eliminated. Feminism's goal must be androgyny.[2] Thus "The Feminists," an influential New York based Radical Feminist group, states: "The sex roles themselves must be destroyed. If any part of these role definitions is left, the disease of oppression remains and will reassert itself again in new, or the same old, variations throughout society."[3]

Many Radical Feminists acknowledge that physiological sex differences will be a major roadblock on the path to androgyny. The solution proposed by many Radical Feminists is straightforward: the physiological status quo must change. Shulamith Firestone is one influential Radical Feminist who insists that only technology can ultimately free women from subordination to men. Technology must keep striving toward the goal of error-free contraception and extra-uterine gestation. Only then, she says, can there be "the freeing of women from the tyranny of their reproductive biology by every means available, and the diffusion of the childbearing and childrearing role to the society as a whole, men as well as women."[4] Radical Feminists such as Firestone want to achieve a world wherein genital distinctions between the sexes would no longer matter culturally.

The so-called "French Feminists" follow this line of thinking. Such thinkers as Monique Wittig, Christine

Delphy, and Luce Irigary maintain that, in the words of Wittig, "one is not born a woman." Central to this thinking is the tenet that the fact that women give birth is central to women's subordination. The ability to give birth is neither good nor natural; women have been systematically bred by patriarchy to do the "dirty work" of reproduction, much as cows have been bred to produce more milk.

Socialist Feminism picks up this thread of women's biology as problematic, and it too locates the source of oppression as women's ability to bear and nurse children. Thus, they claim, the sexual division of labor must be eliminated in every area of life. As Socialist Feminist Alison Jaggar puts it, "The one solid basis of agreement among socialist feminists is that to overcome women's alienation, the sexual division of labor must be eliminated in every area of life.... [W]e must remember that the ultimate transformation of human nature at which socialist feminists aim goes beyond the liberal conception of psychological androgyny to a possible transformation of 'physical' human capacities, some of which, until now, have been seen as biologically limited to one sex. This transformation might even include the capacities for insemination, for lactation and gestation, so that, for instance, one woman could inseminate another, so that men and nonparturitive women could lactate, and so that fertilized ova could be transplanted into women's or even into men's bodies."[5] Jaggar maintains that these developments are already on the technological horizon, and a welcome sight they are, too; as Gayle Rubin writes, "We are not only oppressed *as* women, we are oppressed by having to *be* women."[6]

SOME THOUGHTS ON THE ANDROGYNOUS FEMINIST IDEAL

The worldview proposed by the Androgynous Idealists is problematic. Whether Liberal Feminist, Radical Feminist or Socialist Feminist, the Androgynous Idealist says that she wants a world which mirrors better who women are, but in fact she ends up proposing a world in which only what is male is valuable.   It is precisely this sort of thinking which ultimately denigrates women, and it is also the sort of thinking which leads many feminists to embrace abortion on demand. How so? Allow me to explain.

The Androgynous Ideal Feminists claim that women can never be empowered so long as they are the ones who get pregnant. Until the day of extra-uterine gestation comes (for it is coming, they say), women must at least have the power to get *un*pregnant at will. Women simply cannot compete fairly with men so long as they have so much weightier an investment in procreation. The only path to equality and dignity is the undoing of that tie, so that women will be able to walk away from their sexual encounters as easily as men can already do.   Thus do Liberal, Radical, and Socialist Feminists advocate readily available contraception for all women, as well as abortion on demand and without apology.

One must question whether this is truly feminism at all, or whether this purported "feminist worldview" is truly a "masculinist worldview."   When Simone de Beauvoir claims that "woman's misfortune is to have been destined for the reproduction of life," she is supporting rather than undermining a worldview which points out what is male as what is really valuable. One might well wonder whether "equality" must really mean "sameness," whether there are feminists who envision, rather than an androgynous ideal, a world in which women and men are viewed as distinctive beings, equal in dignity and in nature but blessedly different in important biological and psychological ways. I will return, in the conclusion of this essay to this idea, but at this point I would like to turn to what I take to be the other major strand of thought in feminist scholarship today — those feminists whom I am calling "Woman Ideal

Feminists." Unlike the Androgynous Idealists, the Woman Ideal Feminists propose that it is not women who need changing, but rather the world which needs to recognize the dignity and value which women possess and the unique contributions which only women can make to the world. Like the Androgynous Idealists, however, the Woman Idealists also support abortion on demand. In the following paragraphs, I would like to outline briefly and in general terms what I take the Woman Idealist worldview to be, then state their reasons for supporting abortion, and finally argue that, while the worldview of the Woman Idealists makes more sense of and is more respectful to women's experience than the Androgynous Ideal perspective, Woman Ideal Feminists are untrue to their own foundational principles in promoting abortion.

THE WOMAN IDEAL FEMINISTS

What I am calling Woman Ideal Feminism actually began as a reaction against the sort of Radical Feminism outlined above. Some Radical Feminists in the 1970ˢ became increasingly uncomfortable with the idea that women's own biological and psychological makeup was being blamed for women's oppression. Their solution, however, was to flip the coin to its other face; *women* are not the problem, said these later Radical Feminists, so *men* must be. Thus do later Radical Feminist thinkers such as Mary Daly, Susan Griffin, Andrea Dworkin, and Catharine Mackinnon advocate a worldview which tends to see men as either monsters, necrophiliacs, rapists, torturers, and women-haters. Andrea Dworkin, for example, writes that "Men love death. In everything they make, they hollow out a central place for death, let its rancid smell contaminate every dimension of whatever still survives. Men especially love murder. In art they celebrate it, and in life they commit it."[7] If men would only disappear, say these Radical Feminists, the world would be perfectible. I will not here dwell on this form of feminism, except to say that most women reject it outright and consider it empircally false. Most of us, after all, have either sons, brothers, fathers or husbands whom we do not view as rapists and women-haters. I mention this form of Radical Feminism at all because these thinkers do acknowledge what I think is a real problem with the androgynous worldview it criticizes: there *is* something wrong with a journey toward equality for women which begins by denigrating women's biological and psychological make-up.

Although both women have issued disclaimers, I take this to be one of the central insights of such feminists as Carol Gilligan and Nel Noddings. These feminists are examples of what I am calling Woman Ideal Feminism. In her groundbreaking work *In a Different Voice*, Carol Gilligan proposes a vision of the world which is rooted in *woman's* distinctive ways of being and knowing. Gilligan points out that women tend to relate to the world differently than men do, that women tend to stress relationships and responsibility in their thinking, whereas men tend to stress rules and rights.[8] To so relate to the world is neither inferior nor superior; it is just *different*. Perhaps such difference is a valuable and necessary complement to the more traditional male view of reality. If men typically see the world in terms of justice, fairness, rules and rights, and women tend to see it more in terms of relationships, needs and emotion, then men and women can cooperate to create a complete and harmonious picture of the world.

Nel Noddings has a similar view. She points out that we have lived for all too many years in a world which holds up what is typically male as what is truly valuable. Theory is important, she claims, but so is practice; justice is imperative, but so is care. Any tenable worldview must acknowledge the value of objectivity and universalism, but it must also recognize the corresponding value of receptivity and relatedness. In her most well-known book, *Caring*,

Noddings discusses her philosophy and her reasons for holding it.

In *Caring* Noddings inherits and builds upon the groundbreaking work of Carol Gilligan's *In a Different Voice*. Like Gilligan, Noddings' ideal is a feminine rather than an androgynous one. In her work Noddings suggests that relationships are of tremendous value in human life and their importance has been too long overlooked. Discussions of ethics, she says, have for too long centered solely on abstract principles and not enough on relational values. Human beings are not, she says, isolated atomistic individuals; we live and thrive in communities, in relational units.

Traditional ways of thinking, says Noddings, tend to overlook or minimize the hard work that caring is. All acts of caring concern a relationship between the one-caring and the cared-for. The one-caring attends to the cared-for in her deeds as well as in her thoughts.[9] Caring, then, is by no means simply a matter of holding warm feelings about someone, or of being generally concerned. Real care demands actual encounter with specific individuals; it cannot be accomplished by good intentions alone.[10] Of course, we are most likely to care for our own family and friends, but Noddings encourages us to take seriously the requirement to move beyond our intimate circles and extend our caring to the limits of our energy and ability.

Noddings' focus on caring relationships reveals that for her what truly matters in life is not only rules and principles but also individuals and relationships. For example, there is a difference between teaching my children the virtue of honesty in connection to principles on the one hand and teaching honesty in connection to persons and relationships on the other.[11] To be honest because lying breaks a moral rule is one thing, but to be honest because without honesty I can never form a true friendship is another. Lies distance us from one another, prevent us from knowing and being known. Casting the virtue of honesty in this light, says Noddings, does not just name a principle and describe a violation; it explains why relationships require honesty. The latter approach is too often overlooked, according to her.

Education is crucial if human beings are to cultivate properly their natural tendency to care. Here Noddings agrees with Carol Gilligan's perception that there is a difference between men's and women's moral frameworks. Men speak the language of rights and women the language of responsibility. She points out in *Mapping the Moral Domain* that educators teach girls the language of justice and rights because it is the language they need to function in the world as it is now structured. But educators do not teach the language of care and responsibility to boys; in the world as it is constructed, boys do not need to speak this tongue because it threatens their success in the market-place. Women are predisposed to care, and so could function as natural teachers of how to care. Unfortunately, society is not interested in learning this virtue, and even more disturbing for Noddings, women are increasingly likely to repress their caring tendencies for fear that they will be scorned as "soft," "sentimental," or "emotional."[12]

Noddings believes that we must learn to take caring and relational ethics seriously if we are ever to find our way out of such thorny ethical issues as abortion. She defines abortion as a pregnant woman's decision to end her relationship with her unborn child. Abortion, according to Noddings, is too often construed as a conflict between a fetus' right to life and a woman's right to bodily integrity. All attempts to resolve the problem of abortion through such appeals to rights, says Noddings, are ultimately doomed because they are of no real help to a woman who must decide whether or not to have her baby. No woman ever, she would point out, made her decision whether or not to abort by plotting out a logical syllogism. Rather than approach abortion armed with the language of rights, Noddings suggests that we approach abortion with the language of relations. Whereas rights-talk presumes that what grounds human dignity is reason, relations-talk adds that the ability to reason alone is neither a necessary nor a sufficient criterion for human worth. Also important is another being's ability to call forth my caring.[13]

Shifting our perspective in this way, she says, allows us to see the abortion problem in a new light. I am permitted to abort my child, says Noddings, *not* because my child lacks rights, but because she cannot respond to my caring in a way that I value.[14] There simply is no relationship, says Noddings, when a woman is merely pregnant, especially in the first trimester. Without a relationship of care, there is no responsibility *to* care. Until an unborn child is developed enough to respond to my caring, I bear no ethical responsibility for her. This is why, Noddings claims, "we do not hold funerals for lost embryos."[15] In fact, she says, most abortions occur precisely because the woman does not want a person to exist who will have a "response-based claim" on her.[16] Choosing an abortion, says Noddings, is choosing to end a relationship before it has fully begun.

A RESPONSE TO NODDINGS

As I stated earlier, I find much to recommend in Noddings' philosophy. It is precisely because of her overall philosophy that her stance on abortion is especially astonishing. It is probably true that rights-talk has been less than helpful in society's struggle to come to a consensus about abortion. It is also probably true that the language of relations can be helpful in this discussion where the language of rights cannot. But when Noddings goes on to say that abortion is licit because it ends a relationship before it has begun, she is saying something that is both logically and empirically false. Logically, if no relationship has *begun*, then of course there is nothing to end. The only way I can possibly *end* a relationship if it is has begun; I cannot end non-existent relationships. Empirically Noddings likens early abortion to early miscarriage and argues that we do not hold funerals for lost embryos. In fact, however, study after study reveals that women who suffer miscarriage report a deep sense of loss and sadness. Many psychotherapists currently recommend that such women hold, if not funerals, then some kind of ritual to honor the life that has been lost and the depth of that pain. Similarly, even the most cursory reading of contemporary women's studies literature will reveal a similar pattern emerging with abortion. Even among women who remain putatively pro-abortion, there is a growing recognition of the need to mark an abortion with a ritual, one which allows the woman to acknowledge and grieve for her loss. Loss of what? Loss of what other than her child, and a relationship with that child? Such rituals are popping up all over the West, and Japan even has a name for it: *mizugo kuyo*. Such rituals exist because women know what Noddings denies: when a woman becomes pregnant, whether it be six days or six months, her body has become inextricably wedded to the body of another human being, her own child. Any basic obstetrics text will state that, from the moment conception occurs, a woman's entire body re-orients itself to the protection and nurture of its new companion. Not even Noddings can deny this. What she *does* deny is that a woman has a relationship with this being. She bases this on her claim that relationships require both a one-caring and a cared-for, implying that no such relationship can exist unless the cared-for can acknowledge and even reciprocate care. This notion is a troublesome one. If Noddings is right about this, then it would also be morally licit to withhold care from a hungry child in Romania; I do not even *know* her, so surely she can neither acknowledge nor reciprocate my care. This sort of calculation of benefits and returns is surely *not* the care for which Noddings advocates; it looks much more like a sort of canny bargain that I make. Such quid-pro-quo is in fact the antithesis of caring, and much of Noddings' other work indicates that she *knows* that.

When Noddings claims that it is never helpful to pit the rights of the unborn child against the rights of the mother, she is right, but for the wrong reasons. Such pitting of mother against child is wrong because it misconstrues reality. It is simply not the case that what is good for the mother is bad for the child, or vice versa. Abortion is not *good* for either of them; it hurts them both. This is the truth behind the Feminists for Life bumper sticker: "Every Abortion Has Two Victims: One Dead, One Wounded." Noddings' failure to see this hobbles her ethical vision and lessens her credibility.

CONCLUSION: WHAT'S A FEMINIST TO DO?

Unlike the Androgynous Ideal Feminists, and in line with the broad outlines of the Woman Idealist vision, I endorse a feminism which promotes equality without insisting on sameness. The differences between men and women are not a bothersome accident which technology must overcome, but rather something more profound and valuable. Women, according to this feminism, are not deformed non-male creatures; women are instead co-paradigms for the human race.

Here we can begin to see the outlines of a truly feminist view of woman: not-man, different from man, beautifully, passionately complementary to man. The world, according to this view, needs *not* to ignore or paper over the difference between men and women, *not* to construct bizarre utopias wherein technology will overcome these differences. Rather, the world needs to acknowledge these differences and re-form itself in the image of them, in other words, in the image of both women *and* men. To do so would be truly revolutionary, truly feminist.

The ethic of abortion on demand espoused by both Androgynous Idealists and Woman Idealists actually tells women that they simply cannot be the equals of men unless they chemically or surgically alter their bodies to *be* more like male bodies. The clear implication is that there is something *wrong* with the female body as it is naturally, that it needs fixing somehow. The ethic of abortion encourages (nay, insists) that women must sever their traditional tendency to invest themselves sexually only in relationships which promise commitment and longevity, to take care to offer themselves only to those they can trust with their deepest vulnerabilities. When contraception fails (as all forms do), the abortion ethic offers a woman the "choice" to have her body surgically invaded and her unborn child dismembered and torn from her womb so that she will not have to lose a day in the public, competitive world — the male world. Yet the holders of the abortion ethic call themselves feminists and attempt to silence their sisters who disagree.

When the Androgynous Idealists propose their ideal world, the ability to abort freely is supposed to lead to a fairer, juster world for women. As we move ever closer to the sort of world they envision, are we in fact seeing a "kinder, gentler" world for women? No. In fact, it was only just recently reported that a crisis of epidemic propositions looms on the immediate horizon for China. By the year 2025, men will outnumber women twenty to one. Why? Because China's oppressive policy of forced sterilization, contraception, and abortion has led to large-scale female infanticide and sex-selection abortion of female babies.

China is by no means alone. In India, in provinces so poor that there are no other medical facilities, not even an X-ray machine, there are ultrasound machines so that a woman can determine the sex of her child and abort her if she is a girl. And yes, even in the so-called "enlightened" Western nations, abortion is still done for sex-selection purposes; overwhelmingly, it is female, not male children who are aborted.

What is the source of an attitude toward women which causes such worldwide disregard for female life? What encourages the attitude that female life is cheap and expendable? I believe it is the attitudes of those who imply with their words and their policies that the model of the productive and worthwhile human being is the male model, and strive to make women emulate that model as thoroughly as possible. For this reason I stand with those feminists who aver that women are unique human beings, with a strength and beauty all their own. Yes, women conceive and bear children, and it is sexual intimacy with men which makes this possible. The world, say these feminists, must acknowledge the power and beauty of this possibility and remake itself in the image of this fact.

What would this mean? It would mean a world in which every human being, male and female, took seriously the power and beauty of sexual communion. It would be a world in which humans agreed that violence solves nothing, and almost always begets more violence. It would be a world which valued and held in highest regard the ability to give birth and organized itself around the importance of that power. It would be a world in which both fathers and mothers would be expected to rear their children, and doing so would count in their favor in the marketplace. Never would children be treated as either a burden which society tires of paying for, or a hobby that had best be pursued on one's own time. It would be a world in which all human beings, male and female, adult and child, respected the bodily and spiritual integrity of themselves and those around them.

Feminists need to continue to struggle to secure the rights and dignity of women everywhere. They must continue to demand the creation of a world which respects the intrinsic dignity of women. Women have traditionally been the ones to decry war and violence of all kinds. As co-creators and preservers of life at its most vulnerable, women have historically been the ones to remind the world of the value of life and the cruel futility of all forms of violence. Thus have women often been on the front lines of battles against capital punishment, the destruction of the environment and the fight against abortion. Women have much to teach the world.

I would like to close with a thought from — of all people — the Beatles, the rock group who, in the Sixties, saturated the airwaves of the West with this song among others:

> You say you want a Revolution?
> Well, you know —
> We all want to change the world.

The Beatles to the contrary, not all people want to change the world. A whole lot of people want to change women, though. In fact, they demand such change as the price of a woman's equal status in the world. In order to compete in a world largely shaped and defined by men, such thinkers assume that a woman must re-create herself in man's image and likeness. When confronted with that view, feminists ought to reply with a resounding "No." Feminists must demand a real Revolution — one in which women and men work together, should to shoulder, to re-create the world in the image of women *and* men.

NOTES

1. See, for example, Betty Friedan, *The Feminist Mystique* (New York: W. W. Norton 1963).

2. Alison Jaggar makes this point in *Feminist Politics and Human Nature* (Totowa NJ: Rowman and Allanheld 1983) 86.

3. Quoted in Jaggar 86.

4. Shulamith Firestone, *The Dialectic of Sex: The Case for Feminist Revolution* (New York: William Morrow 1970) 206.

5. Jaggar 132.

6. Gayle Rubin, "The Traffic in Women: Notes on the 'Political Economy' of Sex" in Rayna R. Reiter, ed., *Toward an Anthropology of Women* (New York: Monthly Review Press 1975) 165.

7. Andrea Dworkin, "Why So-Called Radical Men Love and Need Pornography" in Laura Lederer, ed., *Take Back the Night: Women on Pornography* (New York: William Morrow 1980) 148.

8. Carol Gilligan, *In a Different Voice* (Cambridge: Harvard Univ. Press 1982). See also Mary Belenky, Blythe Clichy, Nancy Goldberger and Jill Tarule, *Women's Ways of Knowing* (New York: Basic Books 1987).

9. Nel Noddings, *Caring: A Feminine Approach to Ethics and Moral Education* (Berkeley: Univ. of California Press 1984) 9. See also Chapter Two, passim.

10. A point made by Rosemarie Tong in *Feminine and Feminist Ethics* (Belmont CA: Wadswoth 1993) 110.

11. *Caring* 238.

12. *Caring* 236.

13. *Caring* 151.

14. *Caring* 151.

15. *Caring* 143.

16. *Caring* 152.

ABORTION AND POLITICAL COMPROMISE

Christopher Wolfe

When I wrote the initial version of this paper, it seemed that *Roe v. Wade* was clearly in for substantial pruning possibly even an outright overruling — in the near future, leaving the ball, so to speak, in the pro-life court. As it turned out, of course, in *Planned Parenthood of Southeastern Pennsylvania v. Casey* the Court, with Justice Kennedy's defection, actually *reaffirmed* the central holding of *Roe v. Wade*, though it upheld most of the law at issue. That decision left the final abortion decision to women, subject to regulation at the margin by state and local government.

The recent congressional elections were a remarkable success for pro-life candidates, but it is not at all clear how much that success will be translated into practical political action. The early months of Congress have focused on issues of government structure and process and on the budget, for the most part, with abortion and other social issues very consciously put on a backburner. Republican presidential hopefuls have generally made it clear that they will not provide leadership on the issue, with the exception of Pat Buchanan and Alan Keyes, whose campaign styles, in my opinion, will succeed in mobilizing the party's intense antiabortion minority, but will not appeal (may even put off) the party majority comprised of less intense abortion opponents, those who are ambivalent, and the small but disproportionately influential and growing pro-abortion wing of the party. In the Democratic party, the good news was that Clinton might face an articulate antiabortion opponent, Bob Casey, former governor of Pennsylvania. The bad news is that Casey has opted out of the race for the time being and, in any case, would have

42

little chance of winning that party's nomination.

What the future holds, in both the judicial and the legislative/executive spheres is therefore very unclear at the moment, though I can't say that I'm optimistic. We'll simply have to wait and see how 1996 shakes out.

Nonetheless, I do believe that we must continue to grapple with the question of what we *can* do and what we *ought to* do with respect to the legality of abortion in this nation. This paper is a restatement of an earlier article's thesis that political compromise on abortion can be justified under some circumstances, even for those of us who believe that the direct procuring of abortion is *always* a terrible moral evil.[1]

THE CURRENT STATE OF PUBLIC OPINION

As James Davison Hunter's article in *First Things* (June/July, 1992) reminded us, Americans do not accept the positions of either pro-abortion or anti-abortion activists, but rather they agree with some elements of each. Most Americans agree that what is at stake in abortion *is* human life, and conclude from this that abortions should therefore not be performed for less than a serious reason. They are sympathetic to abortion when it comes to "the hard cases," i.e., life of the mother, serious health problems of the mother, rape and incest, and serious fetal deformity. They also tend to think it more legitimate to have an abortion early in pregnancy rather than later. In other words, they are genuinely ambivalent. One thing, however, seems quite certain: If Americans are given a choice between a pure pro-life position (no exceptions) and a pure pro-choice position, they will certainly choose the latter. In a culture that emphasizes individual liberty as much as ours does, ambivalence on an issue like abortion can easily translate into rhetorical power for a "pro-choice" position — unless, that is, the pro-life movement adopts a flexible political position that accepts the most that prudent action can attain in the present state of American attitudes.

Now it could be said that Americans will not be given such a choice between two "pure" positions, because there will always be different shades of opinion represented in legislatures that consider it, and the result will be some sort of compromise. And if the final result of each legislative battle will be compromise, some might argue that the pro-life movement must be as unyielding as possible in its demands in order to improve the outcome of the negotiating process.

The problem with this argument is that the vote in the legislature (especially after the demise of *Roe v. Wade*) would not be the crucial one. The crucial votes are those cast in elections for the legislators. The key question, then, is how to win enough of such elections to obtain pro-life legislative majorities.

Before *Webster*, the pro-life movement had one tremendous advantage: it could unite people *against* a very extreme status quo. Even people who might favor abortion in a small number of hard cases could be aghast at the almost unlimited right to abortion afforded by *Roe*. With the cutting back of this decision, however, and the expansion of the power to regulate abortion "at the margin" upheld in *Casey*, it will no longer be possible to build a powerful political movement simply on the basis of opposition to the extreme *Roe* position. A larger number of voters will be concerned with the question of what will take its place. Even the withdrawal of the judiciary from this issue — which would, in any event, likely be only a partial one (continuing to protect abortion in some cases, e.g., life of the mother, rape, and incest) — inevitably shifts the focus to legislative battles. And the problem this poses for the pro-life movement is that many of the people who are aghast at *Roe* are no less so at a pro-life position that is completely unyielding on the other side.

Given a choice between someone running on a Planned

Parenthood (or national Democratic party) abortion platform and someone running on a no-exceptions pro-life platform, most citizens will — perhaps even with misgivings — vote for the former. (The term "no exceptions" should be understood to include positions that have an exception only for the life of the mother.[2]) Given a choice between a "pure" position on *either* side and a compromise political position, most of the same voters would choose the compromise. It is harder to say what voters will do if given a choice between two compromise positions. For example, what if one generally pro-life candidate favored allowing exceptions in the "hard cases" and another generally pro-choice candidate accepted a prohibition of third trimester abortions and those based on sex selection? The generally pro-life position would have at least a good shot of carrying the day, though one cannot really be sure.

NO EXCEPTIONS?

But does it make any sense to talk of a "generally pro-life position"? Does not the allowance of exceptions undermine the position by forfeiting its grounds in principle? Moreover, would not such a position be seen as a politically disastrous "waffle," even by those voters who are in the middle themselves? In short, is there such a thing as a morally acceptable political compromise on abortion?

A good way to find the sound affirmative answer to this question is to look at St. Thomas Aquinas' answer to the problem of "whether it belongs to the human law to repress all vices?" (*Summa Theologica* I-II, Q. 96, Art. 4). (Note that "vices" here refers not to personal foibles but to clear moral evils.) St. Thomas says that laws imposed on men should be in keeping with their condition, for (quoting Isidore) law should be "possible both according to nature, and according to the customs of the country." This possibility is related to interior habit or disposition, some things being possible for one who has a virtuous habit that are not possible for others.   "Human law is framed for a number of human beings, the majority of whom are not perfect in virtue.   Wherefore human laws do not forbid all vices, from which the virtuous abstain, but only the more grievous vices, from which it is possible for the majority to abstain; and chiefly those that are to the hurt of others, without the prohibition of which human society could not be maintained; thus human law prohibits murder, theft, and suchlike."   In one of the responses, Aquinas adds that the danger of imposing on imperfect men precepts that they cannot bear is that "the precepts are despised, and those men, from contempt, break out into evils worse still."

On the question of abortion, to be sure, this analysis can cut both ways.   Those who argue for an uncompromising position on abortion could point out that abortion falls precisely into the category which St. Thomas gives as the area where law should repress vice, that is, the area where harm is done to others — particularly, of course, the crime of murder.   Since abortion is a species of murder, it always ought to be repressed.

But to take such a position is not the best way to apply St. Thomas' analysis.   For one thing, the general criterion he offers for determining what vices human law may forbid is those vices that the majority of human beings are able to abstain from.   The quotation from Isidore above suggests that this possibility is defined not just with respect to human nature in general, but also with respect to the customs of the country.   The question of which vices the citizens of a given community are capable of abstaining from is an empirical one.

For another thing, while St. Thomas says that the vices from which a majority can abstain are chiefly those to the hurt of others, without the prohibition of which human society cannot be maintained, that does not necessarily mean that any action involving serious harm to others should automatically be repressed. For example, it may not always be possible to enforce laws against prostitution (II-II, Q. 10, Art. 11), though men's transactions with prostitutes clearly harm wives and children. That acts harming others need not automatically be repressed is especially clear if one gives due weight to the qualification "without the prohibition of which human society cannot be maintained."

Moreover, the reference to murder need not be interpreted as applying to every act that is murder. If we are talking about laws without which human society cannot be maintained, then the reference seems to mean that we cannot forego murder laws *in general*. But there can be laws against murder in general without prohibiting every single form of murder. Even if it is true that any inconsistency on this point "tends" to undermine society, it is nonetheless true that many human societies based on great injustice have been able to maintain themselves for a long time.

This does not mean, of course, that the law should repress only those vices without the prohibition of which human society could not be maintained. The criterion here is that the law should repress those vices which men of imperfect virtue are by nature and by the customs of their country capable of abstaining from.[3] Again, the question here is an empirical one.

Another criterion to be considered is the greater evils that can occur if a particular evil is not tolerated. For one, there is the consequence that the law will be despised and that those who cannot bear the law will, from contempt, break out into worse evils still. It is not hard to see that the inability of society to enforce a law may lead to disrespect for law. While the example is by now overdone, the case of Prohibition in the U.S. illustrates the danger very vividly. It seems very likely that an abortion law with no exceptions would be widely disobeyed. What might be the greater evils to follow from this? One would be the development of a thriving black market for abortions — one that would take all comers (rather than limiting abortions to particular cases), thus resulting in some deaths that might be prevented by a narrower law. An effect more difficult to predict and evaluate would be the effect on the body politic as a result of the disruption, including hatred and violence, that might accompany an abortion law that greatly exceeded what the customs of our country would accept. This hatred and violence, in addition to being an evil in itself, might turn public opinion (especially people with less firm moral views — "the muddled moderates") against the whole effort to prohibit the evil of abortion at all. Finally, perhaps the most obvious "greater evil" of a no-exceptions abortion law would be simply that it would never pass; the law would allow many abortions that might as a result of compromise have been prevented.

Applying St. Thomas' analysis, thus interpreted, one can argue that abortion in general should fall in the category of vices that ought to be repressed (the customs of our country are not so corrupt as to require abortion on demand), but one can also argue that the law would be prudent to withhold criminal punishment of *certain forms* of abortion (since the customs of our community clearly do make a total proscription of abortion impossible).

"COMPROMISE"

At this point, it seems useful to make some distinctions about the term "compromise." It is important to understand that the advocacy of political compromise does not involve compromise on the moral issue of abortion itself. Morally speaking, it is *never* acceptable directly to take the life of an innocent person, which the unborn child always is. ("Directly" means that, in some cases, it may be possible to permit the death of the unborn child as an unintended but unavoidable side effect of another action that is morally good, e.g., the case of removing a cancerous uterus.) "Legitimate compromise" on abortion, then, should always be understood to mean *political* compromise, that is, compromise about when the law should punish abortion as a criminal act.

Political compromise itself can be subdivided into at least two basic types. The first is what may be called "tactical compromise." This involves fighting in the legislature to obtain a prohibition of all directly procured abortion, using all one's resources possible to obtain this end, but when the final vote arrives, accepting something less than that complete prohibition because nothing more is possible at that moment. For example, Henry Hyde has provided admirable pro-life leadership in Congressional battles over the years, working to prohibit any funding of abortion; but on some occasions he has been compelled by political realities to cast a final vote for bills that have allowed funding in some cases, e.g., cases of rape and incest. This kind of political compromise is very limited, for the vote in favor of such a law is occasioned only by immediate political necessity and it simply leads right into the next political battle to achieve complete prohibition.[4]

The second, more controversial, kind of compromise (the one I want to advocate) may be called "strategic compromise." A prudent strategic political compromise on the abortion issue would start with a reminder of what we all agree on: The *political* battle is merely one front in a larger war; the ultimate goal is not merely to obtain laws that will *compel* women not to have abortions, but to form a polity that recognizes the sacredness of human life and whose citizens reject abortion as a violation of that principle. The "cultural" battle is not separate from the "political" battle — there is an intimate connection between the two — but there is a difference. At least part of that difference has to do with the nature and limits of law.

A strategic compromise on abortion would pursue the full moral principle at the level of the cultural or educational battle, while at the political level accepting "for the time being" laws that do not prohibit all abortion, or at least explicitly withhold criminal punishment for some of them, i.e., abortion "in the hard cases." "For the time being" means until public opinion can be brought around to the view that all abortion is wrong. Such compromise therefore goes well beyond the kind of tactical compromise that is forced, say, on a legislator in a given political vote, since strategic compromise amounts to a kind of temporary, political, "truce" on the exceptions.

This truce is limited to the political battlefield — it does not apply to the cultural one. In some ways, policy here might be likened to U.S. strategy in the Cold War, in which the country adopted a policy of containment, accepting for the time being the immoral conquests of the evil empire and looking forward to some day in the future when the Soviet Union would collapse (largely through defeat in the "war of ideas"). And — to spell out one of the less than fully palatable implications of this strategy — just as the containment policy led the United States to avoid using tactical opportunities to make inroads into the Soviet Empire, e.g., as in the case of the Hungarian Revolution of 1956, so the pro-life movement might not for the time being automatically press for the most protective law that short-term political circumstances made possible.

For example, it is easy to imagine a situation in which a series of political "accidents" might give strong pro-lifers a majority in the legislature of a particular state in which at the same time public opinion would not support prohibition of abortion without exceptions in the hard cases. In such a case, political prudence might suggest that a no-exceptions bill not be pushed for in the legislature, even if the votes were there.

A parallel instance of the latter argument is provided by

the recent situation faced by Catholics in Poland. In view of the power and prestige of the Church there, derived from both history and from the Church's leadership in the resistance to Communism, it was tempting for Catholics to push for laws that embodied moral principles as fully as possible. But efforts of that kind — even if partly successful in the short run — seem to have produced a substantial backlash against the Church, with a substantial forfeiting of the Church's influence in politics and in society (which raises the question of the longer-term viability of the laws that were passed).

Closer to home is a recent example from New Jersey politics. In 1992, the New Jersey legislature had a Republican majority that was largely "accidental," a popular reaction to unpopular tax policies of a Democratic governor. Should pro-life legislators in such a situation have pressed to obtain the maximum pro-life legislation that could be passed in that session? Or should a pro-life legislative strategist consider, not just what could be obtained by a vote of the current legislature, but also whether this legislation could be *maintained* and whether it might, due to a backlash, lead to something far worse?

Both tactical and strategic compromise are based on prudential considerations. Since part of the prudential norm is that exceptions be tolerated only as much as and for as long as they *need* to be tolerated, there is a natural tendency to look at things from a short-term perspective ("do we have the votes now?"). That might well be a mistake, especially in a democracy, where elections occur regularly and are often affected by accidental factors. Our prudential evaluation of circumstances affecting how closely we can bring our law into line with the moral law (and in this case, the moral ideal is clearly the political one as well) should consider the ways in which short-term "successes" built on accidental factors might lead to disaster.

The legitimacy of this position turns on an important assumption, namely, that a disputed question of moral philosophy can be resolved in its favor. One of the fundamental principles of morality is that evil may never be done (directly intended) to obtain good, though evil may sometimes be "tolerated" as a side-effect in order to obtain a greater good. Some pro-life moral philosophers are concerned that, when strategic political compromise is used to justify *not* pursuing the full protection of the innocent for which we have the votes right *now*, that refusal to act is directly willing an evil (the injustice of failing to protect some unborn) — not as an end in itself, of course, but as a means to protect other unborn children. Those of us who advocate such strategic compromise are convinced that proper moral analysis will show that it does not directly will an evil (it is not directly willing, even as a means, the refusal to protect those who have a right to be protected), but merely tolerates it as a side-effect.

For casuists, I offer the following analogy. A nation has a moral obligation, in justice, to protect its people from unjust attacks. But when a nation is invaded, strategic considerations may require that, tactically, an invading army be permitted to overrun part of the country (killing some of the citizens), that could be protected more fully, but only at the expense of longer-term success in the war.

Perhaps this is not merely hypothetical. Churchill knew that the Germans were going to bomb Coventry, because the Allies had broken the German code. But, in order to prevent the Germans from realizing that the code had been broken (an invaluable benefit in the long-term prosecution of the war), Churchill decided not to take some of the measures that would have reduced the loss of life in that attack (though, certainly, the nation has an obligation in justice to protect its citizens). I don't think that Churchill was a great moralist, but I think he did the right thing in that case.

THE FEDERALISM CONTEXT

In considering what pro-life strategy should be, I think that it is necessary always to keep in mind that ultimately the resolution of this matter must be accomplished at the national level. Simply returning the issue to the states cannot be a long-term solution. For one thing, some of the states that will probably maintain strongly pro-abortion laws, such as New York and California, account for a large percentage of the abortions in the country. For another, anti-abortion state laws will increase the price and the difficulty of an abortion by the price and difficulty of a bus trip to a pro-abortion state. The increased cost and inconvenience may reduce the number of abortions, but hardly significantly. In the long run, then, the resolution of the abortion issue must be achieved by a Human Life Bill in Congress (pursuant to its power to enforce Fourteenth Amendment "equal protection of the laws") or, more fundamentally, by a Human Life Amendment.

It is, however, necessary to point out that a national resolution is not imminent, to say the least. The national Democratic party is firmly controlled by pro-choicers, and the Congress, while controlled now by Republicans, is clearly ambivalent about even relatively limited forms of restricting abortion. In the near future, then, the pro-life movement must continue its incremental strategy, focusing primarily on overturning *Roe v. Wade*, so as to make abortion restrictions possible at the state level, and then on obtaining whatever restrictions are possible to obtain state by state. These efforts will typically start with the areas that have the strongest support in public opinion, using these victories to educate and to build political momentum for future and broader legislation. Given the considerable variations in public opinion in different states, the legislation it will be possible and prudent to pursue in one or another will vary substantially.

A more difficult question is whether, since the national

battle must remain the ultimate focus, state battles ought to take into consideration the possible effect of state laws on national public opinion. And if highly protective state laws (e.g., those that would allow exceptions only for the life of the mother) would provide ammunition for the national pro-choice movement, then prudence might suggest second thoughts about them.

IS COMPROMISE SELF-DEFEATING?

It could be, and indeed is, objected that the policy of stategic compromise would be morally and politically disastrous. This objection must be taken seriously. How can avowedly "pro-life" candidates, whose position is based on the contention that abortion is taking the life of an innocent human being, compromise on the hard cases, without appearing to be, and being, unprincipled? Besides, voters may disagree with public figures who hold fast to principle but they positively despise those who compromise their principles merely to win political power. Look at the electoral fate of such "wafflers" on this issue as the candidates for governor in New Jersey and Virginia in 1990.

Nevertheless, a strategic compromise that forbids abortion in general but withholds criminal punishment of abortion in the hard cases is compatible both with principle and with electoral necessities.

An example of such a compromise law would be the Utah abortion statute, as amended in 1991. This law would limit abortions to those "necessary to save the pregnant woman's life" or "to prevent grave damage" to her health or "to prevent the birth of a child that would be born with grave defects"— all of these to be determined "in the professional judgment of the pregnant woman's attending physician"— and to cases where the pregnancy is a result of a previously reported act of rape or incest, and within 20 weeks of conception.

Ideally, this law would be reformulated so that instead of "authorizing" abortion for the exceptional circumstances it would prohibit abortion in general, explicitly withholding criminal sanctions in the exceptional cases. (It may also be that leaving decisions to the judgment of doctors may have the practical effect of preventing effective enforcement of the law.)

The above concerns aside, why is a law like this a morally acceptable political compromise? To begin with, the strategic compromise position is in no way based on the contention that abortion, very much including the hard cases, is morally legitimate. Its advocates must emphasize — and unfortunately, many allegedly pro-life Republican leaders who favor certain forms of "compromise" are failing to do this — that their overall position on abortion continues to be that abortion is always wrong because it involves the direct killing of an innocent person. Moreover, they should indicate that they intend to pursue the long-term goal of persuading society that abortion is always wrong, thereby establishing the conditions of a law that fully respects the moral principle of the sanctity of innocent human life. The classic model here is Abraham Lincoln, who was able to favor a compromise solution on slavery "for the time being" while making very clear his commitment to the principle that slavery is wrong.

What then is the basis for such a compromise? It is the limits of politics and of coercive law. The fact that something is contrary to the moral law does not automatically mean that it ought to be forbidden by civil law. When a society is deeply divided on a moral issue, it is not always possible or prudent to try to settle the matter fully by the coercive power of law.

A large majority of Americans think that, as a general rule, innocent human life should not be destroyed. There may even be a majority who believe that human life, in some sense, begins at conception. This by itself would seem to provide a sufficient basis for a law generally prohibiting abortion. Unfortunately, however, there are many of our fellow citizens who believe (1) that the value of unborn human life, important as it is, does not always override other, serious values, and (2) that there are different levels of importance to life at various stages of pregnancy. Until we can *persuade* Americans that it is a mistake to "balance" human life against those other values, it would be imprudent to embody in the criminal law an absolute ban on abortion.

WHAT STRATEGIC COMPROMISE?

One question this leaves for me is whether there is any prudent line to draw with respect to "strategic" compromise.[5] Could strategic compromise justify, for example, tolerating all first-trimester abortions, with strict limits on abortions thereafter?[6] I would argue against accepting this form of legislation, as a "strategic" compromise, on the grounds that it simply gives away too much. One should only "tolerate" an evil if, on balance, the benefits of doing so justify the toleration. I do not think a law that left abortion wide open during the first trimester would, on the whole, be prudent. Perhaps most importantly, such a law would, by its likely "educative" message, undercut the effort to bring public opinion to a deeper awareness of the evil of abortion. A law that compromised on the so-called "hard cases" would be different in that respect, I believe.

The difference with the "hard cases" is precisely that they involve genuine difficulties that make it much harder for most ordinary people to live out the implications of respect for life. Abortion in the case of a threat to the life of the mother is the best example, since it is possible that one of the very highest prices will be exacted from the mother, father, and the rest of the family for adherence to the moral law. Rape and incest, serious health problems for the mother (those that may inflict substantial and irreparable physical harm) and grave fetal deformities (those which, again, are serious and irreparable) also constitute extremely difficult circumstances under which to bear a child.

It is no answer to such problems, politically speaking, that they occur only in a few cases and therefore are not relevant to the abortion debate. Not surprisingly, public opionion would refuse to accept that, and argue instead that precisely if it is "only" a few cases, then exceptions for them ought to be permitted.

One does not want to exaggerate the difficulties of pregnant women in these situations, as is often done; still, it is desirable to avoid a certain kind of obliviousness to human suffering that adherence to principle can sometimes lead to. And I think it is imperative that those who represent the pro-life movement make clear their compassion for those who suffer, even while refusing to concede that sympathy for the suffering can justify the commission of morally evil acts. (Equally important must be the denial that abortion, on the whole, alleviates suffering; rather, it must firmly be maintained that abortion deals only with symptoms, serving as an excuse *not* to deal with the real, underlying causes of suffering.)

None of these circumstances changes the basic moral issue, since such considerations do not justify *doing* a moral evil. They do, however, have an impact on the moral burdens that human beings of "imperfect virtue"— "ordinary people" — are able to bear. This would be true, I would guess, in most times and places. It is especially true of our contemporary culture, in which many of the "customs of the community" — affluence, materialism, sensuality, utilitarian morality — tend to undermine people's fortitude in dealing with moral choices that involve pain or discomfort. This may be a strong argument for using issues like abortion to educate people to a deeper sense of the priority of "the good" over "the pleasant," but in our national circumstances it would not be prudent to try to accomplish this education through the coercive power of the criminal law.

Putting this argument in a somewhat milder, more rhetorical form (it would probably not be advisable for candidates in elections to tell people that most of them fall in the category of "those of imperfect virtue") one can say that human law — especially the criminal law — does not ordinarily demand "heroism" of people.[7]

The pro-life movement can, and ought to, exhort people to respond heroically to difficult moral circumstances. One way in which many pro-lifers do in fact exhort and encourage is by setting an example themselves: helping people in those circumstances, with much self-sacrifice. But to demand heroism *through the criminal law* is likely to breed widespread resentment, disrespect for the law, and illegal action (both public civil disobedience and surreptitious evasion of the law). It is also likely to lead to a political backlash that results in repeal of the law, that discredits those who supported it, and that makes for legislation far worse than the moderate measure that might have been secured in the first place.

Nor would strategic compromise have to appear to be a "waffling" position. Of course, if not presented and defended articulately, it might come across that way. But the "wafflers" who went down to defeat in New Jersey and Virginia in 1990 were not men who clearly and forcefully enunciated the kind of strategic compromise described here; they seemed rather to be trying to duck the issue or push it to the side.

The greatest virtue of this strategic compromise is that it will save many lives that might otherwise have been lost. If a policy of strategic compromise succeeds, it will eliminate a large percentage of our current abortions, numbered these days in the millions.

How many abortions there would be under such a

dispensation is hard to say. It would depend partly on the care with which the policy is drafted, so as to prevent exceptions from becoming large loopholes. (One presumes that at least some in the medical profession will try to help pregnant women to evade the law.) It also will depend on strong pro-life efforts to back effective enforcement efforts.

This justification based on the limits of law would not be readily available for compromise based on the stage of pregnancy, which, as I have suggested, the pro-life movement should avoid, with one (unfortunately massive) exception. Compromise on the basis of the stage of pregnancy would undercut the principle of respect for human life far more than making exceptions in the hard cases, by permitting abortions for something other than "serious reasons," indeed for any reason, however trivial. Obviously, it is lamentable that the law should embody a principle that fails to respect human life (against direct taking) for *any* "reason." But at least requiring a "serious reason" preserves some fuller sense of the principle.[8]

The one, unfortunately necessary, exception to avoiding "stage of pregnancy" lines is at the beginning of pregnancy, i.e., the case of abortifacient "contraceptives." The tendency of many ordinary citizens to say, "If it looks like a baby, it must be a baby" — which helps to provide the pro-life movement with much of its support — also has the effect of depriving the pro-life movement of support when "it" doesn't look like a baby, i.e. the time immediately after conception (and at least through implantation). That factor, plus the deep attachment of American culture to contraception, mean that an effort to prohibit abortifacient contraceptives would be hopeless. It would clearly discredit the pro-life movement with many people.

Unfortunately, the battle is likely to shift to that front. One can see that in Laurence Tribe's exaltation of the principle of "privacy in the home," even as he expresses

some misgivings about *Roe v. Wade*.[9] The misgivings do
not lead him to oppose *Roe* — he supports it by adding an
equal protection argument — but his enthusiasm for the
decision is decidedly muted.   It seems plausible to
speculate that he is hoping the abortion issue can be
resolved by the advent of the "abortion pill" that can be
taken in the privacy of one's home.[10]

But precisely because the future of the pro-life movement
is clouded by the likelihood of such future developments,
it becomes all the more important to try to get as strong a
principle of respect for life into the law as we can now.

SUPPORT FOR PREGNANT WOMEN

Another element in an effective pro-life strategic
compromise would be efforts in the law to support women
in carrying their unborn children to term. Especially where
the temptation to abort children stems from economic
hardship, it is desirable to eliminate this incentive to have
an abortion. Thus, even if criminal penalties are withheld
from abortion in the hard cases, that does not mean that the
law must always be "neutral" regarding such cases. It is
possible for the law to encourage and support pregnant
women in carrying their children to term, whether or not
abortions are prohibited.

A very difficult issue in regard to support for pregnant
women is whether or not it exacerbates the problem in the
long run. Charles Murray and others have made persuasive
arguments that government programs in aid of unwed
mothers help to create a culture of dependency that worsens
the problem by creating perverse incentives. Murray is
generally persuasive, although it is not easy to know what
conclusions to draw from his analysis. But in the instance
of abortion, it is important that one impact of such
programs, intended or unintended, is to show people that
the political community that forbids the "easy way out" of
abortion is not indifferent to their difficulties. Unless some

other way out of the dilemma is possible, this argument, in my opinion, outweighs Murray's.

The current form of that hard question concerns welfare reform. If Congress adopts rules that cut off additional government support for women on welfare who conceive new children outside of marriage, or that cut off welfare for girls under 18 who conceive out of wedlock, there is a likelihood that there will be at least some short-term increase in abortions. (A recent rise in New Jersey abortions may be an example of that.) The National Right to Life Committee and leading anti-abortion congressmen have opposed certain forms of welfare reform on these grounds.

My own view is that pro-life members of Congress should do as much as they can to limit possible incentives to abortion,[11] but that the possibility of some increase in abortions is not a conclusive argument against welfare reform. To say that it is is to defend a form of extortion: "give me more money or I'll get an abortion." It is, moreover, to incapacitate the government from changing incentive structures that have had a profound effect of undermining family formation and stability in the United States.

Of course, if there are other ways to accomplish the goals of welfare reform (family formation and stability, fairness in allocating financial assessments by society) successfully, without any indirect spur to abortions, they would be preferable. But it seems to me that evaluating the likelihood of different effects of different measures would involve difficult prudential questions, and that it would be improper for leaders of the pro-life movement to make one particular position a *sine qua non* for their political support in future elections.

THE NEED FOR COMPROMISE

In the long run, a no-exceptions position is likely to

discredit not only "moralism" but the very source of morality itself. One reason it is very difficult to get Americans to take natural law thought seriously is that historically, i.e. in the Middle Ages, the natural law was articulated in a form that considerably devalued personal liberty, especially in the area of religion. Criminal laws that track the moral law closely (even where there is little in the mores to support such laws) can only serve to exacerbate the suspicion of natural law thinking.

An insistence on no exceptions would doom the pro-life movement to political inefficacy for the foreseeable future. Nor is there any reason to believe that "purifying" the pro-life movement would increase its influence in the long run. The number of Americans who would actively work for a public policy that coincided with the full demands of the moral law is extremely small.

One difficulty here is that a policy of no exceptions would require principled opposition to any and all abortifacient contraceptives. In the short run, that would mean a very small core of activists representing a relatively small portion of the population, serving as "prophets" without political influence. These activists would presumably have a beneficial effect on the lives of some citizens who were persuaded by their advocacy; and however small the number, such an effect should not be dismissed as minor. That is why it will always be good and necessary to have some people in the pro-life movement who represent the "no-exceptions" position.

But the long-term influence of a pro-life movement that, for the most part, accepts strategic compromise would also be valuable, notwithstanding arguments that it would lose its capacity to persuade or transform by its unwillingness to adhere to principle: first, because it could and should make clear its adherence to principle, and second, because it would obtain a hearing from many people who would not bother to listen to those who are completely unyielding on the question of legal prohibitions.

But does not this position, it might be asked, much resemble that of Mario Cuomo — and is not Cuomo's position one that no pro-lifer would be willing to call "pro-life"? Now, it is true that Cuomo's description of general principles is fairly accurate. He is right when he says that the civil law need not always fully enforce the moral law, and that what the law can do is ultimately a matter of prudential political judgment. His problem is that his prudential judgments are poor — so much so that their congruency with political expediency both in New York and in the national Democratic party lead one to certain nagging suspicions about their source.

Cuomo opts for the easy assertion that "abortion is a tragedy." Therefore he limits his anti-abortion stance to saying that we should do all we can to make it easier not to make that choice — by supporting social welfare laws. But "abortion is a tragedy" is too vague and too minimal: It is not only a tragedy, but a terrible injustice as well. In the words of Princeton's Professor Robert George, "A child getting run over is a tragedy; deliberately running over a child is an injustice." Cuomo believes that no restriction on abortion is possible, and even that much opposition to public funding of abortion is impossible. Alas, what he means by "possible" others might be tempted to define as "pussilanimous," in the root meaning of the term.

Finally, he likes to treat abortion as a "Catholic" issue, and then to argue against imposing church morality on our pluralistic society. This is his deepest failure, not only as a Catholic layman but also as a politician. He cannot shift responsibility for moral positions to the Church, and then use that as an excuse not to defend fundamental principles of justice. Abortion is not bad because the Church says so.

The Church says that it is an "unconscionable crime" because it is so — in ways that any person, whatever his or her religion, should be able to see. Cuomo would do well to remind himself that while Lincoln compromised on slavery, in the end he is remembered by all as the great opponent of slavery. Cuomo's so-called "compromise" on abortion is simply to support abortion-on-demand and abortion funding and to beef up government social services and contraception. No one will ever remember him as having been an opponent of abortion.

One of the most difficult problems in pursuing a policy of strategic compromise is how to prevent such a policy from being interpreted as a *moral* compromise. Professor Charles Rice argues that "every time a pro-lifer proposes a law that would tolerate the execution of some unborn children, his pro-life rhetoric is drowned out by the loud and clear message of his action, that he concedes that the law can validly tolerate the intentional killing of innocent human beings."[12] That is, the law does not speak — and educate — merely through its rhetoric. The simple fact of the law is itself profoundly important. No matter how carefully the law is framed in words that respect the ideal of the sanctity of human life, compromise legislation still has as its bottom line the toleration of some abortions. And people being the way they are, some, perhaps many, will conclude from the fact that an act is not illegal that it is not immoral.

THE LEADING EXAMPLE OF MODERATE MORALISM

An example of this impact, but perhaps also an example of the limits of this argument as well, can be found in the case of slavery. Most of the leading founders believed that slavery was unjust and should be eliminated when that became possible. Yet they compromised in the Constitution and tolerated slavery, in the expectation that it was "in the course of extinction" (for reasons related both to economics — it was inefficient — and the spread of enlightened republican principles, such as those found in the Declaration of Independence). Unfortunately, the founders' toleration of slavery made it possible, not long after the founding, for a new generation of Southern leaders not only to defend slavery as a practical necessity (the line generally taken by the representatives of the slave interest during the founding), but also as something positively good, reflecting a natural order.

Eventually, it was necessary for American society to insist on its commitment to its founding principles, and it did so under the leadership of Abraham Lincoln. Lincoln was unwilling to say that slavery was compatible with the principles of our government, arguing that this nation could not long endure "half-slave, half-free." He favored a policy of preventing the spread of slavery any further, trusting that in due time this would lead to its extinction. But at the same time he was willing to accept slavery "for the time being," denying that the federal government had any right to interfere with slavery in those states where it already existed. Indeed, on the eve of the Civil War Lincoln was willing to agree to a constitutional amendment guaranteeing non-interference with slavery within the states.

Lincoln's position, then, was decidedly a "compromise" position. Was Lincoln's approach immoral and/or ineffective because he compromised his principles? Some abolitionists thought so. But in retrospect most of us would disagree. In fact, if the only opposition to slavery had been the abolitionists, who knows how long it would have taken to eliminate slavery? Lincoln, because of his political compromise, was able to win election as President, so that the principle of freedom from slavery eventually guided the prudential decisions of the nation. If the pro-life movement hopes to guide national decisions in the foreseeable future, it will only be possible on the basis of a platform that announces its principle clearly, while accepting prudential limits on it in practice.

Of course, there are some crucial differences between the two issues of slavery and abortion. Among them is the fact that the country was split sectionally on slavery — there is something more like a national "consensus" on abortion, though with some state and regional variations. Abolitionists had considerable influence in the North, where opinion became strongly anti-slavery (enough to elect Lincoln); "no-exceptions pro-lifers" are not likely to be a significant political force anywhere. For the same reason — the sectional polarization — it was possible to "settle" the slavery issue by a war. That will not be the resolution of the abortion issue.

But the slavery issue does show us that compromise — even relatively long-term compromise — is compatible with maintaining political principle. If Lincoln could maintain principle while allowing deviations from it "for the time being," the pro-life movement can do so as well. And that is preferable to letting new generations be "drowned" in the widespread practice of abortion that will result if we do not act in ways that recognize the limits of politics and law in our nation.

NOTES

1. An earlier version of this article appeared in *First Things* Number 24 (June/July 1992) 22-29.

2. For the record, even a "life of the mother" exception raises some serious moral questions that can be resolved only by making careful distinctions. A utilitarian calculus that says the mother is "more important" than the child, and therefore the child may be killed in order to save the life of the mother, is morally unacceptable. On the other hand, actions to save the life of the mother, when they have the unintended but foreseen side-effect of leading to the death of the child, may be morally licit.

3. I do not take up here the question of how law might be limited by its purpose of prohibiting vice that is contrary to the *common* good, and whether there are moral evils whose effects are so much confined to the individual (and whose effects on the common good are *de minimis*) that they should not be prohibited by law. These questions clearly do not apply to any form of abortion.

4. I assume that this form of compromise is legitimate. For Catholics, the issue has been settled clearly by Pope John Paul II in *Evangelium Vitae*, No. 73: "A particular problem of conscience can arise in cases where a legislative vote would be decisive for the passage of a more restrictive law, aimed at limiting the number of authorized abortions, in place of a more permissive law already passed or ready to be voted on. . . . In a case like the one just mentioned, when it is not possible to overturn or completely abrogate a pro-abortion law, an elected official, whose absolute personal opposition to procured abortion was well known, could licitly support proposals aimed at limiting the harm done by such a law and at lessening its negative consequences at the level of general opinion and public morality. This does not in fact represent an illicit cooperation with an unjust law, but rather a legitimate and proper attempt to limit its evil aspects."

5. With tactical compromise, there are fewer questions of line-drawing, since the "line" is set, rather simply, by the strongest form of legislation that you have the votes to get.

6. Mary Ann Glendon, in her thoughtful and provocative *Abortion and Divorce in Western Law* (Cambridge, Mass.: Harvard University Press, 1987), seems to advocate such a position (though, primarily, I think, to "open up" her overwhelmingly pro-abortion audience to some sorts of limits on abortion). On this issue, see my review of Glendon in *The Political Science Reviewer* 19 (1990) 291ff.

7. I say "ordinarily," of course, because in some situations the law must require heroism. For example, a person could not obtain the return of a kidnapped wife by agreeing to the kidnapper's demand that he kill another innocent person. In principle, that heroism is what the ideal law would require with respect to abortion in the hard cases as well. But something short of the ideal may be necessary in the circumstances of a given polity.

8. Such a law would, in addition, be much less likely to reduce

substantially the number of abortions that would occur (the "greater evil" that toleration of the lesser evil attempts to avoid). Planned Parenthood and its allies would simply have to work harder to catch pregnant women earlier in pregnancy — which is in any case when most abortions already occur.

9. Laurence Tribe, *Abortion: The Clash of Absolutes* (New York: Norton, 1990).

10. Not, by the way, RU-486. A pill that often requires a woman to "deliver a dead baby" is not likely to be the abortion movement's "magic bullet." Neater, less messy pills that are variants of today's abortifacient contraceptives are likely to be the answer — at least until easily-reversible sterilization methods become the anti-procreative technique of choice, with abortion pills as a rarer alternative.

11. A flat bonus for lower illegitimacy, for example, without any effort to prevent this from becoming an incentive for states to encourage abortions, would be a mistake. Better to provide a bonus for fewer illegitimate births *less* the number of abortions in such cases.

12. Charles E. Rice, *Fifty Questions on Abortion* (Notre Dame: Cashel Institute, 1979).

THE CHATTANOOGA STORY
HOW ONE CITY REDUCED
ITS ABORTION RATE

Robert H. O'Bannon, Ph.D.

INTRODUCTION

Chattanooga, Tennessee, is now reported by the National Abortion Rights Action League (NARAL) to be the largest city in the United States without an abortion clinic. It is perhaps the only city in America where the prolifers purchased a building housing the city's sole abortion clinic and converted it into a building used exclusively to help young women preserve the lives of their unborn. For those of us who are convinced that abortion is one of the greatest blights ever to curse our society, the Chattanooga story gives us a genuine ray of hope. May it inspire prolifers in cities, towns, and communities across our land to continue in their efforts to curtail this selfish, senseless slaughter of innocent lives.

Since I have been active in the prolife efforts of Cleveland, Tennessee, my own community, just 30 minutes north of Chattanooga, I have been involved only minimally in the Chattanooga story. Nevertheless, I have followed the activities surrounding this issue and am personally acquainted with several of the prolife leaders who have been instrumental in making abortion "taboo" to a large number of Chattanooga residents. Granted that every city has its own personality and that what worked in Chattanooga may not work in every community, it is still my sincere opinion that many of the actions and strategies that were successful in Chattanooga deserve to be considered by prolifers everywhere. After presenting a brief history of the conflict, I will attempt to detail several aspects of the Chattanooga story that might be most helpful.

A BRIEF HISTORY OF THE CONFLICT

Chattanooga is a beautiful, well-known, southern city of approximately 153,000 residents located in the southeastern corner of Tennessee. The greater Chattanooga area has over 400,000 residents. This city is known for Lookout Mountain, Ruby Falls, and, more recently, the Tennessee Aquarium. Several significant battles of the Civil War were fought in and around Chattanooga. The city is again the site of a civil war of a different type. The battle has temporarily shifted in favor of the prolifers, but a lasting settlement is yet a long way off. While somewhat more religious than many communities its size, it has not been immune to the sexual revolution which resulted in a pereived need for a quick fix to end unwanted pregnancies.

In 1973 *Roe v Wade* opened the door to legalized abortions — a door behind which many greedy people stood eagerly awaiting their patrons. That first year 799 reported abortions were performed. In ten years that number had climbed to 2,277 per year. Thanks to active and persistent prolifers, the number of reported abortions performed in the Chattanooga area in 1993 had dropped to 690.[1] How did this reduction come about? Please allow me to give you some of the highlights of the story.

In 1975 the Chattanooga Women's Clinic was opened for the sole purpose of providing abortions on demand. They were challenged by prolifers throughout most of their 18 years of operation. In 1976 clinic owners were charged with performing illegal abortions and practicing medicine without a license. Dr. Harold Hoke was sentenced to ten years in prison, but no records were found of his ever having served that sentence. Owner Tom Cole did spend some time in prison, however.[2]

With the Women's Clinic temporarily closed, Erlanger Medical Center opened its own Voluntary Interruption of Pregnancy Center. As the community became more aware that abortions were being performed, some at taxpayers' expense, public sentiment against abortions began to mount and made its way to the Hamilton County Commission in 1979. It was then that the Commissioners threatened to stop funding for Erlanger Medical Center because the hospital was doing elective abortions.[3]

As is characteristic of most noble causes, there always seems to be some zealots who manage to give a bad name to an entire group of responsible citizens. In 1983 Chattanooga had its own "Bible totin', abortion hatin', street preacher" with vivid pictures of aborted babies used to secure an audience. The prochoice voices in Chattanooga wanted desperately to make this street preacher the spokesman for the entire prolife community. Fortunately, this never happened. Yet the exchange generated much publicity in the media, making the local citizens more aware of the implications of their city offering abortion on demand.

In an effort to insure that responsible prolife voices were being heard, several community leaders in the prolife movement created an umbrella organization called the Prolife Majority Coalition of Chattanooga (ProMaCC). It was, indeed, a coalition of different denominations, different races, different classes of people from all walks of life who had one thing in common: they all believed that abortion was an evil that should be stopped.

One of the most fruitful actions of ProMaCC was to unite forces with AAA Women's Services, Inc., a group which had opened its offices directly across the street from the abortion clinic. Counselors began regular vigils on the sidewalks in an attempt to talk women out of having abortions and to offer them better options. Prayer groups began to meet regularly for prayer. They prayed that God would speak to the hearts of those performing abortions and the employees that assisted. This continued every Sunday morning for nine years. The events that followed are difficult to explain if one does not accept the reality of divine intervention.[4]

In 1989, and again in 1991, Operation Rescue targeted the clinic with dozens being arrested as they attempted to block entrances to the clinics. A few were convicted and sent to jail for short periods. Because the clinic was performing abortions after three months of pregnancy (which they were not licensed to perform), the rescuers were able to use this violation to justify their efforts to "prevent a crime from occurring." Eventually, all charges against the rescuers were dropped.[5]

In 1991 the clinic's owner, Ms. Sue Crawley, died of cancer. The attention then focused on Ms. Fran Muzzacco, the clinic's co-owner. Reverend Bob Borger, president of ProMaCC, reported that "We would call out to Fran and beg her to consider what happened to Sue and to turn from this evil.[6] But she would curse at us. So our prayers continued." In February 1993 Ms. Muzzacco also died of cancer.

Clinic attorney Selma Cash Paty strongly opposed the notion that their deaths were anything but normal. She said, "The clinic closed because Sue Crawley and Fran Muzzacco died of a dreaded disease, not because God cursed them or some nonsense." She defended them by saying that "They were two people with the will power, with the guts to stand up to those who would impose their moral judgments on the rest of us. Had Sue Crawley not died, poor women in Chattanooga would still be able to get an abortion today."[7]

But Sue and Fran did die and Sue's husband became the sole proprietor of the clinic. Mr. Crawley decided not to continue the clinic. Consequently, the owner of the building found it necessary to declare bankruptcy.

Dr. Ed Perry, who had worked at the clinic for several years, made an early bid to the bankruptcy court of $259,000 on the building valued at $220,000. When members of ProMaCC learned of Dr. Perry's bid, they prayed for direction and felt compelled to raise money to bid on the facility. The only problem was that that decision was reached on Thursday — the bidding was to be completed on Monday, just three days later. Getting on the telephone and contacting every one they knew in the community who were sympathetic to the prolife agenda, they walked into court on that Monday morning with approximately $280,000, all raised by word of mouth.[8]

The bankruptcy court judge instructed the bidders to bid in $5,000 increments. Dr. Ed Perry with his earlier bid of $259,000 began the bidding. ProMaCC countered with $264,000. As the bidding went back and forth, it seemed doubtful that the prolifers would be able to make the final bid. Ms. Patricia Lindley, spokesperson for ProMaCC, says that they had decided to bid only the amount that they had. Fortunately, a prolife lawyer who happened to be in the courthouse, learned of the bidding and made a promise of an additional $10,000 to ProMaCC. As the bidding concluded, the prolifers offered $294,000, which was all they had. Had Dr. Perry offered one penny more, they would have had to bail out. But it was Dr. Perry who said, "Enough." He never topped their bid.[9] And the clinic that had performed an estimated 35,000 abortions was deeded over to ProMaCC, which promptly evicted the operators of the clinic. Clinic operators promised they would relocate to another facility within weeks, but it never came about. The State Health Department revoked the clinic's license, and Dr. Perry "packed up his bags and went home." Now in semi-retirement, Dr. Perry remarks: "There comes a time in your career when you just don't need the headaches."[10]

So what impact did this change of ownership have? ProMaCC President Borger says, "We are under no illusions that we have stopped women in Chattanooga from getting abortions. We have taken the first step, which is to keep it from being so readily available and so easy to do.

We want people to think about what they are doing."[11]

In the month before the clinic was closed 145 reported abortions were performed in Hamilton County and plummeted down to only 45 total reported abortions from July through December, 1993.[12]   Neither prolifers nor prochoice advocates are deceived into thinking that Chattanooga women are no longer having abortions. Clinics in all the neighboring states report increases in their clientele from the Chattanooga area.   The total number does seem to be decreasing, and the number of women coming to the AAA Women's Services seeking help to keep their babies is increasing.   The public at large is better informed and more likely to support prolife activities.

Let us then look at some of the key players in the Chattanooga story.   In doing so, I hope to point out some principles or characteristics that have enhanced   each player's role in that story.

PROLIFERS MUST ADMIT AND EMBRACE A RELIGIOUS BASE

In interviewing Linda Keener, Executive Director of AAA Women's Services, she mentioned repeatedly: "None of this would have happened without God's help."[13]   If saving the unborn from premature death is as close to the heart of God as most of us believe it is, it should not surprise us when God responds favorably to the prayers of those who seek to alleviate the suffering of those little ones He loves.

Are there not others that He loves? Yes, of course. But the unborn are the most helpless, least protected members of the American society. Men and women, young and old, in any city of the world, can expect God's grace to be upon them if they seek to help the unborn.

The prolife position should be endorsed by every religious body under the banner of Christianity.   It should be supported by every political persuasion because it is an innately proper human response.

I am convinced that all human life is sacred because each individual bears the image of God. To embrace this concept automatically seems to demand a strong allegiance to the prolife position and a concomitant sense of worship and awe toward one's Creator. You will occasionally find an agnostic or atheist who opposes abortion, but that number is small. Those who deny God's involvement in life will have a weak philosophical argument to support their prolife stance. Thus, small prolife groups in cities where abortions are regularly performed should recruit new members from among those who regard God as Creator and accept His Word as the basis for opposing abortion on demand.

It was from these religious convictions that ProMaCC and the AAA Women's Services were begun. Dr. Nan Pollard, chairperson of AAA's Board of Directors, succinctly demonstrates this religion/prolife relationship in the clinic's 1994 Annual Report:

"There are no choices." The woman entering the abortion clinic told the couple that had intervened to save the life of her baby. "Where else can I go?"

A small circle of Christians felt the leading of the Holy Spirit to give women alternative choices. On their knees, they asked God for His direction. In obedience to His will, they pooled their resources and personal time and opened a storefront crisis pregnancy center across the street from the abortion clinic.

The purpose? To provide women alternatives to abortion, to minister to their physical needs, and to present the Gospel of Christ. And the women came. The small circle of Christians grew.

Ten years later, AAA Women's Services is reaching 3,000 women a year in our office and hundreds more on the 24-hour hotline. We are giving them real "choices" for their babies. Our location? The building that once housed Chattanooga's only abortion clinic — delivered to us in direct answer to prayer.

As more women came, God showed us their needs. We saw their need for healing and started post-abortion Bible studies for those traumatized by abortion. We saw their need for God's plan for sex and developed Why kNOw abstinence programs for schools and churches.

As AAA Women's Services begins its 10th year anniversary, we thank you for your prayers, commitment and financial support — and ask you to join us in thanking God for the privilege of serving Him by celebrating life. . . one life at a time.[14]

The Mission Statement of AAA Women's Services likewise identifies this connection:

> In obedience to Christ
> the mission of AAA Women's Services
> is to lovingly influence women
> to choose life-giving alternatives
> for crisis pregnancies by communicating
> both God's plan for sexuality and
> the sanctity of life of unborn children
> and by ministering to their
> physical, emotional and spiritual needs.[15]

It is also fitting that those who now carry out this Mission Statement should describe their work in the following slogan:

> Together we are ending
> the tragedy of abortion
> one life at a time.[16]

AIM FOR A BROAD BASE WITH A NARROW FOCUS

A general observation regarding the success of Chattanooga prolifers is that they established a broad base of people who all possessed a narrow "abortion is wrong" focus.

From a list of donors to the various prolife activities in the area, it is obvious that the prolife cause found sympathy in nearly every denomination as shown below by the list of supporting churches:

Battlefield Parkway Nazarene   Duncan Park Baptist Church
Bethel Memorial Baptist Church   East Chattanooga Church of God

Bethel Temple Assembly of God
Bibleway Baptist Mission
Brainerd Baptist Church
Brainerd Presbyterian
Brainerd Baptist
Burning Bush Baptist
Calvary Bible Church
Calvary Independent Baptist
Center Point Baptist Church
Central Baptist of Hixson
Chattanooga Chr'n Fellowship
Church of Living Faith
City Gate Church
Clingan Baptist Church
Community Baptist Hixson
Community Bible Church
Covenant Presbyterian Church
Cross of Christ Lutheran
New Life Church
Northside Baptist Church
Our Lady of the Mount
Red Bank Cumberland Presb.
Red Bank Presbyterian
Reformed Presbyterian Church
 River of Life Church
Signal Mountain Bible Church
Signal Mountain Presbyterian

East Ridge Church of God
East Ridge Presbyterian Church
First Presbyterian/Ft.Oglethorpe
Friendship Community
Grace Baptist Church
Green Pond Baptist
Heritage Baptist Church
Highland Park Baptist
Hixson First Baptist
Hixson Presbyterian
Hixson United Methodist
Holy Trinity Catholic Church
Lee Highway Church of God
Lookout Mtn. Presbyterian
Lookout Valley Baptist
Miracle Missionary Baptist
Mountain View Church of God
New City Fellowship
Silverdale Baptist Church
South Seminole Baptist Church
St. Elmo Presbyterian
Valley Memorial Baptist
Varnell Methodist Church
Wayside Presbyterian
Westview Baptist Church
White Oak Methodist
Woodland Park Baptist Church[17]

This may seem a bit skewed toward the conservative denominations, but this is simply a reflection of the community at large.

Individual donors, numbering 2,750, are likewise diverse.

Fund raising activities have been very well designed, appealing to middle to upper-middle class, cross cultural clientele. The major fund raiser for the AAA Women's Services organization is a well-planned, annual banquet. A past supporter of the program agrees to recruit four couples for his/her table and informs them that the banquet is for fundraising. A lovely meal is followed by some outstanding speaker. Washington Post correspondent Cal Thomas spoke at their more recent banquet with approximately 600 in attendance. Personal success stories of local young women who were influenced not to abort their unborn children were also highlighted.

In addition to individual giving, there are a significant number of businesses whose owners or CEO's consider the prolife agenda worth supporting. Listed below are companies who have helped in the success of antiabortion efforts in Chattanooga.

American Communications, Inc.	Hamico, Inc.
BLJ Properties	Hamilton-Roddy Chiropractic
Brainerd Psychological Services	Huffaker and Associates
Brainerd Vending Service	Jeff Locke Sign Company
Chattanooga Area CFC	Knights of Columbus
Chattanooga Coca-Cola Bottling	Ledco, Inc.
Chattanooga Christian Foundation	Lookout Plating, Inc.
Chattanooga Resource Foundation	Maclellan Foundation, Inc.
Cleveland Business Machines	MCM Company of Tennessee
Cyclelex Company	Physicians/Family & Sports Med.
G and M Realty	Pickett, Tarpley & Assoc., Inc.
Gabby's Restaurant	Po Boys Restaurant
Graham Vannoy Construction	Pulmonaire Services, Inc.
Red Bank Athletic Shop	Totten Furniture
Redemptorist Fathers	Unfinished Furniture Expo
Samples & Jennings, P.C.	United Steelworkers Local 3508
Southern Champion Tray	W.C. Teas Company
The Caldwell Foundation	Weld Mart, Inc.[18]
Therapeutic Foot Care	

Another good indicator of support for the prolife position are the thousands of people who line the streets to let passersby know that "Abortion Kills Children" during the annual Life Chain demonstration held in October. Large representations from many different churches make an entire community aware that those who perform abortions are not likely to win or influence people. Nor can they expect to get wealthy by exploiting the sad situation in which a young, single, pregnant girl finds herself. One obstetrician from a neighboring community had this to say: "In Cleveland, it would be professional suicide if I were to be doing elective pregnancy terminations. Personally, I am prochoice. But I work here and I like it here, and the standards and morals of this community are very conservative. I have chosen to stand by these community standards."[19]

Some professors at the University of Tennessee in Chattanooga believe their city to be just as conservative. Medical ethics professor, Dr. Don Klinefelter, had this to say: "There is room in Chattanooga for a courageous debate, but, unfortunately, only one side is speaking out. There is a very strong sense in Chattanooga that abortion should be viewed as the devaluing of human life and evidence of an increase in immorality. To speak in favor of abortion in this town is like saying that you are in favor of sin."[20]

I couldn't have said it any better myself.

SUCCESSFUL PROLIFERS ARE KNOWLEDGEABLE PROLIFERS

The prophet Hosea says of Israel in Hosea 4:6, "My people are destroyed for a lack of knowledge." Many people dedicated to the prolife position have the right motive and worthy intentions but are ineffective as agents of change because they are ignorant of some of the crucial areas in the prolife/abortion debate.

High on the list is one's ignorance of the law — local, county, state and federal law. And divine law, I might add. The prolife folks in Chattanooga were fortunate to have several excellent lawyers with strong prolife convictions who guided and protected them through some difficult situations. If such people are not available, more effort will have to be made to become acquainted with the legal issues that may be faced.

Not only should prolifers be well-informed themselves, they should continually be looking for ways to convince others to join the struggle against abortion. Based upon our Chattanooga experience, one of the more effective ways to do this is by attempting to befriend and convince the media of the validity of our cause and push for the truth to get a fair hearing in the public forum.

I must say that most newspaper, TV and radio newsmen in Chattanooga have been extremely fair and unbiased in their coverage of the prolife/abortion debate, especially when contrasted with media coverage in Washington, D.C. and other national news sources. It was "the media" who hired the Mason-Dixon Political/Media Research, Inc. to gather public opinion on a large number of prolife/abortion issues. Results of this comprehensive survey were published in a six-part series that appeared in the Chattanooga Times and were repeatedly mentioned on both radio and TV. Can you imagine the boost the prolife cause received when the following data appeared as lead stories in the pages of Chattanooga's daily newspaper?

Over 50% of area respondents thought that Chattanooga was better off without an abortion clinic, and that the leading medical center should not provide abortion services.

64% of Chattanooga respondents believe life begins at conception, 59% believe that abortion should be illegal and 84% think there are too many abortions in America.

74% percent regard abortion views of candidates for public office to be an important consideration for deciding one's vote.

82% percent of prolife respondents based their opinion about abortion on religious beliefs, 53% think the Bible condemns abortion, and 69% think abortion is morally wrong.

Prochoice candidates were consistently more willing to pay more taxes to cover uninsured pregnant women, infants born with AIDS, and foster parenting.

85% of respondents recommended that parental or legal guardian consent be required for all women seeking abortions under age 18.

81% of respondents are opposed to government funding of abortion except in cases of rape, incest or to protect the life of the mother.

90% of respondents believe that the act of killing an abortion doctor should be considered an act of murder.[21]

Surely you can appreciate how much more aggressive and confident prolife advocates are knowing that a majority of the community is on their side. We owe a great debt to the media for this highly publicized information.

WOMEN REGRETTING THEIR ABORTIONS MAKE GREAT COUNSELORS

Prolifers have often been accused of talking a young lady out of an abortion only to forget about her once the child is born. And, sad to say, in some instances that may have been true. Because a large number of the personnel at AAA Women's Services have themselves been party to an abortion, their input into the policy and practices of AAA Women's Services have been instrumental in providing a rather comprehensive plan of care for every woman who comes to them. Over 17,000 have been served by one or more of the following services:

1. *Pregnancy Services:* free pregnancy tests, confidential counseling, 24-Hour Crisis Hotline, Shepherding Homes, maternity/baby clothing and equipment, emergency food shelf, Evangelism and Discipleship, "My Baby and Me" Prenatal Program. "In 1994, 3,164 women came through the doors of AAA Women's Services to find compassionate counsel, accurate information and practical help. Last year 45 women accepted Christ, and over 100 women changed their minds about aborting their babies. Over 400 women received help with clothing, food and housing,and 90 participated in our "My Baby & Me" program."[22] Women receiving their services ranged from ages 12 to 52. Each had unique stresses in their lives which made her pregnancy a crisis. And each found love and support at AAA.

2. *Abstinence Education*
AAA Women's Services is also waging a strong campaign to reduce the need for abortions through its abstinence

program. Over 3,200 young people in the Chattanooga area have been taught to save sex for marriage. In 1994, a five-day series was presented in 54 classrooms and in 19 church groups. This emphasis is in stark contrast to school districts that are passing out condoms to curb teenage pregnancies. This "Why kNOw" abstinence program has been well received by both public and parochial schools. It has been featured in *Worldwide Challenge* and WRCB's *Sex on Hold* TV series.[23]   According to Kris Frainie, creator and teacher of the program, the demand for abstinence education by public schools has been much greater than anticipated.[24]

3. *Post-Abortion Support*
   In the post-abortion support groups, even the men are included. The first men's Bible study group began in 1994. "Through these groups, monthly HOPE support meetings, and individual lay counselling, many people found new freedom from the pain of past abortions."[25]
   One of the objectives of AAA is to make a portion of their newly acquired building into a National Memorial for the Unborn who have been aborted. At the very site where over 35,000 babies were aborted, the memorial will provide a place and a way to honor our nation's forgotten children. Small metal plaques giving the aborted child a name, the date of death and a small verse or thought will be placed there by mothers, fathers, grandparents and others grieved by their deaths. It will give those who have lost a child to abortion a place to mourn.
   Tom Klassen, author of *Pro-Life Manifesto*, has said this about such memorials: "The plaque is her personal connecting link to the Memorial, the child's death, and healing. As she begins that simple action, she senses the beginning of new peace within herself."[26]
   The entire staff of women at AAA all have tremendous gifts of service and compassion for the work they do and

render them often with very meager remuneration. The radiance on their faces and the love and compassion in their hearts for the hurting young women is a blessing to observe or experience. In addition to the eight full-time staff, more than 150 other women are among their volunteers.

CONCLUSION

How long will it be before Chattanooga gets another abortion clinic? No one knows for sure. But those who embark upon such a mission should know a host of very religious, well educated, caring, non-violent people will be there reminding them they do not approve of aborting the unborn. Further, they need to know that that host will be extending their hands and hearts to all those experiencing a crisis pregnancy who may be seeking a better alternative than terminating the life of their unborn.

Several years ago, I developed a simple plan to assist my local prolife group in grasping the parameters in their prolife/abortion debate. The Chattanooga folks did not have access to this plan but seem to have lived it out more than I could have ever desired. So I conclude by sharing it with you in hopes that your city, your community may be able to experience the delight of knowing all our sacrifices for the unborn are not in vain.

THE PROLIFE PLAN

R ecognize the sacredness, value and worth all humans possess as a result of their being made in the image of God.

I dentify the social, spiritual, and political forces bent on the destruction of human dignity through the annihilation of the unborn, unwanted, and unproductive of our society.

G ather and disperse accurate knowledge of fetal development and encourage continued research into the long-range effects of abortion on women, families and society.

H elp women with unwanted pregnancies find creative alternatives to abortion by giving love, counsel, friendship, comfort, and support.

T ell the owners and employees of hospitals and clinics performing abortions that legality and morality are not synonymous terms, and their facilities will be picketed until killing the unborn is no longer profitable.

T ranslate the Judeo-Christian ethic into a life-validating, life-saving way of living that convinces others of the merit of the prolife position.

O ppose all views portrayed by the public media that are clearly biased against the prolife cause.

L ink up with all local, state and national organizations dedicated to promoting life, participate in their activities, and support their cause.

I nform political and community leaders of the prolife position, praising them when they are supportive and striving for their replacement when they are not.

F ollow the example of Jesus Christ in communicating God's love to those who have had abortions and those who are considering it by providing better alternatives.

E ducate families, churches, and communities about the abortion issue until respect for all life is restored.

NOTES

1. M. Curriden and C. Patterson, "Driven to secrecy — or another town" in *The Chattanooga Times*, Vol. CXXVI, No. 63 (Monday, February 27, 1995), citing the Tennessee Department of Health.

2. "Chattanooga's abortion fight through the years" in *The Chattanooga Times*. Vol. CXXVI, No. 64 (February 28, 1995).

3. Ibid. (February 27, 1995).

4. Linda Keener, personal conversation, April 1995.

5. "Chattanooga's abortion fight through the years." *The Chattanooga Times,* Vol. CXXVI, No. 64 (February 28, 1979).

6. M. Curriden and C. Patterson, "Clear-cut win" in *The Chattanooga Times*, Vol. CXXVI, No. 64 (Tuesday, February 28, 1995).

7. Ibid.

8. Ibid.

9. Ibid.

10. M. Curriden, "A former traveling doctor now on road to retirement" in *The Chattanooga Times*, Vol. CXXVI, No. 67 (Friday, March 3, 1995).

11. M. Curriden and C. Patterson, "Driven to secrecy — or another town" in *The Chattanooga Times*, Vol. CXXVI, No. 63 (Monday, February 27, 1995).

12. Ibid.

13. Keener, April 1995.

14. Nan Pollard, "Chairman's report" in *AAA Women's Services Annual Report* (1994) p. 3.

15. "Mission Statemen." in *AAA Women's Services Annual Report* (1994) p.2.

16. "AAA slogan" in *AAA Women's Services Annual Report* (1994) p. 2.

17. "List of supporting churches" in *AAA Women's Services Annual Report* (1994) p. 7.

18. "List of supporting businesses" in *AAA Women's Services Annual Report* (1994) p.7.

19. M. Curriden and C. Patterson, "A City's Taboo" in *The Chattanooga Times*, Vol. CXXVI, No. 63 (Monday, February 27, 1995).

20. Ibid.

21. Mason-Dixon Political Research, Inc., Survey of 415 Adults in Chattanooga Area (February 12-February 15, 1995).

22. "Services" in *AAA Women's Services Annual Report* (1994) p.5.

23. Ibid., p.5.

24. K. Frainie, personal conversation (May 15, 1995).

25. "Services" in *AAA Women's Services Annual Report* (1994) p.5.

26. "National Memorial for the Unborn" in *AAA Women's Services Brochure* (1995).

BIOETHICS: THE TWILIGHT OF CHRISTIAN HIPPPOCRATISM

Nigel M. de S. Cameron

Sir Edward Creasy's *Fifteen Decisive Battles of the World*[1] may seem to reduce human history to the military engagements that, since Marathon, have marked the high- and low-water marks of imperial power. Yet there was nothing antecedently inevitable about the victory of Miltiades over Datis, and part of the virtue of this sort of history writing is the lesson it teaches that a well-fought engagement can really make a difference. When our grandchildren come to write their intellectual and social histories there can be little doubt as to the decisive significance of current discussion of bioethics in determining the shape of post-Christian Western society, and it is a thousand pities that the contemporary evangelical movement shows so general a disinterest in serious engagement in this discipline.[2] Widespread recent recruitment of evangelicals to the pro-life cause has had no parallel in the vigorous academic field of inquiry that in the past two decades has taken the leading edge of bioethical thinking far beyond the horizons of the abortion debate. And vigorous it has proved to be. The burgeoning of bioethics as an academic/professional discipline is a recognized phenomenon in the academic world, plainly measurable in publishing, academic appointments, international conferences, and the establishment worldwide of scores of "centers" and other institutional expressions of commitment to this new field. Perhaps the best of all barometers is the appearance of new journals, and here progress has been spectacular, with a constant stream of fresh announcements.[3] Evangelical participation in the mainstream bioethics community has been modest, with a modesty unbecoming those who have such a stake in the

87

outcome of the community's thinking.[4]   Evangelical investment in bioethics institutions has been almost nil.[5]

Explanations are generally elusive, though not entirely so. One factor has been the widespread evangelical unease with philosophy, the lingua franca of the bioethics world. Another lies in the forgivable but ultimately disastrous desire of evangelicals for simplicity at all costs. The pro-life movement offers a necessarily simplistic account of the crisis in contemporary medical-scientific values by fastening exclusively on the status of the fetus as its sole public policy concern (though the question of euthanasia has started to awaken an adjunct interest, if no more). The pro-life movement can hardly be faulted for its political savvy (a single-issue focus is almost required for effectiveness), though a deeper awareness of the public policy issues that will confront evangelicals ten or twenty years down the road would have given a three-dimensional quality to campaigning concerns, as well as helping to prepare the constituency for the next campaign and the next-but-one. Pro-life organizations — evangelical and other — have shown scant interest in sponsoring the kinds of research that would help develop their own thinking beyond the demands of the immediate political agenda.

A further factor, affecting the evangelical constituency more broadly — and perhaps especially its existing educational and other institutions — is the uncertainty and, at points, deep disagreement that have marked its response to key questions such as abortion.[6] There has been some development here, since evangelical opinion was much more divided and uncertain twenty years ago on that issue than it is today. But as euthanasia and the various dimensions of our new capacity for genetic manipulation rise up the political-moral agenda, further division and uncertainty within the community appear inevitable. Indeed, our failure to develop institutions within and among which these questions could be addressed is storing up all manner of difficulty in articulating an evangelical position on issues that have yet to be posed. This is not least among the reasons why such institutional development is now urgent.

But the intention of this essay is no more to explain the parsimony of the evangelical imagination than to lambaste it. There is limited though growing evidence that the situation is at least beginning to right itself, with a handful of evangelicals participating in bioethical debates and interpreting bioethics to the evangelical community. What is particularly urgent, if this development is to be sustained, is the need for appropriate institutions to be established so that a self-sustaining evangelical mind can develop, sketching broad perspectives for its community, defining options on particular controverted questions, and giving effective voice to evangelical concerns in the twin arenas within which the crucial discussions are in progress: public policy debate, and behind public policy debate — and sinisterly and depressingly determinative of it — debate within the international bioethics community.

Yet what of bioethics itself? Its phenomenal growth has been widely observed. As the supremely interdisciplinary discipline, it stands at the confluence of the biomedical sciences, law, philosophy, theology, and, of course, ethics itself as analyst and would-be arbiter of the contested terrain in which most "bioethicists" — who have themselves set out from one of the traditional disciplines — have established for themselves a multidisciplinary bridgehead in the land of values, science, and medical practice. This, of course, is not some arcane country, but the place where a new understanding of what it means to be human is being fashioned and tested. So the Christian stake could hardly be higher.

How then should we understand the establishment and rapid growth of this most interdisciplinary of disciplines? There are two coincident factors that together begin to offer an explanation. The first factor is the "revolution" in medical technology. This is actually not one but a cluster of developments — developments in drug therapy, surgery, the technology of life-support systems, and parallel developments such as the general appropriation of information technology. These developments have combined to lengthen the reach of medical science, and they have also combined to add increasingly expensive items to the menu of clinical options. Expectations have been raised and often met, fueling an inflation of demand. Consequent crises in resourcing have been one result. Attempts at resolution have, of course, taken different forms within different health-care systems, but resultant rationing in such procedures as renal dialysis and neonatal special care has been universal — whatever its method — and has given public focus to ethical conflicts. At other times it is the availability of new biological techniques — supremely, *in vitro* fertilization — that has raised new issues. In other cases, different issues are prominent: abortion, of course, continues for the public and politician alike to be the most significant bioethical issue of our day, and though it is safer and more widely available than ever before, it is nothing new. The next big storm is brewing over euthanasia. Though this question is intersected by special concerns over the use of technology — which enables many patients, whether accident victims or terminally ill, to survive when previously they would have died — the practice, like that of abortion, is as old as human society.

The prominence of these life issues in contemporary bioethical discussion gives the lie to the widespread assumption that the bioethics boom is simply the fruit of revolutionary progress in the development of medical technology and the hard questions it has forced upon us. The second level of explanation is more fundamental, and it lies in the breakup of the ethical consensus in Western society. The medical culture to which we have fallen heir dates back before Christ to the Hippocratic physicians of ancient Greece, though it was early recognized by Christians as congruent with their own special values and came to exercise a mesmeric influence down many centuries of health care in Judeo-Christian (and also, though distinctly, in Islamic) society.[7] Central to that medical culture has been the sanctity of life. (Proscriptions of both abortion and suicide-euthanasia lie side by side in the Hippocratic Oath with principles such as confidentiality and the germ of the idea of what we now call a profession.)[8] Medical values have not been isolated from those of society at large, though the relationship is complex and medicine has maintained — or has been expected to maintain — the highest values held in general esteem.[9] The Hippocratic profession was from the start a moral calling, and its most characteristic feature was its inseparable blending of its distinct moral values and medical technique, strikingly illustrated by the prohibition in the oath from teaching medical skills to any persons who have not already first committed themselves to the Hippocratic values. Part of the special importance of current developments in medical values lies in the role of medicine as an index of wider social change in the double move both away from Hippocratic-Judeo-Christian values and, at the same time, away from *any* consensus values. For it is not that some new religion has usurped the old; the post-Christian society is developing as a kind of anti-society in which consensus values — the substructure of every other society, past and present — have been displaced by a value anarchy that seeks its validation and strives for social cohesion through models of autonomy alone, as if pluralism were a unifying "ism" like any other. Just as medicine once served as standard-bearer of all that was best in the old society, so it is coming to exemplify the new in its ambiguity and growing incoherence.

CHRISTIAN HIPPOCRATISM

The Western medical tradition owes its origins and its character to a striking fusion of pagan and (Judeo-)Christian notions. The enduring association of Hippocrates of Cos and the practice of medicine in the Christian/post-Christian West offers telling evidence of the welcome that the church extended to this product of pagan antiquity. There is some evidence of Christian attempts to bowdlerize the pagan oath[10] (an approach adopted with much success within Islam, where also Hippocratism was welcomed and became the standard of medical values).[11] But it was the original, overtly pagan form of the oath that was adopted into and remained the standard of Christian medicine.

There is much uncertainty as to the origins of the oath and its historical connection with Hippocrates himself. He was the most famous of all the physicians of antiquity, and his name is associated with a considerable library of writings on ethical, clinical, dietary, and other medically related issues, conventionally referred to — with unintended humor — as the Hippocratic *corpus*.   Scholarly opinion locates some of this material after his time, and there seems good reason to believe that, however formal or informal it may have been, there was a Hippocratic "school" associated with the name and memory of Hippocrates of Cos that sought to perpetuate and develop his thinking.[12]

More than one historical reconstruction has been offered,[13] but the most influential (it was actually cited by the court in *Roe v. Wade* in a curious attempt to relativize the significance of the Hippocratic tradition) remains that of Ludwig Edelstein, a distinguished historian of medicine who in 1943 published a monograph on the oath in which he sought a location for its values and its understanding of medicine within the religious and philosophical schools of Greek antiquity. Edelstein searched the religious-philosophical options of the period for one in which the declared values of the oath would find a home. He found it in the school of the Pythagoreans, about whom not much is known, though we do know that they held some distinct opinions on some of the highly controversial issues on which the oath displays a distinctive view (especially abortion and what Edelstein calls suicide-euthanasia, both of which were commonly approved in the Greece of antiquity but forbidden in the oath).

Edelstein's Pythagorean identification of the early Hippocratics may or may not be correct. But the significance of his work has been to repristinate Hippocratic medical values as those of a reforming minority. This is important for two reasons. First, before his monograph there was a tendency for writers to laud the values of the oath as self-evidently true, a collection of statements of the obvious.[14] Second, we have inherited Hippocratic medicine as consensus medicine, for so it has been for many centuries during which few have dissented from its understanding of human dignity and the role and calling of the physician. Edelstein's work reminds us of the highly controversial character of human values, of which the dissonant ethical voices of Greek antiquity offer us a paradigm; and it reminds us of the calling of the first Hippocratics and the challenge they faced as they sought to commend and practice their very distinctive values in a society that marched to a different drum. In other words, Edelstein's thesis repristinates Hippocratism as a dissident medical creed, and the oath as (to use his term) a "manifesto" for the human medical values it advocates. Since the wheel of medical values is set to turn full circle as we emerge into a post-Hippocratic medical culture, this rediscovery is timely.

The readiness with which Christians embraced Hippocratic medicine, and even its plainly pagan oath, underlines its fundamental congruence with a Christian agenda for medical values. That is perhaps most evident in the stress that the oath places on the sanctity of human life. The explicit prohibition on medical killing (whether in abortion or in medically assisted suicide) and the patient-first emphasis (Hippocratic philanthropism) outline a non-manipulative, servant role for medicine and energetically distinguish between medicine as healing and medicine as anything else. The old pre-Hippocratic medicine — like the post-Hippocratism emerging today — did not make these distinctions. Moreover, the context of these distinct ethical commitments was theistic, even if its theism was pagan. The key to the significance of theism for the oath lies in the fact that it was an *oath*. How far we have moved from a medical culture in which the transcendent ethics of Christian Hippocratism set the context for clinical practice is sadly evident in the fact that of the many influential modern restatements of (more or less) Hippocratic medical values, starting with the definitive Declaration of Geneva of 1948, which sought — on behalf of the World Medical Association — to reinstate the Hippocratic basis of international clinical practice after the sorry story of Nazi medicine, not one is actually cast in the form of an oath; and no one seems to have noticed. For the first Christians, this pagan medical ideology, which sought to limit the physician's role to that of healer and which did so explicitly *coram Deo*, was immensely attractive. What is more, by its nature the oath declares medicine to be, first and foremost, a matter of moral commitment.[15] This is made explicit in its own prohibition on the passing on of medical skills to those who have not first accepted its values. The understanding of medicine that is gaining currency today — as essentially a set of skills that may or may not be acquired alongside this or that code of values — is anathema to the oath, which joined together technique and value, the "life" and the "art" of the Hippocratic practitioner, in an indissoluble union that has characterized not simply the idea of medicine but, at its best, the idea of a profession. Thus Hippocratism was adopted into the church, *mutatis mutandis*, as the basis for the Christian practice of medicine. And it is for these same reasons that the Christian stake in Hippocratism is today so great.

It has been common for evangelicals to dismiss the significance of bioethics as simply an intra-professional discussion, important no doubt for physicians, but not more important for the rest of us than ethical discussions within the many other professional communities. But this dismissal arises out of a naive understanding of the significance of medicine. The subject matter of contemporary bioethics is only incidentally related to the professional responsibilities of the physician. That is part of the reason why *bioethics* or *biomedical ethics* is generally used in place of *medical ethics* as the generic term for the discipline (in North America, at least). Bioethics treats of fundamental human values; generally these values involve a medical or medical-scientific component, but at several removes from the "old" medical ethics, which majored in medical etiquette — addressing such questions as whether or not it is proper for a physician to form a liaison with a patient, for example. Not that these areas are unrelated; the Hippocratic Oath addressed them both (and its doctrine of medical confidentiality, for example, remains fundamental and unchallenged). But the farther the center of controversy moves from professional etiquette, the greater is its impact on public policy discussion and matters that affect us all at the most profound level. So abortion and euthanasia are, of course, issues with vital medical dimensions, but none would deny that they are chiefly moral and social questions and that, at the level of principle, they are not for the medical professions to resolve.

This is, indeed, one reason why the discipline of bioethics has developed, and why it has developed alongside and not as a department of medicine. But that leads us to recognize the universality of the questions that are being raised under this head. Rather curiously, part of the reason for and part of the result of the underdeveloped state of bioethical discussion within the evangelical community lies in the conservative character of evangelical medicine in this respect. The medical mainstream has been more open, and has been open for a longer period of time, to non-medical participation in bioethical discussion than has evangelical medicine. In the light of evangelicals' overt religious and moral commitments, this is surprising, and its explanation is probably to be sought in sensitivity in areas like abortion over which evangelical opinion has itself been divided (especially twenty or more years ago, when bioethics was in its infancy and the structure of much later discussion was being decided).

The subject matter of bioethics is humankind; man, male and female, made in the image of God. That is the starting point of Christian reflection, and that is also the point at which contemporary secular bioethical discussion makes contrary assumptions about the nature of the being who is the subject of argument. Human being is made in the *imago Dei*, and while the content to be given to this fundamental biblical concept is the subject of continuing discussion,[16] it is bearing the divine image and likeness that marks off human being from all other kinds of created being and declares human life to be "sacred" or to possess "sanctity." The use of these religious terms to indicate the inviolability of human life (whether in general, or more specifically as technical terms in bioethical discussion) is no accident, and it reflects precisely the Christian theological tradition. The import of Genesis 1:26 — "Let us make man in our image" — is spelled out in 9:6. The capital sentence awaits those who take human life, since is it made in the image of God; human life, that is, is sacred and inviolable because of its intimate connection with God himself, who is its Creator.

Yet men and women are mortal, condemned to death by sin, the effects of which are universal; and it is in this dialectic of sanctity and mortality that the calling of the physician and, indeed, the task of the bioethicist lie. For the believer there is an irreducible ambivalence in his or her attitude to death, the last enemy whose gloomy portal is also the gate of life. Yet for the unbeliever, too, there is ambivalence, and it is the ambivalence of the unbeliever that has dominated and continues to dominate bioethical discussion of issues on the boundaries of life. The unbeliever has no resurrection hope and for that reason may strive to hold on to what remains of life at all costs, since it is all there is. But if there is no resurrection hope, there is also no resurrection judgment, no accountability, no notion that life is God's to give and God's to take away, no confidence in divine providence and comfort. So the unbeliever may move from fear of death to fear of dying — or fear of continuing alive in conditions of distress — and may opt for that control over dying that has always been available in suicide and its medical surrogates.

What is more, unbelievers may take to themselves power over the dying of others, with that same lack of accountability to resurrection judgment and with exclusive concern for comfort in the here and now (whether their own or that of the "other"), whether the "other" is an unborn child or a demented and costly parent, and whether the means is the abortionist's instrument or the withdrawal of the food and drink that sustain the chronic and incompetent sick. Much of contemporary secular bioethics may be understood as a life-and-death struggle between the desire to hold on to life because it is all there is and the increasingly stronger desire to take control of death to make life easier. In some cases the easier life and the eased death are predicated of the same person, and thus it may be the patient who seeks and who takes hold of the keys. But more and more, the life made easier and the death that makes it so are distinct, the keys of death seized not by a patient in anguish (for very, very few now need die like that) but by a relative or a physician or an insurer or an administrator, whose life will be easier (emotionally, financially...) because that other life is over. That is, of course, the typical pattern with abortion (there are some few indicators that could be claimed to suggest that the child herself would be happier dead, but they are few), and that pattern is increasingly becoming the dominant pattern for euthanasia. Life is cheap because death is cheap, and the medical decision-making process become the theater of a power-play in which the race is to the strong, and patients' rights — vaunted as the justification for breaking the mold of rigid Hippocratic values — have become a Trojan horse for the entry of extraneous interests into decisions concerning the life and death of the patient. It has never been plainer that Hippocrates was the patient's friend.

ISSUES IN DEBATE

The list of topics addressed in current bioethical discussion grows every month as technology advances and ethical options open wider. Cryopreservation, fetal brain tissue implants, the immense array of genetic possibilities — clearly this is not a single-issue debate, and for that reason there are questions on which a Christian response will not yet have come to a clear focus. But at the heart of the contemporary scene lies the abandonment of the Christian-Hippocratic conviction of the sanctity of human life. Many of the particular questions being explored around the margins of technological possibility and ethical acceptability are options only because of that denial of the central tenet of our medical culture. So our focus must continue to lie here, in the sanctity-of-life doctrine that imparts such dignity to the individual and that stamps the calling of the physician with such an ideal of disinterested service — without both of which our medical tradition lies in tatters.

BEGINNING-OF-LIFE ISSUES

We have already noted the major, if somewhat belated, evangelical engagement in the pro-life movement. This has not always reflected unanimity among evangelicals on at least some of the abortion options, but it does reflect a mainstream evangelical commitment on one side of the debate rather than the other. In the United States, as in other countries, evangelical medical opinion has been the most divided, both with respect to abortion itself and when confronted with related questions such as that of deleterious research on the human embryo. That does not augur well for the coming round of debate on euthanasia, for which — as with abortion twenty years ago — evangelical opinion is thoroughly ill-prepared, and which is also destined to move rapidly beyond intellectual reflection into the marketplace of public policy and legal change. Indeed, we may well see a rerun of the abortion awakening, in which the intellectual struggle *followed* political-legal decisions and an evangelical mind was achieved altogether too late. We have already noted that among the most striking features of the contemporary debate on life issues is its lack of novelty: the religious-philosophical discussion and the medical practice both go back through classical society into primitive times, and indeed both abortion and euthanasia are practiced today by primitive peoples as well as in technological societies. While these questions may have taken on fresh perspective, in themselves they are unconnected with the new technological and other resources of contemporary medicine. Indeed, it is worth remarking that the Hippocratic repudiation of these practices was in the context of a primitive medical culture; the clinical and other resources available in modern Western society for the care of unwanted children, the handicapped, and the chronic and terminally sick are incomparably greater. Yet it is now that the turnaround in the ethical consensus has taken place.

The abortion argument began as an argument about when life begins, and that is a question on which Christians have a highly distinctive answer. For there is a series of biblical indicators that together come to a particularly — indeed, even a surprisingly — sharp focus in answer to our question. In fact, the debate has moved on, and it is now much more the debate that some of us have feared it would become: a debate about when life, which has very plainly already begun, may legitimately be taken. This is a more logical though also a more sinister debate, in which the continuity of fetal and born human life has ceased to tell against abortion and has begun to tell in favor of euthanasia. The self-evident and substantially Hippocratic assumptions of a generation ago have given place to radical questioning. In the pro-life syllogism (human life is sacred, fetal life is human life, therefore...), the focus has shifted from the minor to the major premise.

Broadly, Christians have taken two kinds of approaches to the determination of a biblical position, both alike recognizing the uniform character of Christian opposition to abortion on all but extreme therapeutic grounds from the earliest days of the church (our first evidence is in the *Didache*).[17] One approach has noted that there is no explicit reference to abortion in Old or New Testament as something to be commended or condemned, though in a famously difficult passage (Exod. 21:22-25) we find casuistic discussion of the penalty due for causing a miscarriage. More than one interpretation of the text is possible,[18] but even on the conventional reading its relevance to the procuring of abortion is very remote; for it outlines a case in which two men are brawling, heedless of the fact that a pregnant woman is nearby, and as a result of reckless but accidental injury to her she miscarries. The result is a fine for those responsible. It is hard to see how they are responsible for anything other than brawling recklessly near a pregnant woman. They are certainly not responsible for procuring an abortion. And, as we need to be reminded, the limited range of criminal sanctions possible in Old Testament society meant that a fine could be an appropriate penalty for a relatively serious offense. The suggestion of some interpreters that if the fetus were fully human the death penalty would have been appropriate is extraordinary.[19]

A very different approach seeks guidance not first of all in the matter of abortion, looking for legislation and arguing from silence, but with respect to the nature of unborn human life.[20] There are several different lines of argument in this approach. First we have the significance of the creation of humankind in the *imago Dei*, as we have already noted. The context of this statement lies in the taxonomy of the created order that is found in Genesis 1. (Whatever else this chapter says, it does set out such a taxonomy.) The implication is plain: wherever humankind is found, wherever this species that we call *Homo sapiens* is met, there is one who bears the divine image. The image is co-terminous with the biological constitution of humankind. This is in truth a very striking statement, for not only does it bear momentous implications for the dignity of both women and men, but it also declares in principle the equal dignity and value of every human life — irrespective of color or creed, moral worth or depravity, age or sickness, mental impairment or genius: all who share in the genetic constitution of the human race bear that inestimable dignity that is bestowed by God in their creation in his image.

A second line of argument picks up the manner in which, within the Old Testament especially, the process of generation is addressed. Abraham begat Isaac. The point at which one generation was succeeded by the next was (surprise, surprise!) the point of generation, the point of begetting. In light of what has been said about the taxonomy in Genesis 1 — and in light of what I shall say next about the incarnation — this argument has particular force. So, from the very beginnings of human biological existence, that being is by definition a new member of *Homo sapiens*, who, in common with all mammalian species begets and reproduces himself and herself — the product of human conception is no *tertium quid* but the next generation of the species.

A third line of argument addresses the incarnation of Jesus Christ. In support of the full humanity of the fetus much use has been made of biblical references to unborn human life, especially in Job, in some of the prophets, and in certain of the psalms. These texts are by no means irrelevant, but they pale beside the narrative of the birth of Jesus Christ. For the point of incarnation is plainly put at the point of his virginal and supernatural conception. There is no separation made between his biological beginnings as Mary's conceptus and the mysterious overshadowing of the Holy Spirit. In the case of Jesus we have an open-and-shut case for the highest possible view of the earliest stage of fetal life. Incarnation took place in embryo. This raises many questions, though in terms of orthodox theology it is straightforward. Jesus' humanity is patterned after our humanity, sin only apart; so the character of his own unborn human life is also the pattern of ours. If we find it hard to imagine a zygote possessing the dignity of one who bears the image of God, we have only to cast our minds to the miracle of the incarnation. The problem lies, not in the unimaginable genetic complexity and completeness of the zygote, but in the altogether limited imaginative faculty that we are able to bring to bear on the subject.

The coupling of these suggestive biblical-theological arguments with the striking fact of Christian opposition to abortion from the earliest days of the church, and until very recently in an unbroken tradition, leads us to an enthusiastic endorsement of the Hippocratic refusal to participate in abortion that was, until lately, the orthodoxy of the Western medical tradition. And if the debate moves on to the possibility of using human embryos for deleterious research, the grounding of our argument against abortion in the decisive character of conception-fertilization already gives us our answer. If human life is sacred right from its biological beginnings, then we stand face-to-face with that which bears the ineffable image of its — her, his — Maker.

END-OF-LIFE ISSUES

No more than a generation ago, euthanasia — however it was dressed up — was regarded as at best the preserve of cranks and at worst as subversive, with ideological overtones of fascism. This issue is now at the very heart of the public policy debate on health care and human values. Although it has not yet been made the subject of a political-legal revolution that compares with *Roe v. Wade* and the abortion legislation that marked a similar path in most industrialized and many other countries during the 1960^s and 1970^s, there is widespread public support for voluntary euthanasia in most Western countries. That support depends critically on fears and misunderstandings, but it has offered cover for a succession of legal and political moves toward a positive euthanasia policy in many countries. These moves have opened increasingly liberal approaches to case law in marginal situations and have prepared public opinion for more general legal change. The high-water mark of these developments in the United States is the so-called Patient Self-Determination Act of 1991, which obliges hospitals and other institutions receiving federal funding to inquire of patients on admission whether they have a "living will"; in Europe it is the *de facto* legalization of voluntary euthanasia in Holland, where statute has still to catch up with a permissive public policy in which prosecuting authorities and courts have conspired with the major medical bodies to give doctors a license to kill their patients.[21] As we have already noted in more general terms, from the standpoint of history the most curious feature of this movement away from the sanctity-of-life doctrine is the degree to which the resources needed to sustain those who are handicapped or chronically or terminally ill have so dramatically increased just at the moment when opinion is shifting round to favor killing. An excellent example of a fundamentally different approach is hospice care, a recent development in geriatric and palliative medicine that has sought "death with dignity" in supportive community care of the dying, joining expertise in drug therapy and pain control with associated medical and nursing skills.[22] Yet euthanasia is cheap, and the central place that cost containment holds in current discussions has given a major fillip to the euthanasia trend, as the Patient Self-Determination Act shows. With the ethical framework of which the sanctity of life was a key element now in flux, the desire to limit costs will place increasing pressure on end-of-life choices and may well be the deciding factor in legislative moves toward voluntary euthanasia. And if the key pressures at the level of legislation will be financial, it seems clear that the Chinese walls that alone separate the "voluntary" and the "involuntary" will not long survive (any more than this distinction has proved reliable in the sub-legal and informal euthanasia context of the Netherlands).[23]

It is important to note some of the distinctions and connections that characterize this discussion before we return to biblical-theological comment. The overt justification for the modern euthanasia movement is that of patient self-determination; patient autonomy is to replace Hippocratic paternalism, as it is perceived, giving patients the right to "medically assisted suicide" or "aid in dying," as its proponents variously term it. In fact, what they seek is a curious amalgam of suicide and homicide; the decision, they say, should lie with the patient, and if the patient requests death the attending physician should be obliged to comply and bring it about. This is not actually assisted suicide but homicide with consent, homicide at the victim's request; it actually partakes of the moral problematic of both suicide and homicide. And its rooting in the patient's act of free decision, on which whatever defense is offered must wholly rest, is deluged in difficulty. For what kind of free choice on this most fundamental of human questions is someone who is by definition a patient able to make? Who can assess the pressures on one who is, say, chronically sick, who is trying to double-guess her relatives to decide whether they would really prefer her dead, who is juggling financial uncertainties and perhaps knows that her children's hope of a legacy entirely depends on her dying sooner rather than later? These are typical of many questions that can be raised about the simple coherence of the euthanasia project, aside from ethical critique.

There is then the question of the alleged distinction between this voluntary, patient-autonomy euthanasia and involuntary killing, which of course most euthanasia advocates seek to disown. Aside from the psychological difficulty of envisaging free choices for and against euthanasia in a family, in a hospital, indeed in a society that formally endorses this as an option, there is a basic logical difficulty. What is to be the ground on which the physician is obliged to bring about death? There are two possible answers: either the simple expressed desire of a person who seeks death, perhaps qualified by its repetition on successive occasions or before successive physicians, or an expressed desire coupled with a certain medical condition. If the latter, the question arises how those who satisfy the medical criteria but do not express a wish to die will ultimately be treated, especially when they are incompetent. The pressure to move from voluntary to "non-voluntary" (in the case of the incompetent) and ultimately to a full involuntary euthanasia policy will be unstoppable. (For example, there might be federal withdrawal of Medicaid and Medicare, insurance exclusions, and so forth if a "voluntary" decision for euthanasia is not made.) On the other hand, if no medical criteria are set down, the policy is simply a charter for suicide: the jilted teen and the postnatal depressive will have nothing to bar their way. The basic problem, of course, lies in the assumption that it can be good to will one's own death and that any community that accepts that proposition as part of its understanding of the rights of the individual can flourish. There is no third way: the acceptance in principle of medical killing will resolve itself either in the encouragement of arbitrary decisions for suicide or in the creation of classes of persons for whom the choice to die is regarded as reasonable; and if the latter, then those in that class who do not choose to die will be marginalized at best, and at worst will be killed for their unreason and their claim on community resources. It is a truly frightening prospect.

Over against this option for death the Christian sets Job's dictum. "The LORD gave and the LORD has taken away: may the name of the LORD be praised" (1:21). Job refuses the urgings of his wife "to curse God and die" (2:9). He lays hold on the providential purposes of the good God who has given him life, and he trusts him for aid as it becomes harder to live and as death looms bitter-sweet on the horizon of his pilgrimage.

This is not to say that there are no hard choices to be faced. One reason why our failure to develop an evangelical bioethics is so serious lies squarely here: we have yet to form a community within which appropriate biblical-theological responses to real, hard questions can be formulated. Yet the beginnings of that culture lie in the old medicine of Christian Hippocratism and in the application of its principles to new situations. In accordance with those principles, futile treatment has never been good treatment. The well-advanced dying process is the place for palliation, not invasive and distressing procedures initiated to please relatives or on the advice of the hospital attorney or to pursue some tacit experimental purpose. How we define futility in a sanctity-of-life context may be radically different from a quality-of-life evaluation, but Christian Hippocratism has always recognized that there is a time to die.

KEY QUESTIONS FOR AN EVANGELICAL BIOETHICS

The agenda is as long as the road is untraveled, yet several key questions stand out that require address from a biblical-theological perspective. First and most broadly, we need to develop a biblical theology of medicine. The field of medicine offers a prime example of the theological-hermeneutical challenges that confront evangelicals today, since the practice of medicine and the questions raised in the discussion of medical values are of prime importance to the church. Yet where Scripture touches on this subject, it does so almost entirely indirectly.

If life is sacred because God has made us in his own image, and if death is nonetheless universal in fallen human experience, what is the place of medicine? The hope of humankind is the hope of the resurrection of the body, and that bodily resurrection — in its imaging yet transcending human experience before the mortal consequences of the fall — gives rich significance to those anticipations of the resurrection of the body that we find in the New Testament, supremely in the healing miracles of Jesus. It is common to see "natural" medical healing as quite other than the healing of a miracle; yet both alike stay the progress of mortality and thereby offer broken and anticipatory witness to the eschatological abolition of death. A biblical theology of medicine will be eschatologically oriented.[24]

Second, we must address the question of health-care provision at the extremes of human existence: the anencephalic baby, for example, or the patient in a persistent vegetative state. The pressure is on (and it has been felt by some evangelicals already) to adopt essentially quality-of-life criteria in these cases that would be vigorously repudiated if they were applied more generally. If we move in just a little from the margins, we stumble over the curious medicalization of the giving of food and drink (symbolized in the use of the labels "nutrition" and "hydration" for these elemental human requirements), a major step — unwittingly or not — in the generation of opportunities for medical killing and a potent threat to the sanctity-of-life position. It is hard to exaggerate the importance of such bellwether questions as the evangelical mind crystallizes in the flux of current discussion.

Finally, the fundamental technological development of our time lies in the field of human genetics. The unlocking of ever great proportions of the genetic code has begun to realize an ultimately enormous range of manipulative possibilities affecting the very nature of the human species. The harvesting of these developments will begin in earnest just as the values of post-Hippocratism have established themselves in mainstream medicine. The generation of appropriate Christian responses will require the resources of a major intellectual community, but such a community in this field has scarcely begun to develop.

THE PROBLEM OF CONSENSUS

Despite the fundamental significance of the sanctity of life for the assumptions that govern bioethical discussion, and despite the central place that beginning-of-life and end-of-life issues hold on the public stage today, there is yet another kind of issue that we must address — that of consensus in medicine. We have already noted that the scene has been set for the incipient breakup of the Christian-Hippocratic consensus. Many particular substantive questions are on the agenda, not because society's mind has all of a sudden changed, but because the prevailing consensus — and with it, the *idea* of a consensus — has begun to crack. Abortion began to be defended, irrespective of the merits of traditional arguments pro and con, as a concomitant of the right of privacy or the rights of women. Euthanasia is on the agenda as an exercise in self-deliverance, the final act of patient autonomy. Curiously enough, academic bioethics has concerned itself less and less with these and other similar substantive ethical questions, and increasingly with questions of procedure. Of course, these questions are not unrelated. Procedural questions may well also, in themselves, be of ethical interest. But the weight that is now placed on the establishment of procedures that will allow individuals of diverse ethical convictions to determine their treatment regime is a declaration of despair. Its implication is that there will be no new consensus and that the only area in which we can seek agreement with one another is in the determination of the procedures of disagreement. This can be illustrated no better than in the title of the milestone congressional legislation of 1991 to which we have already referred: the Patient *Self-Determination* Act. Whatever the cost-containment concerns that may lie behind this and similar legislation elsewhere, the question we must keep asking is this: Why do we need procedures laid down in federal law that assume that we no longer share a community of values in terminal care? Is there no longer a medical *community*, representative of the broader community, infused with the values of centuries of humane clinical experience, whose judgment that wider community can trust? There are many partial answers; but at root we recognize, on the one hand, the undeniable and general fragmentation of community values, though we also recognize, on the other hand, that it is in the interest of a (morally) liberal minority on the leading edge of that fragmentation to give the impression that things have gone farther and faster than they actually have. This in turn is deeply influencing the move to pluralism. The societies of Europe and North America are actually more cohesive — in fact, much more "societies" — than many of their glib interpreters suggest; and that is particularly true in the field of bioethics, where the purveying of half-truths about the significance and state of incipient pluralism is proving catalytic and has actually helped to give birth to the discipline.

So should I have a living will? The answer to this question lies buried in the complexity of Christian-Hippocratic tactics in an age in which Hippocratism is proving to be "biologically tenacious" (a chilling phrase that some bioethicists have applied to patients who refuse to die when they "should"), and yet an age in which, equally certainly, a post-Hippocratic medical culture is in the making. Originally a clever ploy in the armory of euthanasia advocates, this coyly named advanced directive permits the patient to decide ahead of time the principles according to which treatment decisions should be made should the patient become incompetent, so that these decisions are not left in the hands of relatives, physicians, hospital administrators, or — ultimately — the courts. Perhaps our response should be that drawing up a living will offers Christians a wonderful opportunity to ensure Christian-Hippocratic canons of medical care right to the last. Yet, aside from many practical problems that the use of the living will poses, every time someone draws one up another nail is knocked in the coffin of consensus. That may not be an argument against using the living will in the United States, where one evidence of the weakness of the consensus is the degree of involvement of the judiciary in clinical management decisions; but it is an important argument against their general introduction in some other jurisdictions (e.g., in the United Kingdom) where there is still a substantial consensus in medical values and considerable confidence in physicians as interpreters of the best in the humane medical tradition.

This raises the question of tactics. Part of the naiveté of sections of the pro-life movement has lain in the assumption that, with the striking down of *Roe v. Wade* or equivalent watersheds in other parts of the world, all would somehow be well. Liberal abortion is a symptom of the diseased character of contemporary medical ethics; it is not the disease in itself. Political advocacy on those bioethical issues that break surface in public policy discussion is vital, but it must be part of a grand strategy by which political and other initiatives must be judged — everything down to my own initiative or lack of it in exercising patient "self-determination" and drawing up an advance directive.

The key lies in an awareness of the state of fragmentation of the consensus, on the one hand, and a rediscovery of the origins and logic of Hippocratism on the other. Nothing must be done that makes it easier for the bioethics community to point the finger and cry "pluralism"; we must seek to shore up and draw attention to the elements of consensus, which are, incidentally, far more in evidence in our society and in the health-care professions than among bioethicists themselves. And yet we must also begin to look ahead to the day when the prophecies have come true and we enter an age of truly post-Hippocratic medicine. As we focus on this developing situation, we seek to apply our general principles of Christian community and witness. We must be dissident, and we must be prophetic; we must maintain our own distinctive community while never entirely dissociating ourselves and our community from the wider community of which we remain indissolubly a part.

And that is where the rediscovery of Hippocratic origins has a special and challenging relevance. For if the first Hippocratics were dissidents and prophets, protesting the inhumanity of the medical culture of their day and leading the way to a better one, there are footsteps in which we can follow.

NOTES

1. Edward Creasy, *The Fifteen Decisive Battles of the World* (1851), various re-issues.

2. There are notable exceptions, including Carl F. H. Henry himself and, especially, Harold O. J. Brown. Recent writers include Allen Verhey and John Frame.

3. There is a new announcement every few months, though evangelicals have yet to launch a technical journal.

4. Very few evangelicals are to be found at the international conferences that have become determinative of the development of the bioethics community. It is of course true that evangelicals who are interested in these questions tend to be associated with evangelical schools, which in turn may be less interested in funding such participation — which raises the institutional question afresh.

5. Modest exceptions are the Lindeboom Instituut at Ede in the Netherlands and the fledgling Centre for Bioethics and Public Policy in London. Trinity Evangelical Divinity School is in process of launching an M.A. track in bioethics.

6. For example, members of the (British) Christian Medical Fellowship offered two conflicting responses to their government's advisory body on embryo research issues.

7. This thesis is further sketched in my book *The New Medicine: Life and Death After Hippocrates* (Westchester, Ill.: Crossway, 1992).

8. The Hippocratic Oath reads as follows (translation by W. H. S. Jones in his book *The Doctor's Oath* [Cambridge Univ. Press, 1924], with minor alterations and added headings):

THE COVENANT

I swear by Apollo Physician, by Asclepius, by Hygeia, by Panaceia, and by all the gods and goddesses, making them witnesses, that I will carry out, according to my ability and judgment, this oath and indenture:

DUTIES TO TEACHER

To regard my teacher in this art as equal to my parents; to make him partner in my livelihood, and when he is in need of money to share mine with him; to consider his offspring equal to my brothers; to teach them this art, if they require to learn it, without fee or indenture; and to impart precept, oral instruction, and all the other learning, to my sons, to the sons of my teacher, and to pupils who have signed the indenture and sworn obedience to the physicians' Law, but to none other.

DUTIES TO PATIENTS

I will use treatment to help the sick according to my ability and judgment, but will never use it to injure or wrong them.

I will not give poison to anyone though asked to do so, nor will I suggest such a plan. Similarly I will not give a pessary to a woman to cause abortion. But in purity and in holiness I will guard my life and my art.

I will not use the knife either on sufferers from stone, but will give place to such as are craftsmen therein.

Into whatsoever house I enter, I will do so to help the sick, keeping myself free from all intentional wrong-doing and harm, especially from fornication with woman or man, bond or free.

Whatsoever in the course of practice I see or hear (or even outside my practice in social intercourse) that ought never to be published abroad, I will not divulge, but consider such things to be holy secrets.

THE SANCTION

Now if I keep this oath and break it not, may I enjoy honour, in my life and art, among men for all time; but if I transgress and forswear myself, may the opposite befall me.

9. The relation of medicine and society is most helpfully discussed in Eliot Freidson, *Profession of Medicine: A Study in the Sociology of Applied Knowledge* (New York: Harper & Row, 1970).

10. See Jones, *The Doctor's Oath*, pp. 23ff.

11. See M. Ullmann, *Islamic Medicine* (Edinburgh: Univ. of Edinburgh Press, 1978).

12. Little is known with any certainty about Hippocrates of Cos (460-377 B.C. are the years most often suggested for his life; he died old, some say a centenarian). Jones summarizes what we do know in *The Doctor's Oath*, with the authority of the editor of the Loeb edition of the *corpus*.

13. For references see the most recent scholarly study in English of the Hippocratic tradition (though its chief interest does not lie in Hippocratic *ethics*). Owesi Temkin, *Hippocrates in a World of Pagans and Christians* (Baltimore: Johns Hopkins Univ. Press, 1991), p.21 n.16.

14. Jones, *The Doctor's Oath*, offers a good example.

15. For a contemporary echo, see especially the work of Stanley Hauerwas — e.g., his book *Suffering Presence* (Notre Dame: Univ. of Notre Dame Press, 1986).

16. Helpfully and most recently summarized by Gerald Bray in *Tyndale Bulletin* 42/2 (1991) 195-225.

17. The *Didache* is a very early statement of post-apostolic Christian practice, dated to the first half of the second century or before.

18. The New International Version reads: "If men who are fighting hit a pregnant woman and she gives birth prematurely but there is no serious injury, the offender must be fined.... But if there is serious injury, you are to take life for life..." (Exod. 21:22-23).

19. In his influential book *Abortion: The Personal Dilemma* (Exeter: Paternoster, 1972), R. F. R. Gardner introduces this text as the "one clear reference to abortion in the Old Testament" and comments: "it would seem fairly obvious that in any case the text implies a difference in the eyes of the law between the fetus and a person" (p. 119).

20. This line of argument is laid out at more length in my contribution to *Abortion in Debate* (Church of Scotland Board of Social Responsibility; Edinburgh: Quorum Press, 1987), pp. 1-19.

21. See Richard Fenigsen, "A Case against Dutch Euthanasia," in *Hastings Center Report*, Special Supplement (Jan./Feb. 1989); reprinted in *Ethics and Medicine* 6/1 (1990) 11-18.

22. See Cicely Saunders, "Euthanasia: The Hospice Alternative" in *Death Without Dignity: Euthanasia in Perspective*, ed. Nigel M. de S. Cameron (Edinburgh: Rutherford House, 1990).

23. See Richard Fenigsen, "The Report of the Dutch Governmental Committee on Euthanasia," *Issues in Law and Medicine* 7/3 (1991) 339-44.

24. I have developed this theme somewhat in an appendix to *The New Medicine*, cited above in n.7, and in a forthcoming issue of *Christian Scholar's Review*.

POPE PAUL VI — MODERN DAY PROPHET

William F. Colliton, Jr., M.D., F.A.C.O.G.

A presentation of experiences witnessed by an obstetrician-gynecologist practicing three decades in a contraceptive culture

PROLOGUE

Humanae Vitae, the prophetic encyclical on human sexuality by Pope Paul VI, celebrated its 27th anniversary on July 25, 1995. In spite of all its critics have offered, it is a very positive document filled with much wisdom. Of particular interest to the author, a retired obstetrician-gynecologist who practiced medicine for 39 years after medical school, were the prognostications envisioned by his Holiness if a contraceptive culture came to flourish. The marketing of the birth control pill (BCP) and intrauterine device (IUD) has produced just such a culture. What did the Pope say on July 25, 1968? What has happened since?

Paul VI's three main predictions are detailed in his encyclical at #17: "Grave Consequences of Methods of Artificial Birth Control."[1] (1) "Let them consider, first of all, how wide and easy a road would thus be opened up towards conjugal infidelity and the general lowering of morality." The 50% rate of divorce currently being experienced as well as the cultural acceptance of same-sex genital relations as a viable lifestyle option come to mind. (2) "It is also to be feared that the man, growing used to the employment of anti-conceptive practices, may finally lose respect for the woman and, no longer caring for her physical and psychological equilibrium, may come to the point of considering her as a mere instrument of selfish enjoyment, and no longer as his respected and beloved companion." The "philosophies" of *Playboy* and *Penthouse* magazines are examples of this. (3) "Let it be considered

116

also that a dangerous weapon would thus be placed in the hands of those public authorities who take no heed of moral exigencies. Who could blame a government for applying to the solution of the problems of the community those means acknowledged to be licit for married couples in the solution of a family problem? Who will stop rulers from favoring, from even imposing upon their peoples, if they were to consider it necessary, the method of contraception which they judge to be most efficacious? In such a way, men wishing to avoid individual, family, or social difficulties encountered in the observance of the divine law, would reach the point of placing at the mercy of the intervention of public authorities the most personal and most reserved sector of conjugal intimacy." The mandatory one-child policy in force in the Republic of China witnesses the accuracy of this prediction. This policy is enforced through required contraception and sterilization, backed up by compulsory induced abortion when these former methods fail.[2] What other societal by-product has been witnessed as a result of the advance in contraceptive technology?

In the author's judgment, the marketing of the BCP and IUD undoubtedly fueled the sexual revolution of the 60[s], 70[s] and 80[s]. This view is supported by the late Robert W. Kistner, M.D., an obstetrician and gynecologist of Harvard Medical School and Boston Hospital for Women.[3] Speaking to the 1977 Annual Clinical Congress of the American College of Surgeons, he said: "About ten years ago I declared that the pill would not lead to promiscuity. Well, I was wrong." During his presentation he reported that adolescent promiscuity, abetted by access to oral contraception, may ultimately produce a new generation of infertile females. He added, "Anyone who treats patients for infertility must be alarmed at the marked increase over the last five years in salpingitis, tubal adhesions, and virulent gonorrhea. Class III Pap smears in 17-year old

girls who never return to your office are also alarming."
Thus Dr. Kistner confirms the fact that the use of the pill
has led to an increase in sexually transmitted diseases,
infertility, and cervical intraepithelial neoplasia (CIN) in
very young women. The impact of this type of deportment
reaches beyond individual patients.   It touches all of
society.

What has this led to as we view our nation from a
cultural perspective in the 1990s?   A series of rhetorical
questions proposed by Rev. Randall Terry shed some
light.[4] Rev. Terry celebrated the thirtieth anniversary of
his birth in 1990 and was pondering some remarkable
changes that have occurred during his lifetime:

Who, in their wildest dreams, would imagine in 1960 that today we
would live in a country in which vile corruption, rape and lethal
violence would be reported daily by the media? Who would have
predicted an epidemic of teenage pregnancy and sexually transmitted
diseases? Who would have foreseen an outbreak of child pornography
and "snuff" films in which children, after suffering sexual abuse of an
animal kind, would be ritualistically murdered? Who would envision
a society that annually kills 1.5 million of its preborn children and
whose capital records more abortions than live births each year? Who
would have dreamed that this same capital would count over one
homicide every day? Who could envision that our largest cities would
host annual parades featuring gays and lesbians demonstrating for their
rights? Who could foresee a time when representatives in the Congress
would openly profess their homosexuality and several jurisdictions
would consider legislation permitting same-sex marriages? Who would
have foretold a roaring drug epidemic affecting all levels of society?
That we are living in a moral disaster area is not in doubt.   That
Humanae Vitae predicted the possibility of these calamities is equally
true.

INTRODUCTION

In support of the wisdom of Pope Paul, this paper
presents the observations of one who has practiced
medicine for 39 years. After a rotating internship, a year
of active duty as a general medical officer in the Air Force

and a one-year medical residency, the author spent approximately four and a half years as a family practitioner. Beginning July 1, 1955, three years were spent as a resident in obstetrics and gynecology, with the balance of the time consumed in the private practice of the same discipline. The purpose of this paper is to demonstrate that the medical profession, its various organizations and individual physicians have really not thought through the practice of prescribing contraceptives. This practice has helped to generate three significant medical conditions and a social problem. While it may not be possible to demonstrate a crystal-clear cause-and-effect relationship between contraception and these difficulties, the facts, as they evolve, will be consuming in their witness to that possibility that they will display the connection.

What are the issues to be addressed? The first of the problems to be discussed is the teenage pregnancy epidemic, a reality which seems to be antithetical to prescribing contraception. However, numerous studies have been done during the past two decades demonstrating results that fly in the face of human wisdom. In 1971-73 California started with a very modest four million dollar budget to establish an Office of Family Planning (OFP).[5] Spending was increased to 31 million in 1984-85 and subsequently reached a level of 36 million. Data indicated that for each increase of one million dollars spent on contraceptive research, technology and supply, another 200 teenage pregnancies occurred. California has learned its lesson. For FY 1990 they lowered the OFP budget to 12 million dollars.[6] The second problem, the sexually transmitted disease epidemic, is a little bit easier to relate to contraception. Thirdly, an alarming rise in CIN, that is, microscopic tumors on the mouth of the womb that are either pre-cancerous (dysplasia) or microscopic cancer (carcinoma in situ) has been demonstrated. These findings are easily related to the sexual revolution. The final question to be discussed is the epidemic rate of divorce in America. The common etiology of all these problems is the sexual revolution of the 60^s, 70^s, and 80^s, aided and abetted by the advance of contraceptive technology. And what is the cure? The cure is a return to chastity. There is no other cure. Chastity means that a mature and functional emotional relationship between a man and a woman places the sexual act in context, and restores to it the creative and responsible function of sustaining and procreating the family.

TEENAGE PREGNANCY

The first problem to be discussed is the teenage pregnancy epidemic which has been making headlines for over two decades. The figures are deplorable. In 1980 there were a million pregnancies to women under the age of twenty. Some 40% of the girls who are now 14 years old will experience pregnancy at some time before they are 20 years old. One-fifth of them will bear a child. Another 15% will have at least one abortion, and 6% will have at least one stillbirth. In California, adolescent pregnancy is the number one cause of school dropouts among teenage women.[7]

Sex education based on contraception has been routinely offered as a solution. Because of the intrinsic corruption of moral norms that this imposes, because it elevates the sexual act to an end in itself, and therefore robs it of its creative and responsible nature, it is bound to fail. Recent history demonstrates this failure. It is well to remember that 23 years have passed since Congress adopted legislation establishing Title X of the Public Health Services Act. Yet after more than $2.2 billion in expenditures America's teenage pregnancy crisis is not getting better. From 1974 to 1985, the percentage of all females aged 15-19 becoming pregnant each year rose by more than 10%.[8] That contraception isn't the answer was articulated by Peggy B. Smith at the 1986 annual meeting of the Texas Medical Association. "In 1970, I thought I knew the answer. If the pill were made available at no cost and the service(s) were confidential and did not involve parents, I thought we would stamp out adolescent pregnancy. We made this mistake because we considered the facts, the science, but not the art."[9]

What has happened to the teenage pregnancy problem during the intervening 23 years since Dr. Smith thought she had the answer? Henshaw and Van Vort of the Alan Guttmacher Institute (AGI) presented an update on teenage abortion, birth, and pregnancy statistics up though 1985.[10] The information on births comes from the National Center for Health Statistics (NCHS). Abortion data are the results of an AGI survey of all known abortion providers in the country. The national abortion and birth rates are based on population estimates published by the Census Bureau. The figures are low because the numbers are counted at the time of pregnancy outcome rather than the age at which the pregnancy occurred. For example, most women who gave birth at age 20 conceived while age 19. The authors report that women younger than 20 accounted for 26% of all abortions and 13% of all births. The pregnancy rate by age of outcome rose steadily from 104.6/1000 women aged 15-19 in 1977 to a high of 111.2 in 1980. It experienced only minor fluctuations through 1985, the last year of this study. Calculations from the NCHS data show that at the 1985 rates of abortions and births, 9% of young women will have had at least one abortion and another 9% one or more births by their 18th birthday. By age 20 the figures are 18% and 20%, respectively. The latest figures available from the NCHS indicate no improvement. In fact, the 1989 figures document the sharpest increase in the teenage birth rate in over a decade.[11]

Why haven't widely available sex education and contraception stopped this epidemic? In answer to that question, consider the view of Kingsley Davis, professor of sociology at the University of California, Berkeley, whose words are as true today as they were in 1972: "The current belief that illegitimacy will be reduced if teenage girls are given effective contraception is an extension of the same reasoning that created the problem in the first place. It reflects an unwillingness to face problems of social control and social discipline, while trusting some technological device to extricate society from its difficulties. The irony is that the illegitimacy rise occurred precisely while contraception was becoming more, rather than less, widespread and respectable."[12]

SEXUALLY TRANSMITTED DISEASES

The second medical problem area is Sexually Transmitted Diseases (STD's). As far back as 1971, the incidence of gonorrhea in the U.S. was put at two million cases annually.[13] While the reported incidence has hovered around one million per year in recent years and seems to be leveling off, massive under-reporting is a recognized fact. As startling as this figure is, as of 1989 the rate of chlamydia infections is thought to be 4 million cases per year.[14] This infection is very difficult to diagnose, as the offending bacteria only grows in human cells.

Hugh R. K. Barber, M.D., an obstetrician/gynecologist and editor of the periodical *Female Patient*, wrote an editorial about chlamydia trachomatis infection in the female.[15] He was aware of the high rate of infertility that followed this infection secondary to occlusive salpingitis. He said,

Why should we be surprised at these reports? Nature demands a price for everything we do. Just as surgical incision is followed by a scar, sexual promiscuity may be followed by infection. From biblical times, promiscuity has been a self-fulfilling prophecy. The release of our inhibitions and doing one's thing (even in defiance of morality) has been projected as the means to help us become a better adjusted, happier race of free-spirited people. Maybe they have, but we may have paid a high price in physical well-being.

We should recognize that one of the most powerful forces in society, an unbridged revolution, is underway. In the foreseeable future it will not be turned back or controlled. Young, as well as older, people have been affected by the chlamydia epidemic, resulting from 'modern' behavior.

It is obvious that through the sexual revolution we have released an awesome energy, whose final destructive physical power may not yet be foreseen. I am neither a moralist nor an evangelist, but the lessons learned from Sodom and Gomorrah stand out as revelatory of the consequences of unbridled promiscuity. Since we seem powerless to control this monstrous energy, the medical profession must redouble its efforts to protect the population. It is not for us to reason why but rather to treat and cure.

As guardians of the health of the nation, it is our responsibility and duty to meet this challenge and vanquish the enemy. The accomplishment of wiping out chlamydia may give us pride in our scientific excellence and at the same time serve as consolation for our failure or (at best) mediocrity in moral accomplishments.

The author does not agree with all of Dr. Barber's comments, but his reasoning about the cause of the chlamydia epidemic is sound. Less sound is his statement that the human family cannot learn to control the exhibition of the sexual gifts. To the author it is demeaning to suggest that the control of such human actions is located anteriorly in the midline near where the lower extremities join the body in both the male and female of the species. This does not even take into consideration the powerful assistance available through a leap of faith in Jesus Christ and His Father. His suggestion that unbridled sexual activity might lead to human happiness and fulfillment is also in error.

Is there a connection between the STD epidemic and the advance in contraceptive technology? This is the word from King K. Holmes, M.D., an infectious disease expert.[16] He says the rise in ten sexually transmitted diseases is linked with the oral contraceptive. The diseases he cited are gonorrhoea, genital herpes, cytomegalo virus, chlamydia, T-myco plasma, hepatitis B, syphilis, trichomonoas, crab lice, and genital warts. Sadly, chlamydia trachomatis is common among sexually active adolescent women. It occurs more frequently among sexually active female adolescents who use oral contraceptives according to John J. Fraser, M.D., and colleagues.[17] Like other investigators, Dr. Fraser found an association between oral contraceptive use and chlamydial infection. Two possible explanations for the association of chlamydia trachomatis, say the investigators, are increased sexual activity in pill users and hormone induced changes in the cervical epithelium conducive to the growth of the organism.

Perhaps the biggest headlines reserved today for STD's concern viral etiology. The first one is genital herpes. This disease is incurable and has great impact on the child-bearing ability of women. Herpes acquired by the newborn is frequently fatal. If there is any history of herpes in the expectant mother, the labia and lower genital tract must be carefully inspected at the onset of labor. If vaginal delivery is planned, there must be no evidence of active disease. If there is any suggestion of active lesions in the genital area, Caesarean section must be performed in the interest of the baby's health.

Is herpes still prevalent? As herpes is not a reportable infectious disease, one can only give an estimated incidence of 500,000 cases per year.[18] The incidence of most sexually transmitted diseases is leveling off, and in some instances on a decline. This is not because of the discovery of Our Lord Jesus Christ. It is because of herpes and the Acquired Immune Deficiency Syndrome (AIDS), also caused by a virus. Both are sexually transmitted, both incurable, the latter lethal. All the headlines these days seem to be going to AIDS. Medical economists estimate the annual cost of HIV (human immunodeficiency virus) infections would reach 10.4 billion dollars per year by 1994.[19]

AIDS has always been thought of as most prevalent in the homosexual community, and indeed it has been. Results from the largest national sexual survey in over forty years were recently published in the journal *Science*.[20] But findings suggested that many Americans are ignoring the "safe-sex" message. The most egregious denial of risk is occurring among heterosexual Americans who are having intercourse with multiple partners without using condoms. Among heterosexual adults with two or more sex partners in the past five years, 31% were at some level of risk for becoming HIV positive. In some metropolitan areas, such as New York and San Francisco, the risk was 41%. Condom use was 17% among those with multiple partners and 13% among those with high risk partners, such as intravenous drug users. This type of social behavior insures the increasing incidence of this lethal disease among heterosexuals and, unfortunately, their innocent offspring.

With regard to their sexual gifts, declining behavioral patterns among today's adolescents has produced one change. The problem of STD's among teenagers in industrialized countries has gotten so mammoth that people interested in sex education indicate that a change in emphasis is needed.[21] In 1975, speaking at the General Assembly of the "Union Against the Venereal Diseases and Treponematoses" held in Attard, Malta, Dr. K. F. Heinz said, "If people would shield themselves against STD's as conscientiously and efficiently as they do to avoid pregnancy, we might have good reason to expect a decline of VD in industrialized countries similar to that of our birth rate." Dr. Hunger cited data that regular contraceptive use during intercourse had increased from 30% to 70% among West German young people during the preceding 15 years. He added that in that same period the incidence of STD's had risen to epidemic proportions. He blames this on the emphasis on pregnancy prevention in the sex education classes. No mention of the need for change in social behavior was made. This message may be a little slow in becoming widely known, but it becomes obvious if one begins to look at the data.

What single agency is most responsible for the disaster that has been seen here? In the author's judgment, Planned Parenthood. This organization is anti-family, anti-good health and anti-good sense. This organization is supportive of sex education without a value-judgment system, gives contraceptive counsel and provision without parental consent, and urges induced abortion for failed contraception without parental consent or awareness. To anyone who has thought about the problems besetting today's teenagers, the first point of intervention to prevent all of them is before the initiation of sexual activity. There are at least two main courses to be followed. One is premised on strong parental guidance and condemnation of sex outside of marriage. The second casts children as sexual libertarians entitled to absolute freedom in sexual matters and a complete range of rights to deal with the unintended consequences. The Planned Parenthood Federation, which receives approximately $30 million annually under Title X, has embraced the second alternative. Examples of their approach include the following: Alameda-San Francisco told their clients that it is a "myth" that "[y]oung women who have more than one sexual partner are easy. Some people, both men and women, prefer to relate sexually to more than one person at a time. This is an individual preference."[22]

An almost identical theme appeared in a teen pamphlet prepared for the Planned Parenthood Center of Syracuse: "Many people believe that sex relations are right only when they are married. Others decide to have sex outside of marriage. This is a personal choice."[23] Eunice Kennedy Shriver pointed out the crossroads at which our society is poised in a 1987 editorial: "Let us listen to parents, teachers, and teenagers themselves before the vastly increased commitment of resources called for by the advocates of contraception and abortion becomes national policy. There needs to be a recognition by public officials at all levels that there are effective approaches to adolescent pregnancy more in keeping with our traditions and values. Without these, we will only continue to pursue with cold illogic the fantasy of a magic bullet."[24]

CERVICAL INTRAEPITHELIAL NEOPLASIA

Another STD of viral etiology is genital warts. While this condition is not lethal and is treatable, it is evident today that certain varieties of the human papillomavirus (HPV), the offending organism, are responsible for the third medical problem noted earlier, cervical intraepithelial neoplasia (CIN). It is no surprise that the first fallout noted from the sexual revolution was a tremendous upsurge in the rate of venereal disease. Now evidence from several medical centers suggests an alarming second wave of fallout; a sharp increase in the incidence of cancerous and pre-cancerous lesions of the cervix among teenagers and young women.[25]

How bad is this problem? An article which appeared in *The Medical Tribune* reporting on a survey of 2,377,000 Pap smears recognized that there is a connection between sexual activity and CIN. The risk factors noted are early onset of intercourse, arbitrarily age 18 or before, and multiple partners, arbitrarily three or more. But the reality is that the woman, who may be monogamous but who marries or has coitus with a partner who has been promiscuous before she had her loving encounter with him, bears the risk of all of his previous contacts. The studies that have been done clearly implicated the risk factors noted. The cytologist and pathologist who conducted this study were from Cancer Screening Services, a private Los

Angeles laboratory. Of all the Pap Smears analyzed, 118,081 were abnormal. This overall rate of 20 per 1,000 contrasted sharply with the rate for women under age 20. The incidence of cervical abnormalities among them was 50 per 1,000, a 2.5-fold increase in abnormal Paps in young women. The incidence figures rose steadily over the course of the review, but the sharpest jump was registered in those under 20. When the study was begun in 1974, carcinoma in situ, microscopic cancer on the mouth of the womb, was occurring at a rate of 2.5%. By 1977, three years later, the rate was 7.5%, a three-fold increase. In each and every twelve-month period there was a constant increase in the yield per 1,000 of abnormal smears in those under age 30. This was accompanied by appropriate increases in tissue diagnoses of cervical intra-epithelial neoplasia. Two other papers from this same laboratory resource re-affirm these findings.[26] The most recent of these reports on 1,632,847 women from two independent populations. The first is a group of Planned Parenthood patients, which consists of a large population of healthy young women throughout the U.S., and a second a group of private patients, also from throughout the U.S. Condylomatous lesions (HPV infections) were the most frequent cytologic abnormality in women in both the Planned Parenthood and private sector groups (prevalence rates of 18.6 to 19.0 in women between ages 15 and 19).

The epidemiology of cervical neoplasia was first studied by Gagnon, who showed that this disease was absent in a population of Canadian nuns.[27] His study was cited in an editorial entitled, "CIN or Not to Sin" in the *Journal of the American Medical Association*.[28] The author, C. M. Fengolio, M.D., writes: "Since this initial study, it is clear that cervical cancer is related to a number of identifiable risk factors, including early sexual activity, multiple pregnancies, multiple sexual partners, early age at first pregnancy or first marriage, promiscuity, and exposure to a 'high-risk' male sexual partner. When all of the epidemiologic risk factors are analysed, one finds that they have in common the degree of sexual activity engaged in by the women with cervical neoplasia or by their sexual partner(s) and that cervical cancer has many of the attributes of a venereally transmitted disease."

Anna-Barbara Moscicki and co-authors have shed additional light on the causation of this disease.[29] "The epidemiologic risk factors for CIN and STD's have appeared similar, so research has focused on the role of specific sexually transmissible agents in the pathogenesis of cervical neoplasia. Strong evidence indicates that [sic] genital human papillomavirus infection, specifically with type 16, 18, 31, or 33, is a key factor in cervical neoplastic transformation. In addition, STD's, such [as] *Chlamydia trachomatis* or herpes simplex virus infection, cigarette smoking, and oral contraceptive use may increase the vulnerability of the cervical epithelium to HPV infection and neoplasia."

DIVORCE

The final problem to be discussed is social in nature, the epidemic divorce rate in the U.S. A 1981 article in the now defunct *Washington Star* indicated that more American marriages broke up in 1979 than ever before.[30] In that year the number of divorces nearly tripled from what it was twenty years before, according to a Census Bureau report; 1.18 million divorces were granted in 1979, 4.5% more than in 1978. The figure that is most distressing is that more children were involved in broken marriages. The Bureau estimated that 1.18 million children under 18 had parents who were involved in a divorce in 1979. Clearly the family is under attack.

One would think that the decades that recorded widespread cohabitation, "trial marriages" if you will, would improve the outcome of legally sanctioned wedded bliss.   This issue was studied in an article from *Medical Aspects of Human Sexuality* that addressed the question, "Is Cohabitation a Good Method of Spouse Evaluation?"[31] Olday found that cohabitation was not a more effective screening method to make sure one marries a well-suited partner than traditional courtship.   This is in contradiction to the widely held belief that this practice improves the mate-selection process.   In fact, a more recent study by researchers from the University of Wisconsin shows that couples who cohabit before marriage are actually more likely to separate and divorce than those who head straight for the altar.[32]

THE LINCHPIN

As convincing as this data is with regard to demonstrating health and social ills, what leads one to the conclusion that these ills are related to advances in contraception?   It is of interest and very educational to study a graph of the annual gonorrhea incidence rate over time.   Figure 1 represents this data from 1920 until 1980.   The aspects of this curve which deserve particular attention are the spike that occurs in the mid-1940[s] (World War II) and the dramatic upward turn experienced in the early 1960[s].   The incidence is relatively level over the first 22 years of the graph.   For the mid- and late 1940[s] this rate doubles.   This is undoubtedly related to the separation of families and young lovers caused by World War II.   Following the global conflict the rate settles back down to near where it was until the early 1960[s].   There wasn't any war at this time, except an assault on women in the form of the pill and the IUD, which were marketed during this period.   The incidence of gonorrhea rose like a rocket to the moon. This information comes from the Center for Disease Control in Atlanta, Georgia.

Figure 2 presents the divorce rate in the U.S. over the same period.   This graph was developed by the U. S.

Department of Health and Human Services, Office of Health Research, Statistics and Technology, located in Suitland, Maryland. An analysis of the curve allows the exact same interpretation. While no cause-and-effect relationship can be proven, it would be foolhardy to believe that there is no connection between these results and the marketing of the pill and IUD. Paul Weisner, M.D., sadly summarized what is happening in our society in an article that appeared in a 1981 issue of *Urban Health*.[33] Dr. Weisner was Director of the Venereal Disease Control Division of the CDC in Atlanta when he reported "some relatively astounding statistics." He noted that the reported figures for what he called "social indicators" reached a reported incidence of one million per year for the first time between 1975 and 1979. Among these were divorces, teenage pregnancies, induced abortions, and cases of gonorrhea. Sounds like Sodom and Gomorrah revisited.

THE CURE

On a more positive note, the Medical Director for the Center for Disease Control, William Foege, M.D., made these observations in an October 1985 issue of *JAMA*: "The scientific basis for the influence of lifestyle choices on health continues to grow. Lifestyles are changing and it is probably that these changes are already reducing the role of diseases. In the coming decades, the most important determinants of health and longevity will be the personal choices made by each individual. This is both frightening for those who wish to avoid such responsibility and exciting for those who desire some control over their own destiny."[34]

Another pearl of great price was offered by Sam Nixon, M.D., a public health physician visiting Washington, D.C., as a consultant to HELP, a support group for those who suffer from herpes genitalis. He and his wife of 31 years, Elizabeth, were sitting in a coffee shop and being interviewed when he was reported to have said, "I'm just a chicken-eating Methodist, but for me the problems of sexually contagious diseases are very simply handled. The Ten Commandments not only make excellent rules to live by, but they are very good public health laws too." Also impressive was Ted Koppel when he was talking to the 1987 class of Duke graduates which included his daughter. He said, "What Moses brought down from Mt. Sinai were not the Ten Suggestions... they are Commandments. *Are*, not *were!*" (emphasis in the original).[35] Returning to a scientific source, Dr. S. L. Barron, a British gynecologist, states the author's view succinctly: "By offering contraception to girls under 16, doctors are condoning immorality and failing to point out the harmful medical effects of early sexual activity. In this context, early sexual activity should be regarded in the same way as smoking or drinking."[36]

There is little doubt that as we get smarter, we sometimes back away from logic. In 1974 the AMA House of Delegates passed a resolution which favored chastity to prevent venereal disease. The AMA developed policy-positions endorsing abstinence for single people and fidelity and continence for married couples as a means of curbing the epidemic increase in the incidence of gonorrhea.[37] In 1987 Dr. George D. Lundberg, a *JAMA* editor, got some media interest from *The Washington Post*: "The editor of *JAMA* yesterday called for an end to sexual permissiveness to stop the spread of AIDS, saying that changes in lifestyle now do far more than science to protect against a disease that threatens to be one of the great scourges of history."[38]

In 1982 the American College of Obstetricians and Gynecologists came close to this solution, but no action has been seen to date. "In cooperation with a number of national health and educational organizations, the March of Dimes, the National PTA, the American Academy of Pediatrics, The American Academy of Physicians, and the Nurses Association of the American College of

Obstetricians and Gynecologists, ACOG, made plans to explore the need for programs focused on the prevention of sexual involvement of early adolescents and its associated health and social consequences. "[39]

Earlier on Dr. Barber spoke about all of this extra-marital intercourse perhaps being a source of comfort and peace and joy to those who would partake of it. Not so, in the author's judgment. Recent reports indicate that the suicide rate per 100,000 in ages 75-84 was down 75%; in ages 45-54 down 16%; in ages 15-24 up 150%.[40] It should be easy to identify which of these age groups is the most sexually active. The gift you only give once is your virginity. "Go for No" when considering intercourse outside of marriage remains good counsel.

SUMMARY

Pope Paul VI predicted several negative societal by-products of living in a contraceptive milieu. His predictions have been experienced as witnessed by a 50% divorce-rate, rigorous enforcement of a one-child family policy by the Chinese government, and exploitation of women as sex objects by many men in society. This reality and freedom from fear of pregnancy on the part of women as a result of the advance of contraceptive technology led to the so-called sexual revolution of the 60^s, 70^s and 80^s. The author points out the synchronous relationship between the marketing of the birth control pill and intrauterine device and the beginning of the epidemic rate of divorce. This same time-line relationship is noted for the rise in the incidence of gonorrhea. Epidemic rates for teenage pregnancies, other STD's, and other medical problems as well are noted. The author maintains that a return to chastity is the only available cure for all the problems presented.[41]

NOTES

1. Pope Paul VI, *Humanae Vitae*, July 25, 1968.

2. Steven M. Mosher, "One Family, One Child: China's Brutal Birth Ban" in *The Washington Post*, Oct. 18, 1987.

3. Robert W. Kistner, M.D., *Ob. Gyn. News* v.12 n.24 (Dec. 15, 1977).

4. Rev. Randall Terry, personal communication (tape), Address to a 1990 meeting of Christian ministers.

5. The Office of Family Planning: Analysis of a Tragic Failure, Executive Report for Governor George Deukmejian and the State Legislature of the State of California, May 1986.

6. Washington Memo, Alan Guttmacher Institute, 111 Fifth Avenue, New York, NY, 10003, August 2, 1989.

7. See note 5 above.

8. Charles A. Donovan, "Teenage Pregnancy, National Policies at the Crossroads" in *Family Policy* (Nov./Dec., 1989).

9. Peggy B. Smith, Ph.D., cites "'Terrible' Mistakes in Teenage Pregnancy Prevention Efforts" in *Ob. Gyn. News* v.21 n.16 (Aug. 15-31, 1986). This secondary resource is retained because of the value of the quotation used. Phone conversation verified the fact that Dr. Smith, who is an associate professor of obstetrics and gynecology at the Baylor College of Medicine has essentially the same view today. She sent several other references: 1) Peggy B. Smith et. al., "Social and Affective Factors Associated with Adolescent Pregnancy" in *Journal of School Health* (February 1982) and 2) Peggy B. Smith, Maxine Weinman, "Adolescent Mothers and Fetal Loss, What Is Learned from Experience?" in *Psychological Reports* 55 (1984) 775-78.

10. S. K. Henshaw and J. Van Vort, "Teenage Abortion, Birth and Pregnancy Statistics: An Update" in *Family Planning Perspectives*

v.21 n.2 (March/April 1989) 85-88.

11. National Center for Health Statistics, *Advance Report of Final Natality Statistics* v.40 n.8, Supplement (Dec. 12, 1991).

12. U. S. Commission on Population Growth and the American Future (1972).

13. "VD: Gonorrhea Incidence Put at 2 Million Annually in U.S." in *Hospital Practice* (June 1981).

14. "Preventing Pregnancy and Protecting Health: A New Look at Birth Control Choices in the United States" - The Alan Guttmacher Institute (1991).

15. Hugh R. K. Barber, M.D., "Chlamydia: the New Health Menace" in *The Female Patient* 7 (1982).

16. King K. Molmes, M.D., "Rise in 10 Sexually Transmitted Diseases Linked with 'OC Era'" in *Ob. Gyn. News* (June 1, 1976) p. 18.

17. John J. Fraser, M.D., *Pediatrics* (March 1983) pp. 333 ff.

18. Preventing Pregnancy and Protecting Health: a New Look at Birth Control Choices in the United States." The Alan Guttmacher Institute, 1991.

19. F. J. Hellinger, "Forecasting the Medical Care Costs of the HIV Epidemic: 1991-1994" in Inquiry 28 *Fall 1991) 213-25.

20. J. A. Catania et al., "Prevalence of AIDS-Related Risk Factors and Condom Use in the United States" in *Science* 258 (Nov. 13, 1992) 1101-06.

21. "More Emphasis on VD Asked in Sex Education" in *Ob. Gyn. News* v.10 n.18 (Sept. 15, 1975).

22. See Charles A. Donovan, "Teenage Pregnancy: National Policies at the Crossroads" in *Family Policy* (Nov/Dec. 1989).

23. Ibid.

24. Eunice Kennedy, "Rx for Teen Pregnancy," in *The Washington Post* (March 19, 1987).

25. Hara Marano. "Teen Pap Screens Urged as Cervical Cancer Rate Rises Fast" in *Medical Tribune* (Feb. 15, 1978). This secondary resource is retained because of the tremendous volume of clinical material and the remarkable findings it yielded. This article presents details from two separate reports presented at the Pan American Cytology Congress held in Last Vegas in early 1978. A visit to the National Library of Medicine, several phone calls and a round of correspondence with the referenced laboratory failed to locate a printed reference which appeared in a scientific journal. But two other papers with similar findings were supplied by S. B. Sadeghi, M.D., Cytopathologist and Medical Director, Cancer Screening Services.

26. S. B. Sadeghi et al, "Prevalence of cervical intraepithelial neoplasia in sexually active teenagers and young adults" in *American Journal of Obstetrics and Gynecology* 148/6 (March 15, 1984) 726-99. S. B. Sadeghi et al., "Human Papillomavirus Infection" in *Acta Cytologica* 33/3 (May-June 1989) 319-22.

27. F. Gagnon, "Contributions to Study of Etiology and Prevention of Cancer of the Uterus" in *American Journal of Obstetrics and Gynecology* 60 (1950) 516-22.

28. C. M. Fenoglio, "CIN or Not to Sin" in *JAMA* 252/21 (1984) 3012-13.

29. A.-B. Moscicki et al., "Differences in Biologic Maturation, Sexual Behavior, and Sexually Transmitted Disease Between Adolescents with and without Cervical Intraepithelial Neoplasia" in Journal of Pediatrics 115/3 (Sept. 1989) 487-93.

30. "Divorces Set Record, Affect More Children" in *The Washington Star* (June 9, 1981) p.A2.

31. Paul R. Mewcomb and Gerald W. McDonald, "Cohabitation of Young Couples: Answers to Some Common Questions" in *Medical*

Aspects of Human Sexuality 15/6 (June 1981).

32. "'Trial Marriage' No Guarantee of Marital Success" in *Medical Aspects of Human Sexuality* (Jan. 1990) 21.

33. Paul Weisner, M.D., "Future of VD Controls is 'Grim,' 'Uncertain,' but 'Promising'" in *Urban Health* 10/8 (1981) 32.

34. William H. Foege, M.D., "Public Health and Preventive Medicine" in *JAMA* 254/16 (   ) 2330.

35. Ted Koppel, "Commencement Speech at Duke University on Sunday, May 10, 1987.

36. S. L. Barron, M.D. "Sexual Activity in Girls Under 16 Years of Age" in *British Journal of Obstetrics and Gynecology* 93 (   ) 787-93.

37. "AMA Delegates Favor Chastity to Prevent VD" in *Ob. Gyn. News* (Aug. 15, 1974).

38. Christine Russell, "Change in Life Style Urged to Combat AIDS" in *The Washington Post* (June 21, 1985), A2.

39. ACOG Newsletter (August 1982).

40. Gail McCrory, *The Washington Post* (1980 data).

41. The author would like to express his gratitude to the following individuals who helped in the preparation of this manuscript: Mrs. Theresa Barlow, Rev. Winthrop Brainerd, Sr. Teresa Kelley Colliton, and Mrs. Mary Shivanandan.

Figure 1

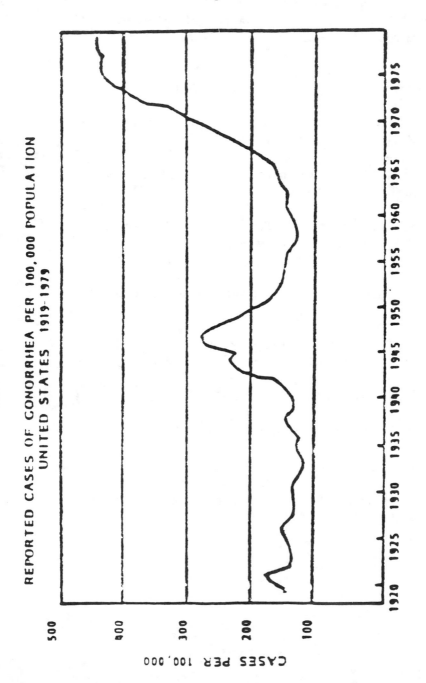

Figure 2
Divorce Rates: United States. 1920-79
Source: U.S. Dept. of Health and Human Services

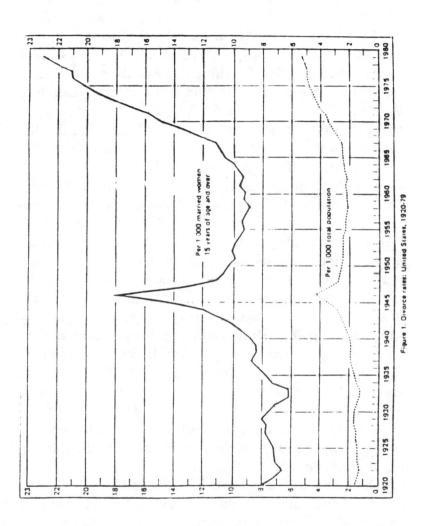

Figure 1. Divorce rates: United States, 1920-79

THE USE AND ABUSE OF THE BIBLE IN THE ABORTION DEBATE

Michael J. Gorman

Some years ago I overheard an argument between two women, one "pro-life" and the other "pro-choice," about what the Bible has to say on the subject of abortion. The pro-life woman appealed to Deuteronomy 30:19 in support of her contention that the Bible opposes abortion: "I have set before you life and death, blessing and curse; therefore choose *life*...." The pro-choice woman responded quickly, appealing to the same verse in support of her belief that the Bible promotes freedom of choice: "That's right," she said. "*'Choose* life.' There has to be choice."

In his keynote address at the University Faculty for Life conference held at Georgetown University in 1992, then-president of Catholic University William J. Byron, S.J., called for pro-life academics to begin to use Biblical language to express and undergird the pro-life position, not only in the church but also in the public arena. In 1982 I myself made a similar plea in print and have written a number of essays in response to my own appeal.[1] But very few other people, to my knowledge, have responded to these calls. One reason may be the difficulty of doing so responsibly, since the Bible does not address induced abortion directly and can be used to support very different, even contradictory, perspectives. The conversation narrated above is a vivid microcosm of the situation confronting those who might want to appeal to the Bible in the abortion debate.

This problem is not, of course, limited to the abortion debate. It was this way with slavery, and is still this way today with such issues as homosexuality. The use of the Bible in the abortion debate is, indeed, just one example of the greater problem of the use of the Bible in ethics, a topic currently receiving very lively attention in theological circles. But the role of the Bible in the abortion debate should not be of interest only to theologians. This is the case for at least two reasons.

First, biblical themes and language — such as compassion, covenant, and hospitality — have permeated many of the ethical debates in this country and in other Western countries, as the work of Robert Bellah and others has recently stressed.[2] Even in this post-Christian age, certain biblical symbols and images are still alive (or are perhaps able to be resurrected) and may have significant rhetorical and substantive power in the discussion of difficult moral issues such as abortion.

Second, the abortion debate in this country is still greatly influenced, if not governed, by religious forces that look to the Bible for moral guidance generally and moral guidance about abortion particularly. Some of the strongest pro-choice groups are religious, including many of the mainline denominations and sub-units within those denominations. Even many secular and political "pro-choice" advocates, including President Clinton, ground or justify their views by appealing to the Bible — either to its silence or to its supposed implicit or explicit pro-choice position. I am convinced that only if these groups and individuals are persuaded that a proper reading of the Bible refutes their position will they alter their stance on abortion. Fr. Byron was therefore right to signal the importance of using Biblical language in the public square.

This paper embodies some of my own reflections on the Bible in the abortion debate. The first part of the paper is an analysis and critique of selected writings of individuals and religious bodies who use the Bible in support of their position on abortion. Included in this analysis are representative statements from pro-life groups and denominations, official position papers of "mainline" pro-choice denominations, essays by pro-choice feminist theologians, and literature from the Religious Coalition for Reproductive Choice (formerly Religious Coalition for Abortions Rights). The second part of the paper proposes a process for using the Bible as a way of understanding, or reading, abortion and for evaluating other, competing readings of abortion. This process is an eclectic one, primarily utilizing commonly acknowledged biblical images and themes rather than traditional abortion proof texts. Some of these images and themes useful for the responsible development of a pro-life perspective are briefly discussed.

PROOF TEXTING: READING INTO THE BIBLE

Some readers of the Bible, perhaps even some who are aware that the Bible has nothing explicit to say on abortion, attempt, by appealing to proof texts, to find the Bible's hidden or *implicit* position on abortion. "Proof texts" are biblical texts that are lifted out of context or otherwise improperly explained in order to prove a point. Some scholars suggest that any appeal to the Bible alone on the abortion issue says nothing about the inherent meaning of the biblical text but merely supports "the ideological commitments of the text's readers."[3]

Proof texting can be done with lesser or greater sophistication. There are, for instance, innumerable printed lists of Scriptural quotations, usually from conservative Christian sources, that are supposed to answer all the important ethical questions ("Is murder wrong?"; "Is the fetus human?"; "Do women have the right to control their own bodies?"; and so on). There is also a significant body of articles devoted to detailed scholarly explanation of such texts as Exodus 21:22-25 ("When people who are fighting injure a pregnant woman so that there is a miscarriage...."). Critics of the religious pro-life movement have often accused that movement of proof texting, but, as we will see, the religious segment of the pro-choice movement uses proof texts, too.

Lurking behind most proof texting in the abortion debate is the soundness, or truthfulness, of the following syllogism (or some variant thereof):

Major premise:	The Bible prohibits the taking of innocent human life.
Minor premise:	The Bible says that the embryo/fetus is innocent human life.
Conclusion:	The Bible prohibits the taking of innocent embryonic/fetal life — abortion.

Because the major premise is relatively self-evident for most people, the minor premise is the key to this syllogism. Its truthfulness is the focus of intense debate. Sometimes this debate is quite simplistic, while at other times it is quite sophisticated, with arguments imported from philosophy about the distinction between "biological life" and "personhood."

PRO-LIFE PROOF TEXTING

The most well-known biblical texts cited in the abortion debate are quoted by pro-life people to buttress their belief that the Bible teaches that the embryo or fetus is a "life" or a "person" and that abortion, therefore, is wrong — even murder. This point of view can supposedly be found in a variety of texts, the most well-known of which are probably Exodus 21:22-25, Psalm 139, Isaiah 44:2, Jeremiah 1:5, and Luke 1 (especially vv. 31, 36, 41, 44).

In 1986, for example, the Assemblies of God approved a paper called "A Biblical Perspective on Abortion" that begins with a section on "What the Bible Says About the Unborn Child."[4] Discussing the aforementioned texts and a half-dozen others, the document concludes that the Bible views (1) the embryo/fetus as a child whose body is being formed and whose life has been planned by God; (2) pregnancy as the work of God; and (3) the child's "quality of life" (handicapping condition, etc.) as an act of divine sovereignty. A similar treatment of the texts — with even less theological sophistication — may be found in Tj. Bosgra's book *Abortion, the Bible, and the Church.*[5]

Apart from a summary of one denominational professor's exegesis of Exodus 21:22-24,[6] the Assemblies of God document — which is representative of much conservative Christian use of the Bible in the abortion debate — shows no concern for the literary or historical contexts of its proof texts. This is the most common and grievous error of those who appeal to the Bible to demonstrate the humanity or personhood of the embryo/fetus. A serious consideration of these issues is necessary for a legitimate reading of the biblical texts, none of which is as straightforward as the Assemblies of God document or Bosgra's book suggests. The questions and difficulties raised by some of these commonly used texts can be explored in some detail at this point.[7]

Exodus 21:22-25 is a legal text prescribing the penalty for causing unintentional injury or miscarriage to a pregnant woman. This text supposedly demonstrates that unborn life is fully human, equal legally and morally to that of an adult, because the penalty for the miscarriage is "life for life," understood by some interpreters to mean "life of the perpetrator for life of the fetus." Although the text is notoriously difficult, it is quite possible that the penalty of "life for life" applies only to the death of the woman and that the unborn child, legally, is more like a limb than a person. If so, then its accidental death is not a capital offense.

Such a view of the *legal* status of the fetus as a non-person became, in fact, the prevalent view later in Judaism. The fetus could not inherit property, for instance, until its head emerged from the birth canal. Legally, it was a part, an appendage, of the pregnant woman. If this view is already implicit here, how would that affect the interpretation of this text with respect to the personhood of the fetus and the penalty for abortion?

Furthermore, one has to consider the possibility that the penalty imposed in this case was motivated by a patriarchal view of women and children as possessions of their husbands and fathers. The penalty imposed would then be compensation to the husband or father. Should such a view of women and children (born or not) be normative today?

Psalm 139 is a well-known psalm that is often invoked as proof of God's creation of the unborn child and, hence, of the immorality of abortion. To be sure, this psalm does beautifully describe fetal development as the act of a loving creator. Many pro-choice readers of the Bible fail, or perhaps refuse, to deal adequately, if at all, with this psalm. On the other hand, however, many pro-life people appeal too quickly to this psalm without reading it carefully. What is the intent of the psalmist?

It has been suggested by scholars that the psalm is primarily a plea of innocence (see vv. 23-24, the last two verses), in which the words in praise of creation function as a proof of God's knowledge of the psalmist — knowledge that should confirm his innocence. To be sure, the *larger purpose* of these verses does not necessarily detract from their significance as an affirmation of God's creation of the unborn, but this is an aspect of the text that must be considered.

Furthermore, even an affirmation of divine creation of the unborn may not be sufficient, in the minds of some readers, to prohibit abortion. After all, according to the Bible, God is also the maker of plants, animals, adult humans, and every other living thing, yet all of these members of creation, according to most people, can sometimes have their life justifiably ended. Moreover, God's creation of living things other than humans is also celebrated in poetry throughout the Bible (Job, other psalms, the Sermon on the Mount), yet few people believe that it is always immoral to kill, say, a deer or a sparrow. So the argument from creation alone, even this creation text, does not completely answer the question of abortion.

Luke 1:41, 44 and related texts in the birth narratives of Luke and Matthew are sometimes said to be proof that the fetus is a "life," i.e. a person with the right to life. It is argued that the pre-natal activity of John the Baptist and Jesus demonstrate this biblical assumption. Further, in a more sophisticated vein, it is also maintained that because the Greek word *brephos*, "infant," is used to refer to the unborn Baptist, the Bible makes no distinction between a fetus and an infant. The moral conclusion drawn from this linguistic argument is that the Bible views the unborn as persons equal in status to the already-born and that abortion, therefore, is as clearly murder as is infanticide.

The logic of these particular arguments might be compelling, if they did not rest on erroneous assumptions about language. The normal use of a common word like "baby" or "infant" does not necessarily reveal anything about one's philosophical or moral convictions. Neither does attributing activity to a fetus. For instance, it is just as possible for a pro-choice woman as for a pro-life woman, seven months into a pregnancy, to say, "I just felt the baby kicking." Such a statement does not reveal either woman's view of the true "status" of the fetus, nor does it reveal either woman's position on abortion. The "pro-life" interpretation of these texts places more weight on a few words than they can bear.

Jeremiah 1:5, which says, "Before I formed you in the womb I knew you, and before you were born I consecrated you," and similar texts referring to the servant of Isaiah 40-55 (Isaiah 49:1, 5) and Paul (Galatians 1:15), are often cited as proof of fetal "life" or personhood and, hence, of abortion's status as murder. It is obvious, this position argues, that God cannot call or otherwise communicate with non-persons.

At least three serious questions about this argument can be raised, however. First, since these texts about pre-natal calling are associated only with prophets and other special servants, does this limitation mean that only prophets or other certain, specially chosen people experience a pre-natal calling and thus possess personhood before birth? Second, is the real point of these texts about the pre-natal prophetic call to affirm the prophet's personhood before birth or the divine authority of his ministry and message in his contemporary situation? Almost certainly, it is the latter. And third, taking the Jeremiah text literally as a message about personhood before birth, isn't one forced to say that personhood begins before conception, "before I formed you in the womb"?

Although one may generalize in response to the first question ("All people are similarly called"), equivocate on the second ("Divine authority is the point, but this could not be had without the pre-natal relationship with God"), and similarly hedge on the third ("Yes, but that's not the main point"), these answers are theological, not exegetical, ones. That is, they are interpretations, revisions even, of the original meanings of the texts, and they are interpretations that have little basis in the Bible. Honest readers of the Bible must at least acknowledge this, even if they feel justified in appealing to these texts as "pro-life" support.

Many other biblical passages can be, and have been, used as proof texts for a pro-life perspective. Prohibitions of murder, injunctions to choose life or to protect the oppressed, and other kinds of texts have all been used. What *all* of them, have in common, however, is that they do not refer explicitly to abortion, and they do not for the most part address the general question of the status of the fetus. Furthermore, many people appeal to these texts without seriously considering either their original significance or the consequences of reading them as commentaries on abortion and/or fetal personhood.

It does not take a professional biblical scholar — only a careful reader — to discern the error in this kind of proof texting. As the abortion debate continues, more and more people are becoming aware of the dubious proof texting methods of the pro-life movement. Indeed, former university professor and journalist-author Garry Wills makes criticisms very much like the ones I have made in his book *Under God: Religion and Politics in America.*[8] Wills has read the religious pro-life literature, noticed the same standard anti-abortion proof texts, and — with the help of a commentary or two — re-examined the biblical texts only to find *serious* problems with the pro-life interpretation. If these problems are so obvious and are clearly spelled out in a book written for the general public, what happens to the point of view that finds its authority in these misinterpreted texts? It is clearly going to be discredited, and its proponents will be edged further toward the periphery of society, out of the main arena of serious public discourse about abortion, both in religious circles and in society at large. Thus the 1974 statement of the Reformed Church in America must be taken seriously:

Scriptural passages often cited as determining the status of a human fetus as fully human, upon careful exegetical examination prove to be indecisive and not clearly supportive of an absolutist position, either affirmative or negative..., and since the above passages are receiving differing interpretations from equally faithful interpreters within the Reformed community, we believe it is not advisable to make the passages bear the weight of an absolute "yes" or "no" position.[9]

All of this is not to say, however, that these quoted but often misinterpreted texts are insignificant, or that they have no relevance to the abortion debate. Quite the contrary: the proof texts cited to defend the position that the unborn are persons and abortion is murder may be very important to the abortion debate. Furthermore, the so-called "pro-life" position may, in fact, be implied by certain biblical texts, especially if they are seen in a larger biblical context. For example, Pope John Paul II's appeal to the traditional proof texts in *The Gospel of Life* is much more convincing than most because it appears in the context of a riveting analysis, in Scriptural language, of our contemporary "culture of death."[10] In a balanced and cautious chapter of his book *The Bible and the Moral Life*, Baptist theologian Freeman Sleeper suggests that the traditional proof texts do contribute to an ethos of the sanctity of life that means a presumption for life and, without compelling reasons, against abortion.[11] However, as one maxim has it, "A text without a context is a pretext." Simply to quote texts or to read unintended meanings into biblical texts is neither honest biblical exegesis nor serious grappling with the moral issue.

PRO-CHOICE PROOF TEXTING

While the "pro-life" position is most frequently defended with biblical proof texts, the "pro-choice" perspective can also be reinforced with proof texts.

One of the most frequent issues that stimulates pro-choice proof texting is the issue of fetal personhood. Just as pro-life people appeal to the Bible to defend the full humanity or personhood of the fetus, pro-choice people can appeal to the Scriptures to deny it. One of the most thorough attempts at this is an article by Paul D. Simmons, "A Theological Response to Fundamentalism on the Abortion Issue."[12] Simmons first deals with Exodus 21:22-25, concluding, with the majority of scholars, that "the woman has been granted full standing as a person under the covenant, while the fetus has only relative standing, certainly inferior to that of the woman."[13] He admits, however, that this text has limited meaning for the abortion debate since the fetal death is accidental.

Simmons goes on, however, to discuss four texts that supposedly reveal the biblical understanding of "personhood": Genesis 2:7 ("dust of the ground... breath of life... living soul"), which demonstrates that a human being is a complex organism of animated flesh; Genesis 1:26-28 ("in the image of God"), which defines a human being as one with God-like powers and abilities; Genesis 3:22 ("has become like one of us, to know good and evil"), which shows that a person is a moral decision-maker; and 1 Peter 2:9 (the "priesthood" of all believers), which shows that a "full person is one with direct access to God and the ability and responsibility to know God's will."[14] The conclusion Simmons draws about the abortion issue, obviously, is that only the woman involved, not the fetus, is a person (the fetus being a potential person).

What Simmons does not say, but should admit, is that such a definition of personhood excludes not only the fetus, but also infants until at least the age of six months, maybe even two years; the severely mentally handicapped; many elderly people with Alzheimer's disease; and probably other members of the human species. It is not at all clear, biblically or otherwise, that these members of the human family should be considered non-persons. But if the criteria Simmons proposes are valid, they must be applied indiscriminately. This situation demonstrates the problems inherent in constructing a full-blown anthropology from a small selection of Scriptural texts.

A similar proof-texting approach to anthropology is found in another pamphlet from the Religious Coalition for Reproductive Choice, "Is the Fetus a Person — According to the Bible?" by Roy Bowen Ward.[15] Appealing primarily to Genesis 2:7 and a handful of obscure texts, Ward contends that the biblical notion of a "person" (Hebrew *nephesh*, often translated "soul" or "life" or "being") is of a *breathing* being and thus excludes the fetus. There are numerous flaws in Ward's argument, but here it is important only to re-emphasize the problem of trying to develop a full anthropology from a few texts of Scripture.

It is especially odd that Ward (and others who appeal to Genesis 2:7 to disprove fetal personhood) fails to realize that a creation story in which human beings appear instantaneously as adults is hardly sufficient to rule out the personhood of non-adults such as adolescents, children, infants, and fetuses.[16]

Other pro-choice advocates have also developed arguments about the biblical definition of personhood, or being in the image of God, that exclude the fetus. Many such arguments take their clue from contemporary theological and philosophical definitions of personhood that emphasize the centrality of *relationships* to human personhood. The basic contention is that the embryo or fetus, being incapable of forming and maintaining human relationships, does not possess personhood. Once again, the principle of logical consistency requires that such a criterion be applied indiscriminately, and once again significant numbers of members of the human family must be labelled non-persons. Is this what readers of the Bible want to be forced to do?

Another issue for which proof texting emerges from the pro-choice side is the importance of "choice" to human and Christian freedom. Some years ago I was invited to present the pro-life perspective at a large denominational conference bringing together pro-choice and pro-life groups for dialogue.[17] The supposedly neutral keynoter, a denominational theologian and seminary president, chose Acts 15 as the text for his remarks. That chapter of Acts relates the controversy in the early church between those who wished Gentile converts to be circumcised and those who did not. The chief lesson to be learned from the passage, according to the speaker, was the principle enunciated by Saint Paul, who opposed requiring circumcision: that there is "no act obligatory for salvation; obligation contradicts freedom in Christ."

Although the keynoter's remarks were intended to initiate

dialogue and reconciliation, and they did not *explicitly*
support either the pro-choice or pro-life side, in a subtle
but powerful way they reinforced the pro-choice perspective and effectively prejudiced conference participants
toward the pro-choice point of view as the *biblical* point of
view. By appealing to a biblical text that condemned a
particular religious/moral obligation and thus, supposedly,
promoted an almost absolute moral freedom, the speaker
implied that requiring *any* religious or moral obligation
from Christians was and is contrary to the gospel. This
implication is suspect, first of all, as a legitimate interpretation of the notion of freedom that Paul embraced and
preached. It is further suspect as a faithful reading of
Acts, because the early church did in fact, according to
Acts, place certain requirements on all Christians, Gentiles
as well as Jews (see Acts 15:20,29 on abstention from
idols, unchastity, etc.). Thus it did not promote an
absolute freedom without obligation.

The implicit comparison of abortion to circumcision is
also questionable. According to the narrative in Acts,
circumcision, unlike unchastity or idolatry, is neither
inherently good or evil, so it cannot be absolutized in any
way.[18] It is not at all clear, however, that abortion is more
like circumcision than it is like idolatry. In fact, early
Jewish and Christian opinion was just as united in
opposition to abortion as to idolatry.[19] All in all, the
association of the circumcision controversy with the
abortion controversy neglects the fuller context of the story
in Acts and does not deal adequately with the moral
difference between circumcision and abortion. In short,
this theologian's remarks represented a subtle, elaborate,
but nonetheless inappropriate proof texting.[20]

Other biblical texts that refer, either explicitly or
implicitly, to "choice," "freedom," and similar ideas, have
also been quoted as proof texts for the pro-choice position.
For instance, the "Choose life" text from Deuteronomy

30:19 was quoted by the woman in the episode narrated at the beginning of this chapter. The 1988 resolution of the American Baptist Churches in the U.S.A.[21] says that while many of its members derive their perspective on abortion from the traditional anti-abortion proof texts, many others appeal to the "biblical principles of compassion and justice... and freedom of will."[22] The document includes relevant supporting texts for these themes, including John 16:13 (which promises the Spirit's guidance into all truth) and Romans 14:4-5, 10-13 (against judgmentalism) to justify freedom of choice.[23] The document fails, however, to mention the issue addressed in Romans — differences about dietary and calendar observance — and thus fails to distinguish between that kind of issue and the much more morally serious issue of abortion.

According to feminist lay theologian Virginia Ramey Molenkott, writing in an essay for the Religious Coalition for Abortion Rights [now Reproductive Choice], a New Testament text that supports freedom of procreative choice, and thus the right to abortion, is the well-known Christ-hymn in Philippians 2. Molenkott's contention throughout the essay is that coercion, especially to the Christ-like self-sacrificial life of motherhood, is always wrong, and that humans should follow the Creator's example in giving free choice to women, even if they think or know that the women will choose wrongly.[24] Writes Molenkott:

It is self-serving and exploitative for people of power to teach powerless people — those trapped in poverty or marginalization — that they ought to lay down any little power they have achieved in imitation of Christ's self-emptying power. According to Philippians 2, Jesus the Christ chose servanthood from a position of tremendous power, laying aside the very form of God in order to die the death of a slave. The lesson for Christians is that Christlike servanthood can only be *chosen* by people who have the power to choose. To deny procreative choice to women is to deny them the opportunity to choose Christlike servanthood — or, conversely, to recognize if and when for various reasons they cannot make the necessary covenant of caring.[25]

While Molenkott's criticism of urging powerless people to be self-sacrificial has some force — both church and society should be servants for, not oppressors of, such people — her use of Philippians 2 is unjustified. While the hymn certainly emphasizes the free choice Christ made to humble himself in the interest of others, the accent falls not on his power to choose but on his self-humbling. Indeed, power is redefined in this text as an act of serving. Moreover, Paul uses this hymn to exhort his readers not to remember the importance of the *option* to serve — or not to serve, if unable — but to practice mutual service within the fellowship in Christ, where each looks out for the needs of the other and the "powerless" are thereby empowered, both by serving and by being served. Citing a text like this in support of procreative choice is misreading the text entirely, as well as avoiding the crucial moral issue — not merely choice, but *what is chosen* (the act itself).[26]

Indeed, the notion of "freedom" advocated by pro-choice people appealing to the texts cited above seems quite distant from other Scriptural texts — to which they do not, conveniently, appeal.   There is, for example, Paul's injunction "not to let freedom become an excuse for the flesh" (Galatians), as well as other texts that connect human freedom to obeying God and serving other people. Scripture, above all, offers no justification for a belief in absolute liberty, in which freedom is defined as unre-strained choice and worshipped as the ultimate goal. With that view, whether consciously or unconsciously, people avoid the real issues in an ethical question, since anything can be defended in the name of unrestricted choice and individual conscience — slavery, domestic violence, rape, apartheid.   Those who wish to claim biblical texts of "freedom" to support their pro-choice convictions must examine those texts much more carefully.

Other proof texts have also been adduced by pro-choice people.   For example, one biblical scholar circulated a paper within his denomination that appealed to Jesus' words in John 10:10, "I have come to bring you life, life in all its fullness," as proof that the "quality" of life is what matters, and if abortion improves that quality, it serves the purposes of God for human life.

THE FAILURE OF PROOF TEXTING

It should be clear from the preceding discussion that "proof texting" can be done by people on both sides of the abortion debate, though it has traditionally been a weapon of the pro-life movement. This, it must be admitted, is due at least in part to the fact that there are more biblical texts that, at least superficially, support the pro-life perspective. There are texts about pre-natal creation and pre-natal calls, prohibitions of murder, calls to help the oppressed, and so on. Pro-choice people are confined largely to scattered, supposedly anthropological texts, the theme of freedom or choice, and perhaps also texts about the "quality of life."

For both sides, however, the pursuit of proof texts no doubt arises from the Bible's silence on abortion and the need — or at least the desire — to hear what the Bible says about what it doesn't speak about and thus to give divine sanction to a particular perspective. In so doing, both sides have been guilty of irresponsible handling of the biblical texts and, to varying degrees, of failure to deal adequately with the act of abortion. Readers of the Bible who wish to use the Bible to help address the abortion question must do so by reading the Bible carefully, not sloppily or ideologically, combined with a serious commitment to grappling with the complex moral issues that our contemporary situation presents. As Freeman Sleeper notes in his book *The Bible and the Moral Life*, "the abortion issue *demonstrates clearly the failure of a proof texting approach to Scripture*" (emphasis his).[27]

GIVING UP ON THE BIBLE

Perhaps in part as a reaction to those who have been guilty of reading into the Bible, some people have given up any hope of finding guidance on abortion from the Bible. Some have (mistakenly) assumed that abortion was unknown in biblical times. Believing that the Bible cannot be forced to address issues that did not exist (so they think) at the time of its writing, they look elsewhere. Others have assumed that the Bible's silence on abortion leaves Christians free to develop their own perspective, independent of biblical guidance, much like they form opinions about other matters on which the Bible is silent, both weighty and trivial, in daily life. Both groups turn, when they feel the need for guidance or assistance, to other religious sources — tradition, experience, reason, clergy, the community — and, perhaps just as frequently, to secular authorities such as philosophers, legal experts, newspaper and magazine essayists, and public opinion.

Still others who have heard the proof texting arguments of the pro-choice or pro-life sides have gone back to the Bible to examine the texts for themselves. An admirably thorough job of this was done a decade ago by Mark Olson, in *The Other Side*.[28] Looking especially at the issue of fetal personhood, Olson concluded that the biblical evidence was inconclusive. Preferring, however, to err on the side of caution, he decided that since the Bible spoke no definitive word that the fetus is *not* a person, it was preferable to think it might be and that abortion should not be championed by Christians.

Olson's cautious approach is commendable. Those who finally give up on the Bible, however, fail to recognize the way the Bible *has* functioned and *should* function in communities of faith. Regarding the past, these people forget that faithful readers of the Scriptures — indeed, even those who actually *wrote* the Scriptures — have always re-appropriated old texts and stories, old themes and truths, for new situations. As for the present, those who think the Bible has nothing to say on abortion view the Bible primarily as a collection of rules or principles with a limited scope of applications, rather than as a determinative revelation or narrative that shapes one's total identity. That is, they neglect the perspective-shaping and character-forming roles of the Bible, both for individuals and communities, that function even when the Bible does not speak directly about the topic at hand.

CRITICIZING AND THUS AVOIDING THE BIBLE

Another approach to the abortion issue criticizes the use of the Bible and avoids it. This approach is reactionary and deliberate, born not out of frustration about the Bible's silence but out of opposition to biblical "tyranny," or "biblicism." Those who choose this approach include self-proclaimed practicing Christians and theologians, but they believe that too many people read the Bible uncritically, without engaging in serious moral reflection, as the final authority on matters of ethics. These people are not simply critical of proof texting — though that, of course, infuriates them — but of giving the Bible an authority greater than one's own ethical thinking and greater than alternative ethical perspectives.

Thus, for example, feminist ethicist Beverly Wildung Harrison, in her widely read book *Our Right to Choose*, is critical not only of how pro-life people interpret the metaphorical theology of Psalm 139 and quote it to prove fetal personhood, but — more importantly — of how they "manipulate"

its [Psalm 139's] status as scripture to obviate any contemporary moral reconsiderations of the nature of fetal life....[,] substitute religious authority for moral reasoning.... [and] falsely portray the past as inherently morally superior to the present by evading the moral inadequacies reflected in scripture."[29]

Harrison continues:

> Biblicists refuse to face the fact that the ancient moral ethos reflected in scripture is not always noble by our moral standards and has been superseded by a more adequate morality at some stages in later human history.... [With respect to abortion,] [a]s in many other matters, scripture at best addresses analogous, but never identical, issues. While we are always well advised to probe these analogies for genuine correspondence, we must remember that we are never justified in simply deducing standards of moral conduct from scripture. On the contrary, we are responsible for bringing biblical norms into dialogue with new circumstances and weighing the relevance of other moral orientations to the development of our value systems.[30]

Harrison's contention, fundamentally, is that although "scripture" contains "positive elements of moral wisdom" and "positive theological values and moral principles... that may have continuing claims to make on us," there are also "distortions" and "moral inadequacies," specifically those that are oppressive to women and represent them as the property of males.[31] She therefore outlines a plan of interpretation for moral issues that includes finding "analogous issues" addressed in the Bible, probing them for genuine correspondence, identifying the values and principles enunciated in the Bible, and evaluating them in light of contemporary value systems. On the abortion issue, this approach means that the biblical theme of God's love for human beings before birth and even conception, which Harrison acknowledges,[32] cannot automatically determine one's view of fetal life or of abortion, since the theme may actually represent an oppressive view of women. Furthermore, even if this theme did not reflect such a view of women but did imply the full personhood of the fetus, and thus the immorality of abortion, Harrison's approach permits a contemporary value such as "women's rights to reproductive freedom" to overrule the biblical theme and its implicit norm.

This position must not be dismissed out of hand.

Harrison, as well as others who share a similar point of view, often correctly perceive the poor handling of the Bible by many of its most loyal readers — of all theological persuasions — and recognize the superficial moral thinking that often accompanies it. But Harrison commits two closely related, grave errors: she forbids the biblical message to challenge the contemporary values that she brings to the text, and she fails in actual practice to follow through on her own proposal to search and use the Bible critically to address the abortion issue.

In rejecting biblical authority, Harrison replaces it with a new authority, the principle of procreative choice, to which all points of view, biblical or otherwise, must now submit. This principle grows out of a more basic view of freedom, power, co-creativity with God, and self-determination as the essential elements of a feminist spirituality and ethic.[33] While there are some elements of profound insight in Harrison's work, one cannot help but suspect that its independent spirit is prompted not only by anger at male abuse of the Bible but also by fear that the Bible, given a dynamic and fresh hearing, liberated from the chains of both chauvinist and feminist ideology, might actually challenge some of the very presuppositions on which her own ideology is constructed. More importantly, it might threaten the moral perspectives and practices to which these presuppositions lead. Harrison's work exemplifies a new "ism" that can be just as rigid, authoritarian, and close-minded as the "biblicism" it rejects.

The second error Harrison commits is her failure to search the Scripture for issues analogous to the issues involved in the abortion debate. After summarily dismissing Exodus 21:22-24 and Psalm 139 as irrelevant to the debate,[34] she proceeds to consider no other biblical text or theme that might correspond to the problem of abortion. The few references to the Bible in her book are passing remarks about such things as the call of the prophets and

Jesus to "serious immersion in real, concrete suffering. "[35]
Her resources and authorities for discussing the issues of
women's rights, fetal personhood, and abortion are other
feminist theologians, secular philosophers, and legal
experts who support *Roe v Wade* — but not the Bible.

Neither deliberately avoiding the Bible in reaction to
proof texting (or in fear of hearing it afresh), nor giving up
on it because of its lack of explicit statements on abortion,
is the most appropriate course of action for those who look
to the Bible for moral guidance. Another approach, which
will allow the Bible to speak to an issue about which it is
silent, must be sought.

THE THEMATIC APPROACH

Unable to accept the proof texting methodology employed
by others, yet unwilling to forsake (or reject) the Bible
completely as a source of guidance on the abortion
question, many readers of the Bible have chosen another
way, a *via media*. They seek to look to the Bible in the
abortion debate by applying more general ethical texts or
biblical themes to the issue. Both pro-choice and pro-life
people have taken this route.

Pro-choice people have primarily focused on the biblical
theme of liberation or freedom, as do their counterparts
who are prone to citing and explaining texts more
specifically. For example, the 1976 study document of the
United Presbyterian church (now part of the PCUSA —
Presbyterian Church in the U.S.A.) found the Scriptural
basis for its pro-choice stance in the teaching of Jesus and
Paul on human freedom:

In several instances [in the gospels] Jesus specifically recognized
women as responsible persons, capable of ethical decisions in the light
of the truth of the good news.... The Sermon on the Mount indicates
that Jesus did not consider any of the commandments absolute in
themselves. Instead he urged persons to review their attitudes and that
attitudes were of sometimes greater significance than the actual

conformity to the law.... [I]n the New Testament, particularly Paul, the covenant is reinterpreted as participation in Christ — as members of Christ's body — as over against being under the law (the Old Testament view of covenant). Christ serves as the model: his ministry, behavior, and teachings are ways in which Christians should model themselves in their decision-making.... Both of these views [Old and New Testament] of the image of God in human beings call men and women to exercise their full capacity for ethical decisions even while subject to the limitations of human error and limitation.... Because the Bible has no direct reference to elective abortion, Christians cannot turn to Scripture for immediate counsel in decision-making regarding problem pregnancies. However, the Bible — particularly the ministry of Jesus — can undergird our freedom, and responsibility as human beings, as well as the ministry of the church and the understanding of God for the human situation. This reinforces the possibility that responsible decisions can be made by women facing problem pregnancies.[36]

The progression of thought is clear: Jesus taught and lived the truth that women are responsible decision-makers; no law is absolute; and freedom to choose is the meaning of being in the image of God. The implicit conclusion, of course, is that freedom to choose abortion is the will of God and Jesus.

The document spells this out further in stating its position vis-à-vis "anti-choice groups" who maintain the "traditional absolutist position"[37] that affirms fetal personhood and right to life as an inalienable right granted by the Creator. Rather, says the paper, a "divine [meaning, one must suppose, attested in Scripture] self-revelation discloses that that the primary aim of Divine Intention is to maximize human choices — so as to endure risk and surmount tragedy. Whenever and wherever human freedom to choose between alternatives is prohibited — where responsibility for such choices is abdicated through cowardice or usurped by external authority-figures — there the Divine Intention is frustrated and violated."[38]

The problem with this line of interpretation of the supposedly biblical theme of freedom is that it sounds much more like certain kinds of modern, secular political or ethical theory than biblical teaching. There is no hint of the self-giving nature of freedom emphasized by both Jesus and Paul, in which one becomes free by "enslaving" oneself in service to God and others. Furthermore, as noted above in the discussion of freedom proof texts, this interpretation of freedom as absolute makes it logically impossible to pronounce any choice or any act — except perhaps the restriction of another's freedom — contrary to the will of God. It is highly unlikely that anyone actually believes in, or wishes to live with, that kind of total moral and social anarchy.

Another biblical theme popular among pro-choice people is "dominion," or "stewardship of the creation." In 1983 the PCUSA issued a document containing two lengthy papers on medical ethics, the latter paper entitled "Covenant and Creation: Theological Reflections on Contraception and Abortion."[39] This paper began by citing and commenting on Psalm 8, which includes the following lines about humanity's "dominion" over the earth: "Thou hast made him [man] little less than God, and dost crown him with glory and honor. Thou hast given him dominion over the works of thy hands." Referring also to Genesis 1:28 to explain dominion as responsibility, the paper asserts that there is a difference between domination and dominion, "power for its own sake" versus "care for that which God has made."[40] Claiming "profound respect for human life,"[41] the paper treats contraception and abortion as an "aspect of our care for creation,"[42] "a question of [the] stewardship of life,"[43] such that abortion can be an act of faithful dominion and stewardship. The paper claims that the decision "to terminate a pregnancy is a question of one's covenant responsibility to accept the limits of human resources." Furthermore, because limiting population growth is "generally understood as caring for the next generation," when a pregnant woman judges that it would be irresponsible to bring a child into the world given the limitations of her situation, this paper [affirms] that it can be an act of faithfulness before God to take responsibility for intervening in the natural process of pregnancy by terminating it.[44]

According to the paper, the difference between abortion, which is frequently a responsible act of stewardship, and murder, which is a violation of the sixth commandment, corresponds to the difference between dominion and domination noted above; abortion can be a responsible choice because a woman "takes seriously the needs of a human child" and, exercising dominion rather than domination, acts responsibly not only for herself but "for the whole of nature insofar as [she is] empowered to direct its design."[45]

This emphasis on the biblical theme of dominion, or responsibility, is connected to the theme of freedom:

Affirming human responsibility for procreative processes is an affirmation of human freedom. The freedom to do what one judges most appropriate in an abortion decision is qualified by the fact that the purpose of such decisions is the responsible exercise of stewardship. Even when we misuse our freedom, God's forgiving grace is offered.[46]

Thus, according to the paper, the Presbyterian position on abortion brings together the Old Testament theme of responsibility and the New Testament theme of freedom, keeping in line with the best of the Calvinist tradition.[47]

The problems inherent in using the biblical theme of "stewardship" or "dominion" as justification for abortion are very serious ones. In the first place, it is striking how the one thing over which humanity is *not* given dominion in the Bible is human life. The animal kingdom, the earth and its resources, yes. Human life, no. Moreover, doing what the Bible did *not* do — placing human life under the dominion of humans — inevitably leads to domination: oppression, murder, genocide. History is nothing if not a testament to this obvious truth. Furthermore, carried to its logical conclusion, the notion of the "stewardship of [human] life" as a function of the "stewardship of resources" could lead to all sorts of future immoralities: refusing to feed a certain segment of the population of a poor country, or even deliberately killing off a percentage of the population, all justified by appealing to the "biblical doctrine" of the stewardship of human life.

What is also lacking in all of the typical pro-choice thematic approaches to the Bible is serious consideration of the biblical texts and themes that might lead to a different conclusion. Themes like God's creation of people in the womb, the gift of children, and other "traditional" challenges to a pro-choice perspective are simply dismissed as antiquarian theological nonsense that is unacceptable to Christians in the modern scientific age who live in a world of diminishing resources.[48]

Among those who have come to oppose abortion but do not find specific abortion-related texts in the Bible, several biblical themes have been suggested as support for their case. Recently, for instance, the United Methodist Taskforce on Abortion and Sexuality, an unofficial band of lay people, pastors, and theologians, issued the *Durham Declaration*.[49] This document, addressed to all United Methodists, focuses on two biblical (especially New Testament) themes — "Our bodies are not our own" and "Welcome the children" — as ethical and pastoral responses to abortion. The choice of these two themes suggests an attempt to address what is perceived to be the fundamental cultural belief behind abortion itself — the right to do as one pleases with one's body — and the responsibility of the Christian church to welcome unwanted children.[50]

The advantages of this approach, and this particular choice of themes, are several: the document refrains from proof texting, moves beyond condemnation to analysis and prescription, calls the church to action, and soft-pedals the issue of fetal personhood. But critics will charge that these strengths are weaknesses: some will say that, Paul's dictum notwithstanding, the right to use one's body as one wishes is fundamental to Christian and democratic freedom, while others will insist that until the issue of fetal personhood is addressed and resolved systematically, the call to welcome unwanted children carries little weight.[51]

Despite the very different themes chosen by pro-choice and pro-life advocates, it should be clear that appealing to broader biblical themes has more promise, more integrity, than simply calling up proof texts. There are many examples today of people addressing other contemporary problems — for instance, suicide — from this kind of thematic approach. They share the conviction that the Bible is capable of speaking *to* issues even when it does not speak *about* them. This method is less likely to read into the text something not there because it is seeking to *re-appropriate* themes for a new day, a new set of problems.

But the problem, of course, especially in the abortion debate, is how to decide which themes and which other kinds of texts — narratives, laws, etc. — to choose. Is there anything that makes "pro-choice" themes any more or less appropriate than "pro-life" themes? In the end, it may well be that our reading of abortion in light of the Bible depends on how we read the Bible more generally. Does it contain a message best characterized as the "gospel of life," the "gospel of choice," or some combination of these?

TOWARD A NEW APPROACH

We have examined several examples of misuse of the Bible in the abortion debate, all of which can be labelled eisegesis, proof texting, or ideologically governed reading. I would like to suggest that most, if not all, of these examples have a common deficiency. They attempt to read the Bible through the lens of abortion. Abortion, in theory or experience, is the starting point. From that starting point, one begins a search through the Bible for a perspective on abortion. Abortion — however that is understood or "named" — becomes the hermeneutical key to the interpretation of certain biblical themes and texts. This not only leads to distortion of the text to make it support one's previously held conviction, but also — and perhaps more importantly — to confirmation of one's understanding of abortion without any kind of re-examination.

I would like to suggest that the process be reversed, that our starting point become Scripture, that Scripture become the lens through which we view and read abortion. In a recent article entitled "Jesus and Ethics," New Testament scholar Pheme Perkins claims that in doing Christian ethics by using biblical materials, we ought to "seek to inculturate the inherited [biblical] images [of God and human life] by *reading our own times in their light*" (emphasis mine).[52] Applied to abortion, this means that we must seek to "inculturate," or re-appropriate, the image-rich words of Jesus and the biblical writers by reading, or interpreting, abortion in light of those image-rich words. We are to read Scripture, through its narratives, themes, and images, as a means of reading abortion. Ethicists such as Stanley Hauerwas have already been advocating and doing precisely this when considering abortion.[53]

I recognize, of course, that a hermeneutical circle exists between the text and the contemporary issues and situation we wish to address. Nevertheless, if we must choose a starting point, a place that will be more definitive than any other, it must be Scripture rather than the contemporary situation.

Several implications follow from the fundamental method I have suggested.

First, this approach will take the historical-critical method seriously but will see the method as its servant, not its master. The appeal to Scripture for moral wisdom assumes that it has "an ability to transcend the particularities of time and culture."[54] Careful exegesis protects us from misusing Scripture, but it must also free us to use it creatively. As Richard Hays says, "[t]he task of hermeneutical appropriation requires an *integrative act of the imagination*."[55] *Second*, this approach will be textually and thematically broad. Many different themes and images from Scripture must be employed to "read" abortion, not just the traditional pro-life or pro-choice proof texts. It will be particularly important to appeal to commonly acknowledged themes, images, and narratives. In reading the various ethics within the Bible, and in doing ethics with the Bible, we need to discern and then utilize a "cluster of master images to govern our construal of New Testament [or, I would add, biblical] ethics."[56] *Third*, the resulting reading of abortion will be holistic. Because abortion will not be interpreted by one, narrow set of texts, it will be read and addressed within a more comprehensive Christian ethic rooted in a wide variety of biblical images and themes.

Fourth, this approach actively engages any and all understandings, or readings, of abortion in order to re-read these readings in the light of Scripture. These contemporary readings of abortion include abortion as murder, the shedding of innocent blood, termination of pregnancy, an exercise of freedom, a rite of passage, a tragic necessity, an act of desperation, a result of poverty. As a matter of procedural principle, no reading of abortion is excluded from consideration, and any reading may prove partially appropriate and partially inappropriate in the light of Scripture. *Fifth,* this approach will be prophetic, or critical, vis-à-vis status-quo readings of abortion. Because this approach takes Scripture, not abortion, as its normative starting point, all readings of abortion — those that are labelled pro-life, pro-choice, and anything else — are subject to intense scrutiny. Abortion must be, so to speak, *deconstructed and then reconstructed.*

Finally, this approach assumes a community of moral learners who take Scripture seriously as their hermeneutical key to reading abortion and to ordering their lives in accord with that reading.

WHERE DO WE GO FROM HERE?

The approach to reading Scripture as a reading of abortion, and as a reading of competing readings of abortion, that I have outlined will not provide easy answers to the complex moral and social problem that is abortion. Nevertheless, there are several commonly acknowledged themes, narratives, and images in Scripture that have significant potential for becoming a "cluster of master images" (Hays) to undergird and express a responsible pro-life perspective. I have chosen the biblical number of seven, appropriately, to discuss briefly.

1. *Shalom*. One of the most promising biblical themes or images is captured in the Hebrew word *shalom*. This image figures significantly in contemporary theological ethics on a host of topics. The word *shalom* connotes wholeness and the restoration of broken relationships; it is often described as eschatological peace and justice for all creation and is symbolized in the image of the lion and lamb lying down together. Since the time of the New Testament, Christians have believed that the Hebrew vision of *shalom* is inaugurated by Jesus and continued in the ministry of the church in the world.

In a 1986 essay, "*Shalom* and the Unborn," I outline various dimensions of the biblical vision and their relevance to the abortion issue.[57] *Shalom* means peace, justice for the defenseless, security for all, and violence toward none. It is thus a comprehensive image and central to a consistent ethic of life. *Shalom* means that we protect and provide for *all* human life, both born and unborn. *Shalom* creates a secure place for women and children in need.

2. *Covenant.* Another promising theme is that of covenant. Covenant means a binding relationship of love and faithfulness, expressed in the Hebrew word *hesed*. Relationships of *hesed* are the norm in Scripture and underlie many texts even when the word "covenant" (*berit*) is absent. The notion of covenant figures not only in the Judeo-Christian tradition but also in the tradition of American social and legal thought. It has the potential to describe the many personal and societal relationships that are jeopardized by abortion and how covenant faithfulness can be actualized or restored through acts of mercy, justice, and sacrifice.

3. *The feminine metaphors and similes for God.* In my 1994 University Faculty for Life conference paper, "Abortion and the Biblical Metaphor of God as Mother,"[58] I suggest that feminine images of God, found largely in the Hebrew Bible, constitute a hermeneutical circle of theological affirmations about God and corresponding moral demands on people. If God, as feminist theologians have especially reminded us, is like a birthing and nursing mother, full of life-giving power and eternally compassionate, then abortion, no less than infanticide, betrays the character of God. Moreover, it is the responsibility of the faith community to act on God's behalf to provide the care and compassion needed by child and mother.

4. *Freedom/liberation.* According to the Hebrew Bible, the people of Israel were liberated from slavery into a relationship of covenant love and faithfulness with their liberating God. In the New Testament, Christians are described as liberated from the power of sin to worship

God by living for Christ and others in the power of the Spirit.

The scriptural vision of freedom, as Pope John Paul II has frequently pointed out,[59] is a prophetic critique of our culture's captivity to hedonistic autonomy, whether of the right or of the left. The scriptural vision of freedom is one of personal and communal responsibility for others as the "horizontal" expression of one's "vertical" love of God. Freedom is thus freedom *for*, not merely freedom *from*. "Freedom to choose," in the scriptural vision, is, paradoxically, an interdependent freedom, a freedom to choose love that is dependent on the love of God channelled through the loving actions of other human beings. "Freedom to choose abortion" is thus a contradiction in terms; freedom to "choose life," on the other hand, can be exercised only with community support. A Christian vision of freedom does not compel a woman to face an unplanned pregnancy alone; rather, it allows for the kind of love in community that liberates, that allows a crisis to be survived and new life to be birthed and nurtured.

5. *Hospitality, including welcoming children.* The mandate of hospitality to the stranger, widow, and orphan permeates the Hebrew Bible and New Testament. Hospitality was not only an essential mark of ancient middle Eastern culture; it was perceived as a divine command. Hospitality to those afflicted by the temptations, and possible effects, of abortion is no less an implicit mandate of the biblical texts.

The well-known gospel text, "Let the little children come to me and forbid them not, for of such is the kingdom of heaven," is an extension of the hospitality mandate to those who were, and are, often marginalized. This text challenges us in many ways. What are the attitudes and structures we have created — not just individually but corporately — that compel people to turn away from the gift of children? What personal and corporate revisioning and restructuring are necessary to discourage abortion and other impediments to the life and welfare of children?

6. *The Good Samaritan.* This well-known parable begins with the ordinary human question "Who is my neighbor?" and ends with the prophetic question "Who was a neighbor to the person in need?" This transformation suggests that the old question of "personhood" (or "neighbor-hood"), construed as the establishment of criteria for membership in the human community, is the wrong question. The text of the parable suggests that even those who might not be considered fully alive or human according to human perception or status-quo biological and social criteria, are in fact worthy of our compassion.

The right question, then, is how I can *become* a neighbor, on the assumption that membership in the human community is inclusive rather than exclusive and therefore that the other — specifically anyone in danger or need — is *already* a neighbor. Thus the issue of "personhood" is transformed from a philosophical or social construct into a moral imperative. It is not the personhood of the fetus that is ultimately at issue or at stake, but rather the personhood of the person or persons who refuse to acknowledge and appropriately respond to this member of the human community.

7. *"Choose life."* It may be appropriate to conclude this essay by returning to the text from Deuteronomy 30:19 with which the paper opened: "Choose life." Ultimately, our reading of Scripture as a reading of abortion and of competing readings of abortion may hang on the issue raised by this text. Does Scripture offer a message that is best characterized as the "gospel of life" or the "gospel of choice"?

As a Protestant theologian, I would agree wholeheartedly with Pope John Paul II, that the fundamental posture of

Scripture is toward life rather than choice. Referring to Moses's invitation in Deut. 30:19, the pope says that in the present "enormous and dramatic clash between good and evil, death and life, the 'culture of death' and the 'culture of life,' we have the inescapable responsibility of *choosing to be unconditionally pro-life*" [emphasis his].[60] This is not to deny human freedom but rather to suggest that human freedom is ultimately slavery unless directed toward the way of blessing, of life, of God.

The Jewish tradition of the "two ways," one of death and curse, the other of life and blessing, which was born in this text from Deuteronomy, was taken over by the first Christians.   When it was so, they specifically included abortion and infanticide as part of the way of death that Christians had abandoned and must continue to abandon. This, it seems to me, captures the heart of the moral vision of Scripture when it comes to the issue of abortion. This, in other words, is how Scripture "reads" abortion. But the expression of that vision, the embodiment of that reading, must be done creatively and consistently by those who appeal to Scripture.[61]

NOTES

1. *Abortion and the Early Church: Christian, Jewish, and Pagan Attitudes in the Greco-Roman World* (Downers Grove, IL and Mahwah, NJ: Paulist, 1982) 91-101; "*Shalom* and the Unborn" in *Transformation* 3/1 (1986) 26-33; "Ahead to Our Past: Abortion and Christian Texts" in Paul Stallsworth, ed., *The Church and Abortion: In Search of New Ground for Response* (Nashville: Abingdon, 1993) 25-43; "Abortion and the Biblical Metaphor of God as Mother" in Joseph W. Koterski, ed. *Life and Learning IV: Proceedings of the Fourth University Faculty for Life Conference, June 1994* (Washington, DC: University Faculty for Life, 1995) 253-270.

2. See Robert N. Bellah et al., *The Good Society* (New York: Alfred A. Knopf, 1991).

3. Kathy Rudy, "Abortion, Grace, and the Wesleyan Quadrilateral" in

Quarterly Review: A Journal of Theological Resources for Ministry 15/1 (1995) 75.

4. In J. Gordon Melton, *The Churches Speak On: Abortion* (Detroit: Gale Research, 1989) 29-33.

5. Toronto: Life Cycle Books (1987) 4-17.

6. See Melton 31-32.

7. In the interest of space, I have chosen in the following paragraphs not to document every question and difficulty mentioned. It will be readily apparent to careful readers of the biblical text that these are legitimate interpretive problems.

8. New York: Simon & Schuster (1990).

9. Melton 151.

10. Pope John Paul II, *The Gospel of Life* (Papal Encyclical): *Evangelium Vitae* (Mahwah, NJ: Paulist, 1995).

11. Louisville: Westminster/John Knox (1992) 151.

12. Paul D. Simmons, *A Theological Response to Fundamentalism on the Abortion Issue* (Washington, DC: Religious Coalition for Reproductive Choice [formerly Religious Coalition for Abortion Rights], 1987, rev. 1990).

13. Ibid. 10.   14. Ibid. 10-12.

15. Washington, D.C.: Religious Coalition for Reproductive Choice (formerly Religious Coalition for Abortion Rights), n.d.

16. For a fuller critique of Simmons and Ward, see my "The Sounds of Silence: Abortion and the New Testament Canon" in *Proceedings of the Second University Faculty for Life Conference* (Washington, DC: University Faculty for Life, 1993).

17. Because the proceedings of this conference were not, as far as I know, made available to the public, I have decided not to name the specific individuals or denomination involved.

18. The more Jewish Christians thought circumcision necessary, the more Gentile Christians thought it superfluous or contradictory, and the two groups seem to have compromised by finally classifying it with the "indifferent matters" (what the Stoics called *adiaphora*).

19. See my *Abortion and the Early Church*.

20. For a similar use of Acts 15 and related texts to justify, by analogy, "the acceptance of 'nonabstaining' homosexual Christians," see Jeffrey S. Siker, "Homosexual Christians, the Bible, and Gentile Inclusion: Confessions of a Repenting Heterosexist" in Jeffrey S. Siker, ed., *Homosexuality in the Church: Both Sides of the Debate* (Louisville: Westminster/John Knox, 1994) 178-194. Curiously, editor Siker concludes the book on "both sides of the debate" in a way not unlike the keynote began the conference on both sides of the abortion debate (though Siker is more explicit). Interestingly, the conference ended with an odd worship service in which the main point of the sermon, based on a biblical story about Hebrew women, was that the only bad choice for women is a coerced "choice."

21. In Melton 25-28.　　　　　　22. Melton 26.

23. Exodus 21:22-25, John 8:1-11 (the woman caught in adultery), Matthew 7:1-5 ("judge not..."), and James 2:2-13 are used to illustrate compassion and justice.

24. Virginia Ramey Mollenkott, "Respecting the Moral Agency of Women" (Washington, DC: Religious Coalition for Abortion Rights, 1989).

25. Ibid. 4.

26. The similar theological criticisms of modern understandings of moral freedom made in the 1993 papal encyclical *Veritatis Splendor* are relevant at this point.

27. Sleeper 149.　　　　　　28. *The Other Side* (June 1980).

29. Beverly Wildung Harrison, *Our Right to Choose: Toward a New Ethic of Abortion* (Boston: Beacon, 1983) 70. Because Harrison does not capitalize "scripture," I have not capitalized it in quoting her or in restating her position.

30. Ibid. 71.   31. Ibid. 70-71.   32. Ibid. 69.

33. See ibid., chapter 2, "The Morality of Procreative Choice," pp. 32-56, and chapter 4, "Toward a Liberating Theological Perspective on Procreative Choice and Abortion," pp. 91-118.

34. Ibid. 68-70.   35. Ibid. 92.

36. *Problem Pregnancies: Toward a Responsible Decision* (New York: Office of the General Assembly, The United Presbyterian Church in the U.S.A., 1976) 23-24.

37. Ibid. 27.   38. Ibid. 28.

39. *The Covenant of Life and the Caring Community and Covenant and Creation: Theological Reflections on Contraception and Abortion* (New York and Atlanta: The Office of the General Assembly, Presbyterian Church in the USA, 1983). For a critique, especially of the document's use of Scripture, see William S. Kurz, "Genesis and Abortion: An Exegetical Test of a Biblical Warrant in Ethics" in *Theological Studies* 47 (1986) 668-680.

40. Ibid. 31-32.   41. Ibid. 32.

42. Ibid. 32.   43. Ibid. 36.

44. In J. Gordon Melton, *The Churches Speak On: Abortion* (Detroit: Gale Research, 1989) 29-33.

45. Ibid. 47.   46. Ibid. 33.

47. Ibid. A similar appeal to "the biblical doctrine of stewardship," in which "[c]hoice, not chance, becomes the divine mandate" (especially regarding genetic deformity) may be found in Simmons, *A Theological Response* 7, 11.

48. See, for example, especially *Problem Pregnancies* 29-30; also *Covenant and Creation* 43-48.

49. For the text with notes, see Stallsworth 11-16.

50. For a similar approach, see also Terry Schlossberg and Elizabeth

Achtemeier, *Not My Own: Abortion and the Marks of the Church* (Grand Rapids: Eerdmans, 1995).

51. It should be pointed out that I served as a consultant for the writing of the *Durham Declaration* and have, therefore, a natural bias toward it despite some possible weaknesses in it.

52. Pheme Perkins, "Jesus and Ethics" in *Theology Today* 52/1 (1995) 49-65 at 64.

53. See, most recently, his "Abortion, Theologically Understood" in Stallsworth 44-66.

54. Perkins 64.

55. Richard Hays, "Scripture-Shaped Community: The Problem of Method in New Testament Ethics" in *Interpretation* 44 (1990) 45.

56. Ibid. 45.

57. See note 1 for bibliographical information.

58. See bibliographical information in note 1.

59. E.g., throughout the encyclical *Veritatis Splendor*.

60. *Gospel of Life*, p. 50.

61. I wish to thank the interdisciplinary group of members of University Faculty for Life who heard this paper for their feedback. Special thanks goes to Sue Abromaitis, Professor of English at Loyola College in Maryland, for her comments.

HEALING POST-ABORTION TRAUMA

Susan Stanford-Rue

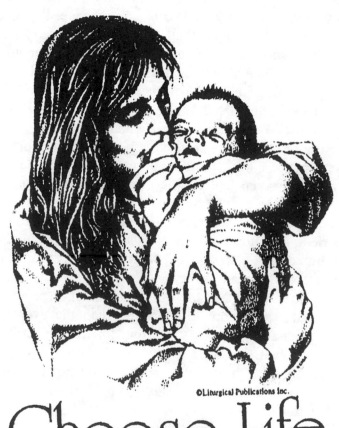

©Liturgical Publications Inc.

Choose Life

This is an image we would all identify as a picture of "motherhood." It is a woman holding a child. What are the first three words that come to your mind? There are many which might surface: nurturer, giver of life, defender, caring, loving, protector, encourager, taking responsibility.... Almost all are words of nurturance. It is my belief, strongly backed by my practice, that we now live in what Pope John Paul II calls "a culture of death," one that constantly gives conflictual messages about even so basic a factor in human life as motherhood. Instead of those nurturing images of motherhood, women are given a perversely manipulated image by being told that "Motherhood must be a matter of choice and abortion is a choice. The use of our bodies must be a matter of our choice." In my practice, this conflictual message produces great ramifications, far beyond the event of the abortion. This is true for women who have had an abortion in high school or college, before marriage, but later want children when married. But it is also true for those who have unplanned children during marriage and want to go back to raising the children they already have.

My message is that the ramifications of these abortions are greater and more long lasting than the event itself. They persist for five years, for ten, for fifteen, for twenty. In my current practice I am working with a woman who had an abortion thirty years ago, and yet just recently she shared something with me she had never told anyone else all her life.

Let me speak about theory first. Then I'll supply some anecdotal stories to convey an understanding about just how conflictual a message is being given to women in our society. On the one hand they are to be nurturers but on the other hand it is acceptable to take the life of your unborn child.

FIGURE 1
POST ABORTION SYNDROME: DIAGNOSTIC CRITERIA[1]

A. *Stressor:* The abortion experience, i.e., the intentional destruction of one's unborn child, is sufficiently traumatic and beyond the range of usual human experience so as to cause significant symptoms of re-experience, avoidance, and impacted grieving.

B. *Re-experience:* The abortion trauma is re-experienced in one of the following ways:

1. recurrent and intrusive distressing recollections of the abortion experience
2. recurrent distressing dreams of the abortion of the unborn child (e.g., baby dreams or fetal fantasies)
3. sudden acting or feeling as if the abortion were recurring (including reliving the experience, illusions, hallucinations, and dissociative [flashback] episodes including upon awakening or when intoxicated)
4. intense psychological distress at exposure to events that symbolize or resemble the abortion experience (e.g., clinics, pregnant mothers, subsequent pregnancies)
5. anniversary reactions of intense grieving and/or depression on subsequent anniversary dates of the abortion or on the projected due date of the aborted child

C. *Avoidance:* Persistent avoidance of stimuli associated with the abortion trauma or numbing of general responsiveness (not present before the abortion), as indicated by at least three of the following:
1. efforts to avoid or deny thoughts or feelings associated with the abortion
2. efforts to avoid activities, situations, or information that might arouse recollections of the abortion
3. inability to recall the abortion experience or an important aspect of the abortion (psychogenic amnesia)
4. markedly diminished interest in significant activities
5. feeling of detachment or estrangement from others
6. withdrawal in relationships and/or reduced communication
7. restricted range of affect, e.g., unable to have loving or tender feelings
8. sense of foreshortened future, e.g., does not expect to have a career, marriage, or children, or a long life

D. *Associated Features*: Persistent symptoms (not present before the abortion), as indicated by at least two of the following:
1. difficulty falling or staying asleep
2. irritability or outbursts of anger
3. difficulty concentrating
4. hypervigilance
5. exaggerated startle response to intrusive recollections or re-experiencing of the abortion trauma
6. physiologic reactivity upon exposure to events or situations that symbolize or resemble an aspect of the abortion (e.g., breaking out in a profuse sweat upon a pelvic examination or hearing vacuum pump sounds)
7. depression and suicidal ideation
8. guilt about surviving when one's unborn child did not
9. self devaluation and/or an inability to forgive one's self
10. secondary substance abuse

E. *Course:* Duration of the disturbance (symptoms in B, C, and D) of more than one month's duration, or onset may be delayed (great than six months after the abortion)

The above chart depicts the various symptomatic aspects of Post-Traumatic Stress Disorder (hereafter PTSD). It was only in 1980 that the American Psychiatric Association recognized the trauma Vietnam veterans were chronically suffering and diagnosed it as PTSD. One of the most unhappy aspects of PTSD is the intrusive re-experiencing of traumatic memories.

In the case of post-abortion women, many of the women suffer from this same type of intrusive re-experiencing of memories of their abortion. These painful and sometimes horrific memories are part of their on-going trauma.

Many women try to "cope" with these intrusive memories by not feeling them. Avoiding their painful feelings at all costs becomes a persistent goal. For some women this manifests itself by becoming workaholics; they keep themselves so busy that they do not have time to feel anything. Some women find they need several drinks at night to unwind. Still others find "help" by asking their doctors for more tranquillizers to help their chronic anxiety. And some turn to illegal drugs to escape their pain or self-hatred.

Unfortunately, what many people do not recognize is that all abortion is a death experience, and all death experiences need to be grieved and mourned. Women frequently complain of feelings of sadness, guilt, and shame. Abortion can cause tremendous shame and guilt. The memory of the event, if not properly grieved, acts as a "pus-pocket" inside the psyche. We can never get free of it. It is always lingering there in the background. We can try to run from it psychologically in many ways, but it is always there ungrieved, needing to be addressed.

If the abortion experience remains ungrieved and unhealed, a woman will have a sense of "re-experiencing" the abortion in any number of ways: a recollection or memory may come to her while at work or driving down the street. During sleep she may have nightmares or fetal dreams that recur. Such re-experiencings could be triggered by an unexpected resemblance, e.g., a suction-machine like a vacuum-cleaner, or a person who resembles the doctor or nurse from the abortion. Anniversary dates of the abortion or the would-be due date can be another trigger.

In my practice I am currently seeing a woman who presented her concern as one of thinking about changing careers, but in the course of taking an inventory of her history, it came out that she had had two abortions. I asked, "Do you feel resolved with these or need to work some things out?" She cut me off abruptly, "I don't want to talk about it." I noted that she had unresolved issues. One day two months into our work she came in very angry and upset. When I asked why she was so upset, she answered, "It's the anniversary of my second abortion.... Maybe I do need to talk about it." She had no faith-experience to help her deal with the abortion. Apparently the anniversary always triggered a flashback she had just tried to run from.

It is very common for women to want to avoid these painful feelings. The problem is that they will not be resolved on their own. Feelings that are repressed over a long time can become a serious problem. Our defense-mechanisms work well in the short run, but they can become extremely dysfunctional in the long run. We can become very conflicted and torn. We just can't deny our sad and painful feelings across the spectrum. In fact, someone who tries to deny her feelings will "feel" less and less, even about day-to-day matters. She will have less interest in daily life and even feel "frozen" or just shut down. This is true of all grief experiences that have not been mourned. Ungrieved loss can become a slippery slope. She can eventually slide into a deep depression. Some may reach out to get help. But others think of getting out of life, i.e., suicidal attempts. Many women, however, seek no help and even take a stab at suicide. Some are found after their attempts and may finally get help then.

One aborted woman I have known had repressed her grief for an extremely prolonged time and suffered some horrific experiences as a result. She lived a very fast life-style. She was a professional skier and had had five abortions. She "coped" by using lots of recreational drugs. And she kept running from her feelings. But she had a persistent, repetitive nightmare. She dreamt of a tree with many branches, and on each branch was a fetus without limbs. Finally, unable to deny this horrific dream and act normally, she had to stop running from her grief. She had been suppressing the pain and the sadness. Like the Vietnam veterans after the war, she experienced a kind of "survivor guilt." We have heard many Vietnam survivors report the feeling "How come I lived when my buddy died? Could I have done more to save him?" When my client began to deal with her feelings, she felt excruciating guilt that she was alive but her "babies" were all dead.

Today even Planned Parenthood acknowledges that some women have grief from their abortions. So many clients I have seen ask, "How come they never warned me that I would have to deal with these feelings? I have so much sadness. Much more than I ever expected. Even more than I know how to deal with." For most women grief takes at least a year to get over, sometimes more. Even in a crisis pregnancy they have lost a loved one. Our society acts as if they should simply make a decision and get on with their lives. But it is not that simple. Abortion's aftermath is very conflictual, and the woman persists in great pain and sadness that is not dealt with. So she goes through the next weeks and months often very unhappy. She may in fact be relieved from her immediate pregnancy crisis, but there is no one there to help her deal with this loss. Many women will tell no one, or just one person in their whole lives. They tend to cry alone, or use drugs alone. They try to live with the pain alone. When they come into our office, they only want to know how to live with the pain. Many feel they do not deserve to be healed. Sadly, our society does nothing to prepare women for this tragic grief. The abortion industry certainly does nothing, and the print and television media never report stories on a woman's need to grieve her abortion. Just a few stories in the media would give permission for thousands of women to seek help.

Let me share a couple of other examples from my practice of the conflictual message about motherhood and abortion and its consequent repercussions long afterwards. My first example is Jeannie (not her real name), now aged 40, who had an abortion during her sophomore year of college. She had been raised a Catholic. She told no one except her boyfriend about her decision to abort, and she promised herself that "no one will ever know." She went to New York for the abortion. She now "feels frozen" and remembers only the whirlwind of that time. There was no discussion of the risks, no help to deal with the grief. She remembers the abortion as painful, including the doctor yelling at her, "You'll hurt your kidneys if you don't stay still." In the recovery room she made a vow: never to let anyone get too close to her. Her husband knows the history, but she told no women friends. She had had a very successful career in real estate. Six years ago, at age 34, she decided to get pregnant. At first she had much difficulty in doing so but now has a little girl and stays at home with her. Her motherhood has been much affected by her abortion. She is utterly unsure of herself as a mother. She is always second-guessing herself. How odd this seems, given her prior successful career in a business with complicated negotiations and her experience of dealing with "all kinds of people." We have spent so many sessions on simple, small decisions. Today her daughter is very strong-willed and tests her mother all the time.

Jeannie had postponed motherhood for so long because she was so unsure of herself in this area. She began counseling by "presenting" issues about her child, but eventually she told me about her abortion. She has not begun the grieving process for that child. It is indicative of how far the shame goes that recently she let a woman friend into her life, but only so far! Jeannie told me she wanted to refer this friend to me for counselling when the friend had asked whom she was seeing. But she couldn't bear to tell her my name because she couldn't stand the idea that someone she knew would talk to someone else who knew her story, and all my explanations of how entirely privileged and confidential such information always is made no difference to her. She still has a long way to go to forgive herself and be set free from her shame.

The next example is Lee, who had an abortion six months ago. She is now 36, the mother of two children, one ten, one seven. It is a very complicated story. Faith is not a strong part of her life. She was raised a Catholic but has been lukewarm with respect to religion in her life. She couldn't decide about whether to have a third child, so she started praying "If it be God's will." Her husband seemed satisfied with two children. She had had an abortion during her freshman year in college and said that it took her four years "to get over it." She had always said to herself, "I'll never do that again."

Unexpectedly she found herself pregnant after an occasion of unprotected sex. Initially she felt a sense of joy, that her prayers had been answered. Her husband seemed pleased and kissed her when she said to him one morning as he headed off to work that she had a hunch she was pregnant. Then her panic set in: "I don't know if I'm ready to do this again. Can I handle a little baby again?" When asked for counsel, her physician would give her no more help than to say "It's your choice." In her panic she asked her husband, "You have to tell me if it's okay to have an abortion." He vacillated, and further panic set in for her. They were strained financially, but not at a breaking-point. In her panic she made an appointment for an abortion. When she came home, she went to bed and slept for 12 hours. But when she awoke, she began sobbing and couldn't stop. She couldn't face her two kids. She was angry with her husband, whom she had badgered until he said "It's your decision, do what you want." In shock this woman now sits in my office saying, "I am... a nurturer. I love kids." She feels alienated from all that she now does for her two kids. She seems utterly dumbfounded why she had the abortion. She says she thinks it is far too easy to get an abortion today. "Somebody should have stopped me." But nobody said, "It's just panic. Relax, you'll be okay." She has now had two abortions, the second one out of panic, and she feels terrible guilt. She hates herself for what she's done, and she can't believe that she did it. She calls herself "stupid" and asks "where was my brain?" She is now cold to her kids, and her husband spends most of the time tending to them. She cries a great deal. She is very conflicted in her concept of herself as a mother. She is very angry and full of sadness.

In summary, the women described above are typical of many thousands of women today suffering from "impacted grief." They suffer because: 1) There is lack of awareness of the grief to be expected and the need to mourn it. 2) In abortion there are no images and visual memories the way there are in other types of death. These images are always part of grief-work, but in abortion there are no memories, no pictures of the child. 3) Lack of awareness that she needs to do the catharsis-work, to deal with her pain. Consider, for example, a woman whose abortion was thirty years ago. She only recently told me what she'd seen in her toilet after coming home from her abortion: part of the fetus was floating there, the face looking up.... She has never before told a soul about this, and never forgiven herself. There are hundreds of examples of how women "cope" with their pain, e.g. by eating disorders, staying in abusive relationships, substance abuse, etc. More than anything they need to deal with their loss and then to seek forgiveness from God and to forgive themselves.

There are many stages a woman needs to go through as she heals from the pain of abortion. If she is Catholic, I encourage her to seek the sacramental gift of absolution in the rite of reconciliation. She will most likely need to see a trained professional to help her work through her guilt and shame. Many women find it helpful to write a letter to the baby that speaks of their love for the child and their regret at what happened. These letters really turn into love-letters and are a very cathartic tool toward healing.

Finally, when I feel the woman has adequately processed her grief and forgiven herself, I end my work with her by a "guided prayer" to Jesus. Almost all the women I have led through this prayer receive real peace and feel God's love amidst their tears. This guided prayer follows.

HEALING OF THE ABORTION MEMORY[2]

I begin the healing of the memories experience by asking my client, "Jane," to choose a comfortable posture, close her eyes, bow her head, and relax so that the details in her memory can unfold. I start the healing journey by expressing God's desire and power to heal us of our sins and our pain. Then I employ the psychological tool of directive reflection to lead the client back to the painful memory of her abortion.

"Healing Father, we thank You for Your promise that when two or more are gathered in Your name, You are in our midst. We thank You for Your presence here with us, and we ask You to guide us as we journey toward healing for 'Jane.' In the name of Jesus, I bind any spirits of darkness that would try to disrupt the healing process. Jesus, I know You to be the one true Healer from whom all total healing comes, whether through medicine, psychology, or divine healing. Guide us now, Holy Spirit, so that 'Jane' will receive total forgiveness and healing from her abortion. May al the glory be Yours, dear Lord."

"I would like you now, 'Jane,' to let yourself journey back in your memory to that time around your abortion experience. Allow the Holy Spirit to run the projector of your memory. Perhaps some particular part of the event will stand out to you, like the abortion clinic, or where you were when you made the decision to have the abortion, or perhaps your feelings after you had the abortion. It is different for each individual. Just allow your mind to open up and visualize your memories." After a few moments' pause I then ask: "Can you tell me what has come to your mind at this point?"

Pause for client to share the memory that has come to her.

"Fine, 'Jane,' that's very good. Now I would like you to allow yourself not only to get in touch with the facts and the circumstances around your decision, but more importantly, to start to sense the breadth of feelings that were present at that time. Spend a few moments now concentrating on your emotions. If you want to cry, let the tears flow." Usually the client will begin to cry by now, and this is an important part of the grieving and healing process.

"Now, 'Jane,' in your memory I'd like you to look up from wherever you are sitting or lying and look over to the nearest doorway. I'd like you to see, standing at that door, what you would imagine a loving, forgiving, and healing Jesus to look like. He may be tall or short, He may or may not have a beard, but I want you to imagine Him as you think Jesus would look. He may have deep dark eyes that hold your attention immediately. He seems to be radiating a deep warmth and love, and there appears to be no judgment or scorn anywhere on His face.

"Then you also notice as you see Him standing there that He is holding something in His arms. It is something wrapped in a blanket, and after a moment or two you realize that He is holding a little baby. He is holding your baby, 'Jane,' and He loves this child even more than you would if that baby were right here on earth with you. Now I want you to get up and go across the room in your memory and face Jesus where He is standing. You look straight at Him, and He holds your gaze with His forgiving eyes. You realize that Jesus is not condemning you. He is only living you. His death on the Cross was to atone for all of our sins, so He stands there offering you forgiveness and love. So the debt for your sin has already been paid. The gentle smile on His face never leaves, and you begin to feel His permeating love flowing deep into your heart and mind. I want you now just to drink in His love and allow it to come inside your whole being.

"I am going to be quiet for a few minutes, and I want you to dialogue with Jesus in silence. Give Him all of your pain. Tell Him about all the feelings and emotions that you have — every single one of them. Lay all of your hurt and sadness at His feet; give Him every feeling that is present for you.

"After you have poured out your feelings, you need to ask for God's forgiveness. In your words express your regret to Jesus for taking the life of your child and ask Him to forgive you. Tell Jesus you forgive all those who were involved in your abortion. If there is one or more particular individuals that are difficult for you to forgive, ask Jesus who is the essence of forgiving love, for the help to forgive them.

"You realize that the pain you have experienced is not punishment from the Father, but only a real consequence of the grieving of your child's death. As we take our pain to the Father through Jesus, whose greatest desire is for us to receive the Father's love, we are drawn closer to Him, and His forgiveness becomes the very foundation of your healing.

"When you are finished sharing, I want you to remain quiet and listen to what Jesus has to say to you. He has some specific things he wishes to say to you particularly. He may say just a word or two, or He may give you several sentences. You will come to realize His words are full of healing power. They are His healing touch to you. Just as He healed through touch during His life here on earth, His words to you will provide the healing for your abortion. As you are journeying in your dialogue with Jesus, I will be in silent prayer, interceding for you with our loving Father.

"After you have heard all that Jesus has to say to you, I want you to see Jesus giving you your little baby to hold. This is likely to produce some tears, but this is all part of the healing process. Please share with your child all that you would like to say regarding your love and how you regret what happened. Let your heart share fully as you hold your child. Do not be afraid to ask him or her for forgiveness."

After waiting ten minutes in quiet prayer, I then move to the committal prayer.

"Lord Jesus, we know that 'Jane's' baby is with You now in heaven. 'Jane' can see her baby being held in Your arms. Lord, we thank You for the love You have for this child and for how You love each one of us individually on this earth. We want, now, Lord, to commit this baby of 'Jane's' to You forever."

I now stop my prayer and ask 'Jane' if she has any sense of what the sex of her child might be. I then ask her if she has any hint of a name the baby might be called. After hearing these two vital pieces of information, I continue my prayer.

"Heavenly Father, Lord Jesus, and Holy Spirit, we come to you at this point in our journey, and we wish to dedicate this child to You for all eternity. We know, Lord, that You love this child more than any earthly parent can comprehend. But 'Jane,' as the earthly parent of this child, wishes now to commit little 'Janie' to You, Heavenly Father, to be with You in heaven, to be loved by You, and to be with Your host of angels for all time. Thank You, Father, for the love that You have for this child. We are confident, Lord, that one day the souls of 'Jane' and her daughter 'Janie' will be joined together in heaven, and we look forward to that day. We praise You, Father, and we thank You for all the healing that You are doing at this very moment."

I then conclude by asking 'Jane' if she has anything she would like to add to the prayer and committal service for her child, either out loud or privately. Finally, I close the service with this prayer.

"Lord Jesus, we praise You and we thank You for all that You have just done to heal 'Jane' of her abortion. We thank You for little 'Janie' and for Your taking care of her for all eternity. We thank You also, Lord, for how Your death and resurrection have set us free from all our sins. We thank You for the new freedom 'Jane' feels. Father, I ask You to carry 'Jane' in the palm of Your hand for this week until we meet again. Continue her healing. Help her to continue to see the power of Your love and Your healing forgiveness. We praise You, in Jesus' name. Amen."

NOTES

1. Developed by Vincent M. Rue, Ph.D., from diagnostic criteria for "post traumatic stress disorder" in *American Psychiatric Association, Diagnostic and Statistical Manual on Mental Disorders Revised* [DSM III-R: 309.89] (Washington. D.C.: American Psychiatric Press 1987) 250. The American Psychiatric Association in no way supports the existence of, nor does it find any clinical evidence for the basis of the diagnosis of "post abortion syndrome." The DSM III-R does not reference nor include the diagnosis of "post abortion syndrome," but the DSM III-R does identify abortion as a type of "psycho-social stressor" (p. 20).

2. Taken from Susan M. Stanford-Rue, Ph.D., Will I Cry Tomorrow? Healing Post-Abortion Trauma (Old Tappan, N.J.: Revell 1986) ch. 12: "Healing Steps for Post-Abortion Trauma."

RIGHT TO LIFE IN LITERARY THEORY:
THE SILENCE SCREAMS

Jeff Koloze

Recently, at Kent State University, I had the pleasure of being introduced to a foreign language. Well, not really a foreign language, but an alien language: English literary theory. I will be the first to confess publicly — as the other students in the literary criticism class thought — that most of the material discussed was irrelevant, obscure, or offensive.

But I came away from the course thinking how grand it is that now I know something of the critical vocabulary needed to tear apart anti-life writing and to bolster the status of pro-life writing.

Certainly, given the hostility most literary critics have towards the pro-life movement, one would think that established literary criticism would use whatever tools are at hand to promote an anti-life agenda.

This may indeed be the case. Literary theorists bring their various approaches to the study of literature to argue for the inclusion of women's experiences — except that the unborn woman is excluded. Literary theorists bring their approaches to literature to validate the experiences of marginalized groups in society such as homosexual men, lesbians, minorities, non-Western authors, etc. — a good thing to do, basically. But pro-lifers who are marginalized by an anti-life media or an anti-life academic power need not apply.

Pro-lifers, their viewpoints, their writings are left out of the discussion. The silence that literary theorists heap on our views offended me then when I had to read their works. The silence burying our issues offends me now. And now it is time for us, in true feminist literary critical fashion, to speak out.

While there is a pervasive silence in current literary theories regarding the right to life issues, each of the major contemporary literary theories can be utilized to explicate pro-life truths embodied in our literature.

I will discuss pertinent aspects of these literary theories and interweave the applicability of the theory to the discussion of pro-life issues in literature. Since the theories will be presented in alphabetical order, I ask that you think of the acronym CDFMNRS. Senseless and meaningless, I know... as senseless and meaningless as why theorists would exclude the pro-life view from our literature.

In the final portion of this paper, I will document specific instances in literature where a pro-life viewpoint can be excavated (a word which I selected after great deliberation). Moreover, I believe that there is an emerging body of as yet noncanonical pro-life literature.

C IS FOR CULTURAL CRITICISM

The history of Cultural Criticism as a literary theory began with research among the working classes of Britain after the Second World War. In essence, Cultural Criticism attempts to incorporate surrounding aspects of a work of literature into its appreciation. While books as textual artifacts are an important element of the culture to be studied, other items in the culture to be studied include videos, photographs, print advertisements, televised commercials, political publications, etc.

The appreciation of elements in one's culture is not meant to be a static study. Regarding Cultural Criticism, the Right to Life movement may have been given its marching orders with the following statement by Jonathan Culler in his essay "Literary Theory":

The desire of many critics and theorists [is] to make literary and cultural criticism politically progressive. This desire has stimulated work on noncanonical writings, especially those by members of groups that have been oppressed by or within Western cultures.... (217)

I think immediately of Jean Blackwood, who is certainly not part of the official canon — yet, that is, since Blackwood is a pro-life poet, one of those writers who have been marginalized by fellow feminists who, unlike her, are anti-life in philosophy. Blackwood's understanding of the forces behind abortion makes us aware of who is oppressed — and who oppresses — within Western cultures.

Taking a cultural studies approach, we can immediately justify the use of pro-life videos and pictures, as well as written texts, in the study of literature. All of these texts function to help the student understand a particular work. The photograph of the nearly 750,000 people who marched on Washington in 1990 should be as iconic as that of the 1963 civil rights march on Washington. Similarly, *The Silent Scream* should be as iconic as the famous photograph of the mother who died from her illegal abortion.

Equally important, the pro-life student reading a particular work which may be hostile to pro-lifers can incorporate into her critique of the work her own cultural artifacts which may disprove the anti-life intent of the author. An author who tries to convey an image of pro-lifers as uncaring or ultraconservative will have the rhetorical effect of his or her intention frustrated by a student who knows that the opposite is true. More forcefully, the suasive effect of anti-life writing can be frustrated by the pro-life student who can demonstrate that there are items in the catalog of the culture which show that pro-lifers are caring and may not necessarily all be stereotyped as uncaring political conservatives.

D IS FOR DECONSTRUCTION

To put us in the right frame to understand this theory, let

me quote literary theorist Stephen Bonnycastle who claims that "You don't need deconstruction unless you are feeling oppressed" (90).

Deconstruction maintains that nothing expressed in language can be absolutely true (Bonnycastle 93). While deconstruction as a literary theory should not be reduced to mere word play, it does aim to demonstrate how the substantiation and fixed meaning of any term in a text can be replaced by a term in a subordinate position. Thomas Fink in a recent essay states

Deconstruction seeks whatever latent rhetorical or other power may exist in the marginalized term, and this power almost always subverts the centrality of the previously privileged term. (241)

The rhetorical games which deconstructionist authors may play in their works conceal a profoundly serious philosophical goal. As Sharon Crowley demonstrates in her book, deconstruction wishes to achieve nothing more than the "obliterat[ion of] the doctrine of presence in Western metaphysics" — an important mission, without which deconstruction's further goal of displacing and replacing the objective meaning of specific terms is futile (x). In opposition to reader-response theories, deconstruction stresses the importance of the text over that of the author.

Deconstruction seems to me to be a great paralipsis. If deconstruction is a system where the text is shown to say "something other than what it appears to say," then this is a contortion of language which leads to paralipsis. Is this methodology a reading into the text? Possibly. However, if deconstruction questions the veracity and stability of each and every word in a text, then we who are pro-life can apply the same methodology to current texts dealing with the life issues.

Was an author correct in using one word instead of another when describing pro-lifers? Is the pejorative term used by an anti-life author to describe pro-lifers or a pro-life activity actually the superior term which commands our respect? Is "picketing," for example, such an inferior term? Why? Why is the woman seeking an abortion not correctly called what she is — mother to an unborn child?

Finally, if deconstruction aims to subvert the privileged term of binary opposites, then we can work with the privileged terms of the anti-life movement to frustrate the political intent of those terms. Why should abortion necessarily be linked with "rights" when "wrongs" would be more proper? Why should the term "fetus" be used negatively as though designating a non-human entity, when it represents merely a stage in a human being's development? Our students can be empowered through deconstructive techniques to replace the privileged terms of an anti-life media or literature with the subversive (and correct) pro-life ones.

F IS FOR FEMINIST LITERARY CRITICISM

It is this theory which would seem to be the most fertile area in which pro-life academics could argue their case that literature conveys essential pro-life themes. Those who read feminist literary tracts are, of course, disappointed that protection of the unborn child is not included in the agenda of feminist activists. It is understandable, however, when one considers that feminist literary theory strives primarily for the validation of women's experiences, previously neglected by what was perceived as a male-dominated (strictly patriarchal) mode of viewing the world.

Currently, it seems, the venom spewed forth comes from women who have been oppressed by men and who think that abortion is a means toward their liberation. Pro-life women are only now having their voices heard.

Despite efforts to show how feminist studies will aid men in understanding their role in society, an anti-male bias still pervades the theory, evidenced by the extreme concern with not merely sexist stereotypes, but the dominance of patriarchy (which is always considered negatively) in women's lives. In fact, Naomi Schor emphatically reiterates this distrust of patriarchy in a recent essay when she shows that research in homosexual male studies "collaborates in feminism's unveiling of the phallus and the hierarchies it underwrites" (264). This gives new meaning to the phrase "Hey, fella, your zipper's down!"

Schor further argues that "the crime of rape has occupied a central place in feminist theory" (272). The pro-life professor would ask why abortion, which is at the center of the political hurricane of anti-life feminism, is not as aggressively mentioned as rape of women or rape of the environment (which feminism also chastises in its promotion of environmentally correct principles).

However, despite some objections to the explication of feminist viewpoints, pro-lifers can utilize specific aspects of the theory. *A Feminist Dictionary* can inspire us to create a pro-life dictionary, where words are truly inclusive of all viewpoints, including our own.

Feminist literary criticism can be used to validate the experiences of pro-life women. Much of feminism's experiences are anecdotal and are justified as literature — and correctly so. Everybody has a story. Everybody has a right to live. Everybody has something to say — including pro-life women.

Therefore, pro-life women should document their experiences and create a body of literature equally potent with (in fact, superior to) anti-life experiences.

What is it like for a pro-life woman to march outside an abortion clinic knowing that her sisters are passing her by, going inside?

What is it like for the mother losing a baby by miscarriage to receive a phone call from somebody asking for help to persuade another young mother not to have an abortion willfully?

I think that the anecdotes of mothers suffering from Post-

Abortion Syndrome (PAS) qualify immediately as vital new forces in the pro-life feminist canon. The stories of these women may be ignored by social scientists who may have political reasons not to admit that the performance of an abortion has consequences on the body and the psyche of the mother. These women's stories, however, cannot be ignored by other women, even anti-life women, because they are real. Since we pro-lifers have not ignored the accounts of abortions perpetrated by greedy and unsanitary abortionists, then all women — especially anti-life women — should give PAS mothers an equal respect.

Finally, adopting the view that the right to life position is as liberatory as feminist thinking will eclipse the power of the anti-life faction within feminism. It is empowering for a student to know that her pro-life beliefs are important. It is empowering for a student to know that her beliefs have been transmitted through literature for centuries.

M IS FOR MARXIST LITERARY THEORY

Terry Eagleton, the premier Marxist literary critic, states that

> Marxism is a scientific theory of human societies and of the practice of transforming them; and what that means, rather more concretely, is that the narrative Marxism has to deliver is the story of the struggles of men and women to free themselves from certain forms of exploitation and oppression. (vii)

Marxist literary theory strives for opening one's consciousness so that modes of production become evident in literature. Marxist literary theory can assist pro-lifers by helping us explicate what circumstances could possibly operate to permit some mothers to think of abortion as an "option." In fact, a pro-life analysis of the means of production within society can help a student understand how some mothers are forced to consider abortion as the only option forced on them.

Moreover, pro-life faculty can demonstrate another aspect of the anti-life movement, which embraces all three issues of abortion, infanticide, and euthanasia. To what degree do economic motives operate in literature for the killing of an unborn child, a handicapped child, or an elderly person? We do not need to whip out references in the *Wall Street Journal* to have our students recognize that abortion is big business. Carol Everett will tell us that. We similarly do not need to refer to the *Journal* to document how the killing of a Down Syndrome child alleviates not so much the physical pain of the child, but the embarrassment of the parents who don't want to be burdened with a less-than-perfect child. Of course, our students will understand that the use of the term "burden," in a Marxist literary sense, always implies a financial aspect. It does cost money to care for a handicapped child or an elderly person.

Furthermore, Marxist literary theory focuses on the dominant ideology operating within a work and how the reader can free him- or herself from that ideology. A point which is frequent in discussion of contemporary literary theory is especially enunciated in Marxist literary criticism. Often it is what is not said in a work which indicates the dominant ideology which it embodies. "A work is tied to ideology" Eagleton writes

not so much by what it says as by what it does not say. It is in the significant silences of a text, in its gaps and absences, that the presence of ideology can be most positively felt. (34)

We can find ample evidence of what is not said on behalf of the pro-life viewpoint in contemporary literature. More importantly, we can use Eagleton's words in the above quote almost verbatim to represent the struggle we pro-lifers must engage.

The key word for Marxism is struggle. We must struggle to have our pro-life voices heard. We must struggle to include our pro-life writings for discussion. It is this theory, with its emphasis on struggle, which I think has the most potential for pro-life literature. I'm willing to stand or sit corrected on this one.

N IS FOR NEW HISTORICISM

In a recent essay, Brook Thomas appropriates a quote from Christopher Lasch who argues that the problem with American culture is not narcissism, but amnesia. The inability to recall the past history of one's culture "is a precondition for what has been called a New Historicism" (86). This theory attempts to reintegrate historical study with explication of literary passages, two elements which were separated by New Critical pedagogy. This separation, Thomas further argues, "did not provide more solid ground for judgment but led to the deconstruction of all ground for judgment" (99).

A New Critical approach can be useful; it is certainly fun to have a student squirm over the meaning of a poem without knowing its historical context. It is the approach of New Historicism, however, which will make our students' appreciation of literature even richer.

Thus, if explicating Blackwood's poem "Generation," we who are pro-life academics are empowered to parallel the civil rights movement with the first civil right movement. I will defer specifics of this approach until we examine Blackwood's poem later.

R IS FOR READER-RESPONSE CRITICISM

As Richard Beach argues, reader-response theories share "a concern with how readers make meaning from their experience with the text" (1). While Romanticism seemed preoccupied with the status of the author, and New Criticism seemed preoccupied with the text, literary critics are now concerned with how that text "works" for the reader. Reader-response theories can work for a student, can affect him or her, in five modes: the textual, the experiential, the psychological, the social, and the cultural.

Those who read Beach's work will be turned off by his demeaning patriarchal values, his seeming to find sexist meanings everywhere, and his apologetics for being a male, but his thoughts are interesting, especially because they can be useful for pro-life educators.

This shift in focus to the individual reader is itself a very pro-life concept. It is appropriate that we affirm the right of the individual to an interpretation of literature. To emphasize the individual once again is important for another reason. Within feminist literary discourse, for example, it is proper to speak of a feminist "subject" as opposed to the feminist "woman." The feminist "subject" is a combination of the representation of "women" (essence) and "woman" as an historical being. Similarly, the homosexual "subject" as opposed to the homosexual "man" or "woman" is a construction of the representation of "homosexuality" (essence) and the homosexual "man" or "woman" as an historical being.

Many of us will not be satisfied with considering our students as "subjects," the current term which is used by literary theorists in place of the human being who reads a text. I teach the particular subject of English to particular human beings named John, Laura, Leslie, Omar, Pat, and Scott. I do not teach the subject of English to other subjects.

Another aspect of reader-response theories should serve the pro-life movement well. In discussing Jane Austen's *Emma*, Beach considers that which is missing from literary works. Readers can take issue with Austen's portrayal of genteel English life at the end of the eighteenth and the beginning of the nineteenth centuries in that the lower classes, the ones who work to support the English aristocracy, are rarely presented. Pro-lifers can similarly ask from a contemporary work, especially if it is anti-life: what's missing? Why does Mary Logue omit favorable characterizations of pro-lifers in her anti-life novel, *Still Explosion*? Why is no pro-life character sympathetically portrayed? Why should the pro-life activists in her diatribe be involved in bombing abortion mills instead of, like real-life activists, working for pregnancy support groups?

S IS FOR STRUCTURALISM

As developed from the work of the Swiss linguist Ferdinand de Saussure, structuralism defines language "as a system that offers you a set of categories for understanding the world" (Bonnycastle 61).

The first function of structuralism is to designate the polarities operating within a text. Its attention to paradigmatic elements demonstrates that a work will reference an overriding paradigm; attention to syntagmatic elements in a work helps the reader understand why a particular term in the series of the grammatical construct was used instead of any other.

Bonnycastle in his *In Search for Authority* points out that literature has undergone a paradigm shift over the last few decades, much like those discussed by Thomas Kuhn in his work with scientific paradigms. Dr. Nigel M. de S. Cameron, in his work with medical ethics, demonstrated last night how a shift in the appreciation in and application of the Hippocratic Oath similarly occurred only recently in human history. Unfortunately, all three shifts have brought about the present situation in academia where absolute truths are doubted. "Once you become aware of the existence of paradigms," Bonnycastle asserts, "and how they influence the way people think about the world, you can see that the 'truths' about the world — about religion, politics, and even science — are not absolute truths; they depend on particular paradigms" (42).

The application of structuralist principles can be liberating for the pro-life professor. No longer are we bound to adopt an anti-life interpretation of a literary text, if we understand the paradigm being used in its formation. If an author uses a paradigm of a world where women have an absolute right to kill their unborn children, or a world where the elderly have an absolute right to have themselves killed by assisted-suicide, then we can question the literary work which espouses these actions since the absence of absolute rules, according to anti-lifers, do not apply.

PRO-LIFE ELEMENTS IN THE CANON

While literary theorists have formed and based their theories on certain works and trends in literature, there should be recognized also the emergence of an increasing pro-life canon.

The canon of pro-life literature can — indeed must — be constructed archaeologically.   Our work as pro-life educators is truly an excavation: we must first sift through the various theoretical layers covering a text, much like archaeologists uncover an ancient city.   Having sifted through the various theoretical layers, our task is to reaffirm the importance of a literary work.   Literary archaeology is not new. Naomi Schor states that "Woolf undertook through an archaeology of women's writing to theorize and valorize a specifically female subjectivity and textuality, and that specificity was bound up with the maternal" (266). As feminist literary theory was compelled to dig into past literary works to show that women's writing was not only being produced, but important, so we who are pro-life educators must archaeologically recapture our literature.

▪ James Fenimore Cooper's *Deerslayer* can be viewed by the student as just a weighty novel written in thick nineteenth century language depicting life on the frontier of colonial New York.   It is also a battleground of values concerning what constitutes valued life. Hetty, described negatively as a "retarded" woman, is further described as one who has been "struck by God's power" (15).   The striking is apparently positive, for Hetty refines the way other characters view life.

■ Nathaniel Hawthorne's *Scarlet Letter* may be viewed in contemporary terms as a prototype of the dysfunctional family, modeled on contemporary sexual values. A pro-life reader-response application of this novel, however, would have our students identify with Hester Prynne, Arthur Dimmesdale, and Roger Chillingworth as actors in the great drama of a woman who chose a pro-life course of action: giving her baby life in the face of obstacles from her lover, her husband, and her community. After all, the relief promised and often performed by characters like Mistress Hibbins (a follower of the Black Prince) was available to Hester. True to a reader-response methodology, our students' own experiences with single parenthood are validated by the actions of these characters.

While I am unfamiliar with characteristics of your student populations, I can comment on those of students at Cuyahoga Community College. According to statistics generated by the College's Office of Academic and Student Affairs, most students usually entered the college between the ages of 20-24: in 1994, 6,876 students. The second highest age category is the 25-29 year old age group: for 1994, 4,153 students. The average age of the CCC student, dominantly a woman, is, due to the general aging of our population, increasing towards the age of twenty-nine years.

Many of these young women who are either unmarried with children, or divorced, or who have been abandoned by their boyfriends/husbands/lovers can identify with Hester's situation. They can come to understand intellectually and, perhaps more importantly, to feel the significance of Hester's pro-life action.

■ George Eliot's *Adam Bede* addresses the pro-life issue of infanticide. Hetty Sorrel is accused of "a great crime — the murder of her child" (389).

■ Clyde Griffiths in Theodore Dreiser's *American Tragedy* was well aware that in killing his lover, Roberta Alden, he would be responsible for "the death of that unborn child, too!!" (477). I think that Dreiser's punctuation was an extra signal to the reader. Why use that seemingly superfluous exclamation mark? Of course, the pro-life mind suggests that the exclamation marks represent Roberta and her unborn child.

■ Ernest Hemingway's "Hills Like White Elephants." As demonstrated in a recent University Faculty for Life newsletter, Hemingway does not favor an anti-life position in the story, as if abortion were a positive value in the relationship between the man and the woman. The abortion is devastating to their relationship ("Bibliography" 3).

■ John Dos Passos' *U.S.A.* similarly depicts abortion as a factor which contributes substantially to the failed relationships not only between union activists Ben and Mary, but also assorted other characters.

■ Richard Brautigan's *The Abortion: an Historical Romance 1966* is another text which does not ultimately seem favorable to abortion, since the confusion of the text replicates the confusion in the minds of the characters regarding whether the main character, Vida, should have the abortion.

■ Walker Percy's Father Simon in *The Thanatos Syndrome* is a character with whom all pro-lifers can sympathize. Set in the future, the world of *The Thanatos Syndrome* has legalized abortion, infanticide (called "pedeuthanasia" at 333), and euthanasia. Maybe the best thing to do in such a world is to move beyond political action, beyond education, and, like the good priest given the appropriately-generic name, Smith, hole yourself up in a tower and wait. Waiting for what is the mystery of Percy's novel.

OUR OWN ADDITIONS TO THE CANON

Moreover, the pro-life canon can be constructed by

additions from our own people. I think immediately of Stephen Freind's narratives. His *God's Children* is a fictionalized account of the passage of the Pennsylvania Abortion Control Act which can be a useful tool in the literature classroom. In one section of the novel, Freind has his main character, Kevin Murray, debate an anti-lifer. This section relies on ancient rhetorical redefinition to assist the reader in understanding how anti-life terminology has corrupted a language which formerly was pro-life. This passage illustrates a Marxist literary application of the struggle between a pro-lifer and an anti-lifer extremely well.

I was fortunate to discover another pro-life author here at this conference. Carl Winderl of Eastern Nazarene College is able not to compose, but to construct poems on the theme of the right to live. Besides its mastery of onomatopoeia, I think that "Dead in the Water" can be analyzed from the structuralist perspective quite well.

I remember when I presented Jean Blackwood's "Generation" before my fellow students in a Recent American Poetry course. I wanted to present "a pro-life poem" for this show-and-tell portion of our seminar, hoping to excite substantial discussion not only about the poem, but also the issue. Of course, except for one openly pro-life fellow student who advocated it, the poem was attacked as either being deaf to the concerns of women who wanted abortion or, in the opinion of the professor, not even "good poetry" after all. The poem aroused no anger. Despite the strong opinion of the professor, the supposed discussion which I had hoped would bring out the animal in all my fellow students never materialized.

Here is Blackwood's poem which did, however, "generate" silence:

> Is this the generation
> That Marched in Birmingham and Selma?
> That spoke for free speech in Berkeley?

That sang of love in San Francisco?
That swelled the Peace Corps ranks?
Whose hearts responded when he cried,
"I have a dream!"
Is this the generation?

Are these the flower children
Who called for peace in Vietnam,
For justice for the Indian nation,
An end to hatred, prejudice, and war?
Are these the flower children?

Does it mean the freedom ride is over,
When the dream is half fulfilled and half forgotten?
When we trade songs for screams and love for violence,
Where does the ride take us now?

When we put away the agent orange
     to brandish prostoglandins (sic);
When scalpels replace the bayonette,
And People's Park has no children left to play in it...
Then, old friends,
You are indeed past thirty,
Not to be trusted again.
Guess I'll throw in my lot
With another generation. (12)

While it is beyond me that some in academia schizophren-
ically advocate certain humanitarian and animal rights
causes yet ignore the first civil right to life, Blackwood's
poem is a litany of questionings of an activist of the 1960[s]
who sees through such schizophrenia. The persona looks
at the paradigm presented by his or her own experience of
rights and finds that it does not compare with current
history; it contrasts.

I think this poem would most immediately benefit from a
New Historicist approach. Our students, as is supposed to
be typical of American students, may not be familiar with
things which happened in ancient times — that is, thirty
years ago. Certain elements of the poem's contrasts will

need to be explained ("People's Park" and "agent orange" for example).

After settling these historical concerns, students may be made aware of the power of the pro-life message in the poem through a Marxist or a Cultural Criticism approach: the former to delineate the power structures operating in society now, and the latter to encourage questioning regarding why the deplorable situation of killing babies is tolerated when it contradicts civil rights.

Finally, the pro-life canon can be constructed by the emergence of a pro-life faculty. Let's see. If I finish Ph.D. coursework this summer, learn a foreign language in autumn, take comps in winter, then I'll be one of those ABDs and can get me a job at a college or university, teaching students about the glories of the pro-life perspective in, on, and through literature.

Seriously, though, just as the current crop of literature professors reached their positions carrying their anti-life baggage with them, so future professors of English — especially those who are pro-life — will have a chance to apply the archaeological method of pro-life work to literature. Such pro-life future professors need to be encouraged, certainly; more importantly, they need to be hired.

Henry Louis Gates, Jr., premiere advocate of African-American signification in literature, recalls that he was once asked, quite seriously, "Tell me, sir, ... what *is* black literature?" As a partial response to that, Gates stated:

It is a thing of wonder to behold the various ways in which our specialties have moved, if not from the margins to the center of the profession, at least from defensive postures to a generally accepted validity. (289)

We who are pro-life in the academy must ask and answer a similar question: what is a pro-life literature? The future of our students and the fate of our culture depend on our answer. If we in the humanities cannot find evidence for the pro-life viewpoint, then what justification can we provide that we are a people who have exercised freedom of choice and chose life?

Think of the analogy with legislative history and its importance in judicial decision-making. Often courts will not only refer, but defer to legislative histories created while a law was progressing through a legislature. How much more important is it for us to emphasize the pro-lifeness of our literature?

I look forward to that time when a pro-life perspective on the canonical works will be as valid an approach as a feminist or a Marxist one. I look forward even more to the inclusion of what are now non-canonical works by our own poets and authors.

WORKS CITED

Beach, Richard. *A Teacher's Introduction to Reader-Response Theories*. Urbana: National Council of Teachers of English, 1993.

"Bibliography: 'Hills Like White Elephants': Hemingway's Abortion Story." *UFL Pro Vita* 5 (1995) 2.

Blackwood, Jean. *Beyond Beginning and Other Poems*. Rolla: Low-Key Press, 1982.

Bonnycastle, Stephen. *In Search of Authority*. Peterborough, Ont.: Broadview Press, 1991.

Brautigan, Richard. *The Abortion: an Historical Romance 1966*. New York: Simon and Schuster, 1971.

Cooper, James Fenimore. *The Deerslayer*. Philadelphia: Macrae Smith, [n.d.].

Crowley, Sharon. *A Teacher's Introduction to Deconstruction*. Urbana: National Council of Teachers of English, 1989.

Culler, Jonathan. "Literary Theory" in *Introduction to Scholarship in Modern Languages and Literatures*, ed. Joseph Gibaldi. New York: Modern Language Association of America, 1992.

Dos Passos, John. *U.S.A.* Boston: Houghton Mifflin, 1960.

Dreiser, Theodore. *An American Tragedy*. Cambridge: Robert

Bentley, 1978.

Eagleton, Terry. *Marxism and Literary Criticism*. Berkeley: Univ. of California Press, 1976.

Eliot, George. *Adam Bede*. New York: New American Library, 1961.

Fink, Thomas. "Reading Deconstructively in the Two-Year College Introductory Literature Classroom" in *Practicing Theory in Introductory College Literature Courses,* eds. James M. Cahalan and David B. Downing. Urbana: National Council of Teachers of English, 1991.

Gates, Henry Louis. "'Ethnic and Minority Studies'" in *Introduction to Scholarship in Modern Languages and Literatures*, ed. Joseph Gibaldi. New York: Modern Language Association of America, 1992.

Hemingway, Ernest. "Hills Like White Elephants" in *Men Without Women*. Cleveland: World Publishing, 1944.

Logue, Mary. *Still Explosion*. Seattle: Seal Press, 1993.

Percy, Walker. *The Thanatos Syndrome*. New York: Farrar-Straus-Giroux, 1987.

Schor, Naomi. "Feminist and Gender Studies" in *Introduction to Scholarship in Modern Languages and Literatures*, ed. Joseph Gibaldi. New York: Modern Language Association of America, 1992.

Thomas, Brook. "The Historical Necessity for — and Difficulties with — New Historical Analysis in Introductory Literature Classes" in *Practicing Theory in Introductory College Literature Courses*, eds. James M. Cahalan and David B. Downing. Urbana: National Council of Teachers of English, 1991.

ONE POET'S JOURNEY
AS ARTIST, CITIZEN, AND FATHER
TOWARD THE RIGHT TO *LIVE*

Carl A. Winderl

I'm not the first writer to assert that life is a journey, nor will I be the last. From Bunyan to Bellow and Dickens to Twain, from Homer to Faulkner and Dante to Updike, writers have indeed dealt with the notion of a journey, literal or figurative, physical or spiritual, emotional or intellectual, as moving the traveler from a state of innocence to experience, from ignorance to intelligence, even from bestiality to grace. But of those above cataloged writers few considered the issue of abortion as a social concern, and fewer still have dealt with that issue in their literary works. I, however, stand before you as an artist who has lived with it both as a social malaise and as a theme in my poetry. To be sure, I do not so readily include myself in their company as literary lions; nevertheless, young pup that I may be, I *am* here. And they are not.

The journey that *I* have taken — the journey that I am *on* — is a journey of awareness in the Right to "Live" Movement, as a member of society, as an artist, and as a parent articulating what I believe into what I create artistically.

Typical of journeys, mine reveals to me an awareness that increases the longer I travel, the more travelers I meet, and the more I contemplate the significance of my travels. My record, my journal, if you will of this travelogue, is the poetry I write along the way, espousing my beliefs into my creations.

In particular here, I have chosen four poems spanning eighteen years of this journey, beginning several years before the adoption of our first child, almost fourteen years ago, and continuing to the very real present. The voices of three of the personae in the poem are women, revealing, I sense, the state of their lives as determined by the world of men, and the persona in the fourth poem is the voice of an unborn child aborted by a saline injection. In all four poems the voices speak of their futility in a male-ordered and dominated society, and all of the voices consider what could have been, what could not be, or what might yet be.

"How" I'm going to reveal "all" of this is a somewhat atypical format, to be sure. But it's one that has worked several times before. I will present chronologically these four poems that I have written at intervals in my adult life, focusing my discussion and revelations on and around them. Before but mostly after each poem I will discuss, explain, and reveal aspects of my creative process, my value system, and my role as a citizen, as a poet, and as a father in these last few years of the 20th century. In the revealing, I will discuss what I sense is my responsibility and my vision for influencing in some way an audience to see this issue as a malaise. It is also my intention to express in some very personal way my concerns about abortion-on-demand's long-term effect.

It is an atypical format, I know. Writing about myself — as the subject. Telling what it's like to write a poem — the process; talking about what the poem means to me — the producer; and the product. It is an audacious mode of inquiry, to be sure. And yet, I proceed wholeheartedly, confidently, even boldly, with the advice of Edgar Allan Poe and Henry David Thoreau rallying me. Bold and brazen as I might appear, as a writer who is *alive*, I offer a look at the process and the product from the inside-out, or from the "other" side. It's almost as if the voice of Edgar Allan Poe urges me forward. In his essay on "The Philosophy of Composition," he said, "[H]ow interesting a magazine paper might be written by any author who would — that is to say who could — detail, step by step, the processes by which any one of his compositions attained his ultimate point of completion"[1] (and so on, for a *very* full 19th century paragraph). I do not intend to reveal all the step-by-step decisions and "machinations" of my creative process for the poems that follow, but I will discuss some. More importantly, I think, I will reveal more about *how* I think and *what* I think about this topic of abortion. To some readers I might really be pushing the standards of boldness and brazenness now, and perhaps I am, but I also feel urged on by Henry David Thoreau. Remembered best and most for writing about himself and what he thought, often just about himself, Thoreau reasoned in *Walden*, "I should not talk so much about myself if there were any body else who I knew as well."[2] It seems rather hard to argue with that.

Thus, I should proceed, confidently and boldly, and yet because I am the only creature of my kind represented in this volume — that is, I'm a poet, an artist... among theologians, philosophers, physicians, lawyers, scientists, historians, who all speak a different language from me, I am perhaps not quite so confident. But I *am* bold, because the words of my mentor, now friend, Neil Postman, ring in my ears. He said, "[A]rt is much more than a historical artifact. To have meaning for us, it must connect with those levels of feeling that are in fact not expressible in discursive language."[3] That, I think, is why I'm "here" ... to offer an alternative to the otherwise purely discursive expressions in this volume. That is, what *I* have to say about the topic of abortion I "say" in a truly divergent way.

Other writers in a volume such as this may address the topic in ways like this, for example:

In 1979 there were 82,788 abortions in West Germany, in a population of 60 million. This works out roughly to an abortion for every 723 people. In 1980 there were almost 1.3 million abortions in the U.S. in a population of 226 million. This works out roughly to an abortion for every 173 people. Comparing these numbers one can see that the

West German rate per population is less than one-fourth the American rate.[4]

In fact, that was stated exactly that way at last year's conference at Fordham University by John J. Hunt. And "what" he said is *very* important.

It is, however, an extreme way of discoursing, using statistics, just as I no doubt offer an opposite extreme by using poetry. And yet Hunt tells the reader something I can't, while I, through poetry, tell the reader something Hunt can't. Perhaps more importantly, I can make the reader "feel" something about abortion that he can't. He could maybe make the reader feel something that I can't, but I don't think that's likely. For, as I perhaps oversimplify in my creative writing classes in making the distinctions between prose and poetry: I say prose is about "knowing," poetry is about "feeling"; prose appeals to the "rational," poetry to the "emotional." Pure and oversimple.

To be sure, I do heed Paul's admonition, "not to think more highly of myself than I ought,"[5] but I likewise heed Walker Percy's injunction that "writers are in the front line of sensibility, like the canaries miners take down in the shaft to test the air."[6] That should be a familiar scenario: the canaries are to "squawk" — "tweet"? — when things get bad. If things get worse, the canaries die; if things keep getting worse, and are ignored, then the miners die.

It *is* an interesting analogy, and if I extended it, I could come up with an explanation for why so many poets commit suicide. But that's from a different paper and a different time....

For now, though, I am prepared to divulge the wherewithal of how I use poetic language to "discourse" upon this topic of abortion. And so, the first poem I present is "the CICATRIX."

the CICATRIX

he said
no one would ever know

that
it's like having your appendix
or your tonsils
removed
or maybe even a simple extraction

he said
women have done it
for years
with coat hangers
knitting needles and sometimes even
crochet hooks

that
it's not any
really big deal;
i wouldn't even have
to leave
the state

he said
that there wouldn't be a mark
no telltale after effects
at all
that
it'd only be a pin
prick

said he[7]

   The form and structure of this poem is simple and
straightforward, as most poems seem to be presented,
particularly mine. And because of that, its accessibility is,
I think, perhaps one of its strengths. The reader gains
entrance to this poem and its "issue" rather quickly and
easily. The "experience" in this poem is related in

retrospect by a nameless, faceless, but universal female narrator. Her recounting the experience is brief, terse, almost clinical, possibly like the event itself.

The very fact that the "event" is easily, candidly discussed through such day-in-day-out details, simple outpatient procedures, and cold, clinical terms reveals society's and this man's attitude toward abortion: it's something that can be fixed, quickly, easily, no-muss-no-fuss. That's a fact which Pope John Paul II bemoans in his *Gospel of Life*: that abortion "is an idea of society excessively concerned with efficiency."[8] The Pope's pronouncement actually aligns itself not too coincidentally with one of the themes in Postman's *Technopoly*, his work I quoted from earlier. And that's the point of this poem: the situation can so easily be dispensed with, as if a man closing his lid over the gleam in his eye is employing a form of contraception.

In the poem the limited use of traditional literary devices and few vivid images is intentional, to underscore and reinforce the narrator's attempt to objectify her experience, to depersonalize it if possible. And yet as Shakespeare's tragic heroine Gertrude[9] observes that her alter ego doth protest too much, so too does this "heroine" objectify too much, revealing down to her very core the searing subjectivity of her "time." The very reversal of the speech tag in the last line of the poem not only turns the beginning and ending ironically into a palindrome, but especially allows, at last, the persona to evince finally a twinge of her remorse, disgust, even anger.

The next to last stanza of the poem, where the narrator's doubt and disgust seems to reach fulfillment, reveals an ambiguity, with "pin" and "prick" placed on separate lines without hyphenation. This typographical placement allows the persona to turn the male's advice to her on himself as she divulges aspects not just about his personality but perhaps his anatomy as well.

I wrote this poem in 1976, and I think it reflects my then naive but growing concerns about abortion. Like many things in life, my awareness of the ramifications of abortion did not spring forth fully headed and maturely developed. Instead it has been a gradual process, a continuous journey, including this conference. And so I mark this early, concise, almost didactic effort, as evidence of me as least "listening" to a voice that could tell me what I was thinking and trying to know, about myself. That's a curious process, I know, but for "outsiders" to best understand that, I defer to Robert Frost's thoughts on this idea. He said, "For me the initial delight in writing a poem, is discovering something I knew, but didn't know that I knew before I wrote the poem."

Thus, what I think *I* came to know and realize was that I was thinking and feeling that there was a very basic conflict going on at that time in society, as typified between my "it's-no-big-deal" male and my "it's-my-body, God-what-am-I-doing" female. And so to illustrate that, the poem has a very physical, external focus to it.

(Some time ago I talked with a college girlfriend of mine, who had an abortion instead of giving birth to a fourth child, because it would have complicated hers and her husband's professional lives. They felt that three children were enough; he, in fact, insisted she get the abortion, but wouldn't go with her. So she took a "personal" day at work, went in alone, and came home late that afternoon. But her husband didn't even ask her about it, how she felt, etc., nothing, ... until days later, when he rather offhandedly asked her how it "went." To her grave, though, she said, she will wonder if that would have been her daughter; her other children are all sons. I could respond in many ways to this personal anecdote, but I will here simply note that Aristotle is purported to have said, "Art imitates life." But I, on many occasions, suggest that "Life imitates art.")

This "anecdote," as well as the poem "the CICATRIX,"

puts me in the mind of something else John Paul II deplores: "[G]rave and disturbing is the fact that the conscience itself, darkened as it were by such widespread conditioning, is finding it increasingly difficult to distinguish between good and evil in what concerns the basic value of human life."[10]   Whether I apply the Pontiff's remarks to the poem "the CICATRIX" or to the anecdote of my college girlfriend, I cannot but *have* to see how true and real Pope John Paul's concerns are: for either the "life" in a poem, or the "life" in a life.

Lastly about the poem is the title. Denotatively, "cicatrix" is a botanical term, referring to a scar left where a leaf or branch was severed. Anatomically, it refers to scar tissue, especially connective tissue on a healing wound. Of course, *I* intend graver implications. I started by capitalizing the entire term, for emphasis; and by using a term that ends with a "t-r-i-x" suffix I intend also to bring to mind other terms used today to equalize women's roles and capabilities: aviatrix, executrix, directrix, and so on. And naturally I intend connotations far beyond mere dictionary associations; that's why I juxtaposed the term with this woman: so that she comes to be identified symbolically as *the* FEMALE SCAR. The wound may go away, but not the remembrance of it, just as with my old college girlfriend.

Before I attend to the next poem I would like to point out that my comments and discussion of my poems is not in any way meant to be exhaustive nor all-inclusive; on the contrary, what I do say can only be representative of much more that I could say. What I'm trying to briefly address then are those aspects particularly germane and illustrative of why we all are even at this conference and for what all else it is we believe in the rest of the year.

And so, on to the next poem.

Dead in the Water

My anchor's umbilicus severed
I float
(brought about to be
by coming)
adrift
foetus-like

while my ship-to-shore
transmits no more.

Cast off
, or about to be
cast out
, I await the salt seas' shudder

to be engulfed;
I gulp --

       death by strangulation
or by asphyxiation
no, by drown-ing
supposedly the worst of ways
to go -- so
as sea billows roll
awash, I breathe such thick
air? ... gag -- gu - guhg

So much for sailing!
in the amniotic sea

I, suspended
  colloidal-like,
(should have kept clear of
the debris at sea:
flotsam, jetsam, & jism)
          thus
am about to be: precipitated.
But the catalyst?

The salt sea waves surge, froth,

submerge,
rush o'er
me -- I khack ... xxxch
guggle -- guggle -- gugguggug
guch-uh -- guck
guck, guck, cuck, cuck, cux
x -- x -- x -- kt-kt....k.

Death in a puddle:
98.6° bathwater

and me. Swell,

now I'll never get to suck
at the milky fount of

amnesia.[11]

This poems rather demands more, of the reader, and the writer. For me the writer, I was challenged to penetrate the persona of the narrator, at once more anonymous and yet more universal, I think. Or to be more to the point, the persona penetrated me, permeated me in essence, so that I could propound those series of onomatopoeic and gustatory images. I literally went through the choking, coughing, gagging spasms of the "victim" to sense what I could figuratively replicate. I used my phonetic and phonemic background as a linguist to supplement and echo throughout the poem the various and multiple voiced and voiceless stops, especially in the velar and alveolar regions of the articulatory apparatus: "anchor's," "umbilicus," "cast off," "cast out," "strangulation," "engulfed," "surge," "submerge," "suck," "thick," "milky," and "gulp." These I used to emulate and underscore the tension of the "guggle--guggle--gugguggug" passages. The repetition was intentional, if not devious. No, call it "subliminal." But if, as in this one technical instance, the poem is more demanding and challenging for me, as writer, it is also more rewarding. As I hope it can be for the reader, on both counts.

As a poem, this is a more sophisticated and complex effort than was "the CICATRIX," but then "Dead in the Water" is also probably less accessible for the reader. And yet the readers too can have their rewards, because I have placed clues within the text. For example, the phrase "about to be" appears three times. This persona *is* "about to be," but something happens, some catastrophe: a saline solution is injected into "the amniotic sea," and some readers no doubt know far better than I the horrific results that follow. Clinically, they may know better than I, but aesthetically I have my suspicions... as I have attempted to demonstrate.

I also used more figures of speech to make my point in this poem: alliteration, allusions, metaphors, especially in extending them into an analogy, and some irony. Perhaps most revealing and rewarding for me, as poet, were specific word choices. Two in particular are: "amniotic" and "amnesia." Though similar in form, they are different in origin. Today "amniotic" biologically means "a watery fluid in which the embryo of a mammal, bird, or reptile is suspended."[12] But "amniotic" has evolved from the Greek "amnion: a sacrificial plate to hold a victim's blood, during a sacrifice."[13] That is a crucial point to consider: my using of that term ... in this poem ... about this topic.

The other word, "amnesia," much more familiar, has also evolved from the Greek: *a (not)* and *mnesthai (to remember)*.[14] It is the last word of the poem, with its own line and its own stanza. Solitary. It's left there alone, for emphasis.

Its use is meant to be ironic, even tragic, because I project, at the end of the poem, that this persona, this person, and millions of others, will never drink what will help those who *were* born to forget: being born. Therefore, because this persona was not born, this "victim" will always remember *not* being born.

I wrote this poem in 1982, shortly after my son's adoption, and it displays more thought and concern in a slightly global way and in certainly a more visceral, personal way.

The poem reflects too from that time my growing concern and more mature understanding of how abortion affects the individual "soul." I admit that only as far as a poet can go do I feel as if I myself understand the soul. But I am alert enough to rely upon what others more knowledgeable than I have to say about this matter. Again I turn to the Pontiff for insight and wisdom here. He said,

After all, life on earth is not an "ultimate" but a "penultimate" reality; even so, it remains a *sacred reality* entrusted to us, to be preserved with a sense of responsibility and brought to perfection in love and the gift of ourselves to God and to our brothers and sisters.[15]

Maybe that's what I was getting at in writing this poem then; as for now, I sense that what this persona laments is those missed opportunities: to live, for God and for brothers and sisters, literal and figurative ones.

The supreme irony in the poem, for me, is that as civilization seems closer than ever to the pinnacle of medical technology, society may actually be approaching an abyss instead. Technology enables a woman to abort a child so relatively pain-free, to herself, with a saline injection. Pure and simple.

(I have a poster on my office door at the college where I teach, of a baby girl aborted at twenty-two weeks by just such a simple saline injection. It is not a pretty sight. And it is not for the faint hearted, as generations of my students can attest.)

Walker Percy, not just a novelist but also a physician, had similar thoughts on medical technology and technology in general. He said, "You don't have to be a sage or a prophet to point out the fact that the 20th century, which should have been the greatest triumph of all time — the triumph of science, technology, consumership — has [instead] been the most murderous century in all of history."[16]

Those very same thoughts and ideas Pope John Paul II, himself a man greatly admired by Percy, also addressed and articulated. As recently as this spring the Pontiff stated, "The twentieth century will have been an era of massive attacks on life, an endless series of wars and a continual taking of innocent human life."[17] In the early 80's that is what I sensed was happening wholesale, thus the emphasis of my poem "Dead in the Water" and thus the urgent need I sensed for a poem to intensely, if not literally, hit at the viscera of the reader, especially since appeals to the heart and head seemed to be futile.

A decade later I was taking my poetry in different directions and using different personae, but I returned occasionally to the topic of abortion, as I still do. In the next poem, written in 1992, I was using a very specific persona for a sequence of poems I call "femme fatalities 14." The voice of that persona is Mary, the Mother of Jesus. In the next poem, "femme fatalities: 14.h," she is the narrator.

femme fatalities: 14.h

if he came to me today
how he did so long ago
unannounced

to pronounce
The impending conception
I would instead
be expected
in this day and age
to scream "RAPE!"

... would the painters
then portray

me
for ever after
locked in some dyspassionate
struggle
with my Gabriel-like assailant,
thus:

in full grapple his
knife'd
be at my throat
with my blue sweat-
shirt
hiked up half off of
my head,
my panicking stick-fingers

groping to gouge his eyes (as
    instructed in my
    'Attack-the-Attacker Seminar')

but because the illustrators
are always male
from their perspective

they'd detail
how his celestial knee
deflects my desperate would-be
kick into
his sacred, sanctimonious
crotch

or,
probably they would
picture me
as taking it --
lying down

passive
submissive
even introspective, pondering

in my heart

> "Why me, Lord?"
> praying just to
> survive
> the immaculate violation
> so that
> early in the term then, I'd simply
> abort Him
>
> go for counseling, and
> get on with
> *my* life
> and never after think twice forever
>
> how I would save my son
> from the Cross
>
> what a loss[18]

In many ways, this might be the most divergent of the four poems in this paper, and it might just be the most disconcerting too, because I give voice to a *persona* who typically in art is just seen and not heard: for she is Mary, the Mother of Jesus.

To give voice to such a *persona* can be a stretch, for both the reader and writer. But as a poet and a practicing Believer, I have been indoctrinated to listen for the still, small, quiet voice. And not just listen but *hear* what that voice has to say.

And so I make demands upon the reader to put aside the usual expectations of what a "poem" is like and to put aside the notion of who can speak in a poem. What I'm asking the readers to do is, to paraphrase Samuel Taylor Coleridge, "willingly suspend their disbelief,"[19] and listen to what this fictional Mary has to say.

When we listen to her, what do we hear?

What I have provided is actually a contemporary verbal version of what painters have longed to capture on canvas for centuries: the Holy Spirit visiting the Virgin Mary and placing within her the seed that will enable her to give birth to the Son of God. That is what is happening in this poem, but in very late 20th century terms.

Times have changed, not just for a Baroque, or Renaissance, or Neo-Classic Mary, but for one living in a Post-Modern Era. What *are* her responsibilities, if she is a truly modern woman...? She tells us. And we learn of the consequences, for her, and for us.

No doubt Mary did wonder about ways to save her son from the Cross; after all, she was only human, and she was a mother. We ought never to discount that. But the resulting loss ... how to gauge, how to measure what the world would have missed... that is incalculable.

And yet, today the world out-Herods Herod. Thus, what is the pressure today for modern virgins, former and otherwise, to ponder in their hearts: "Why me, God?" Who's to tell them what to do? ... How are they to know in this country how to act, how to choose ... and for whom?

When did it all start, this loss of the sacredness of life, this lost *sacred reality*, as Pope John Paul II referred to it? I have my ideas, and so does Walker Percy. He was asked by an interviewer if he believed that we are living in "the century of death." Percy responded:

I guess I do. I have referred to that in past books and essays. In *The Thanatos Syndrome*, a character states the death century began with the battle of Somme and Verdun, where in two months two million young men were killed — all from the same civilization of Western Christendom. At the end of these two horrendous battles, I think the lines changed a few hundred yards. That's as good a place as any to begin this dreadful post-modern age, this century of death.[20]

And in that war, twenty million people were killed. But in World War II between forty and fifty million were killed. Since World War II, however, more babies have been aborted than human beings were killed in all of World War I, and I am told that before this century is out abortions in this country alone may eclipse the total souls killed in all of World War II. That indeed is something to consider.... By the way, poets occasionally use statistics. But mostly poets use poems, and so I turn now to the last poem. It's titled and begins

in the Temple of the Lord I'm

committing in cold blood because
of you and your
fucking intrusive self violating
all I'd ever sortuv learned
in Sunday School, yes, even
no, especially that Golden Memory
verse --

What are the Wages of Love?

-- murder;
that's what it's come
to be
cause you've made this temple of the Lord
into an outhouse
for your excrement

the only birth you'll ever know
anything about: you squat

and you laugh,
you think you're giving birth
in your parody of me
(in your oh-so manly way),
to your daily shit
and thus trespass against me,
encasing your seed

you Shit, expecting me
instead of
me expecting

oh, if only "if" my middle

name was Judith

and yours
first *and* last was Holofernes
why then your head'd be
at my belt instead

but, it's not

so that
the essence of us is flushed
out of me
down my so-called drain

flotsams, flow
-ing beneath bridges never been crossed
nor will be

let alone
ever will need to be burned,
under which specimens of life (the fruit
of our loins
from that one-night covenant) pass-
over the Spillway of Love toward

the Delta of my Miasma
where icebergs enshrine the fetal
futilities (the ark of
our selves, yes, the supposéd Spirit within)
and so adrift,
awash
unto the deadliest of Bering Straits,
coolly certain

-- So, ... --
it is just as my old Sunday School teacher
once upon a time catechized me

-- the Gift of Love Is

"For the wages of sin is death,
but the gift of God is eternal life."   Romans 6:23[21]

This too is not a very easy poem. For the reader, or the writer. It's still not easy for *me* to read, even though I wrote it, although the writing was more like taking dictation. Really.

The speaker, "narrator," here too is a definite persona; her name is Alice Brooks-Smith. She's a fictional voice I've sort of "created," maybe "listened to" is more to the point. She has a definite voice, definite opinions, and a definite style. I mean, she's me, and she's not me ... as much as any fictional character in a novel or short story is the same for its author.

This poem of the four is, in many ways, the most demanding and most strident, while in most respects it is also the least accessible, perhaps because of the definite persona. Her speaking "style" reveals fractured syntax, minimal punctuation, line and stanza breaks between words and phrases, and she relies heavily upon symbols and stockpiled imagery, "superpositioned," as Ezra Pound would describe it; and literary, religious, and historical allusions abound.

It is a dense piece. Taken together, these devices and strategies all force the reader to keep up or catch up. But ideally not give up.

For example, the many scatological references that become distorted and perverted symbols can be very offputting, even unsettling, but that's the point, *I* think. As I tell my linguistics students, on what has become historically known as "Dirty Word Day," swear words don't carry meaning; they convey emotion. They hit at a very low common denominator, the absolute physical nadir of human experience, *and* expression, for shock effect. That the "male" in this poem would parody the birth experience with the elimination of his solid waste is a frightening perversion indeed. And yet isn't that what a specific sector of society sees an aborted baby as — human waste? "That" indeed is something to think about....

The stockpiled, "superpositioned" images in the seventeen lines from "flotsams, flow" to "coolly certain" combine and range from multiple biblical images and ideas to the female anatomy to geographical locations to homely homilies and to current practices for waste removal. It *is* a bit much, I agree, but the density and complexity compounds the urgency and the plight of this woman's situation. And her "to be aborted" child.

Allusions point especially to the Bible, to specific passages in the scripture: in Romans, the Lord's Prayer, and to Bible stories, especially ones containing arks (at least three different ark stories are alluded to). The specific historical allusion could bring to mind the tale of Judith severing the head of Holofernes,[22] the man who murdered her son; and it is Holofernes' decapitated head Judith attached to her belt as a gruesome reminder of her son's death, as a warning, and as a testament to her vengeant power. That Alice wants to wear this male's head on her belt reveals her knowing association of the heinous deed she's about to commit and what course of action she considers "appropriate" following the murder of her child, inside herself, "in the Temple of the Lord" that she's otherwise been instructed to keep holy and upright.

That's part of the irony of this poem. Even Alice seems convinced, almost, so far, to commit this "crime," as enjoined by her male counterpart. To me this "situation" seems so endemic in our society today, a place where, as observed by Pope John Paul II, there is "the tendency, ever more widely shared, to interpret ... crimes against life as legitimate expressions of individual freedom, to be acknowledged and protected as actual right."[23] This tendency leads to our "facing what can be called a 'structure of sin' which opposes human life not yet born."[24] These quotes should remind the reader of the Pontiff's earlier observation about the "darkened conscience" that finds it increasingly difficult to distinguish between good and evil, especially concerning the basic value of human life.[25] That is certainly the case in this poem. And just as importantly, it is not just the "about to be aborted" child whose life is going to be trampled.

I could continue discussing in more detail the specific aspects that make this poem so disturbing. I hope it's disturbing. But I would prefer to reveal what *my* voice says: that people today *must* be confronted with the Truth of this issue in a straight-up, no-holds-barred, in-your-face fashion.

I wrote this poem about a year ago, and I think it indicates, clearly, how I feel more and more strongly that I as artist must stand up and be counted and must make myself heard. My motives in this poem, quite frankly, are to horrify people. And yet I'm afraid, as Walker Percy said, "The twentieth century might be described as a century of horror in which no one is horrified."[26] No, I take exception with Percy. Some *one is* horrified. Me. I am often horrified by those who are *not* horrified at what takes place, every day, and every day, and every day, across this "Great Land of Ours."

And so, to combat it, as much as I can, as often as I can, whenever I can, I make the absolute most of my beliefs and attempt to instruct and model them practically and aesthetically. In situations like this, with readers of a volume like this one, I think I can be and have been successful, by appealing to the shared and granted sensibilities, humanity, emotions, reason, intellect, even to the souls of such like-minded readers.

But in some situations, with some people, none of those appeals succeed. And it is at those times, with my back to the wall, when I feel cornered by the foes of woe who would wail and assail me, and when I've exhausted the limits of empirical evidence for defending my position on this issue, then I rely upon my two irrefutable, undeniable, and indefatigable reasons for being wholeheartedly, wholesale against abortion: I refer to my two adopted children, Zach and Allie, both of whose fourteen-year-old biological mothers made the only true and real Pro-Choice: those young girls chose to give life to my children ... by giving Zach and Allie birth and by giving them to my wife and me. Therefore both of my children enjoy the Right to *LIVE*.

Originally, that was to be my clincher, my emphatic conclusion to this paper. But in keeping with the spirit of my "poetic" presentation and with further reliance upon my sources, I would like to defer one last time to the words of our Pontiff and appropriately conclude with them instead. The poetic entreaty that ended his encyclical *The Gospel of Life* is...

> O Mary,
> bright dawn of the new world,
> Mother of the living,
> to you do we entrust the *cause of life*:
> Look down, O Mother,
> upon the vast numbers
> of babies not allowed to be born,
> of the poor whose lives are made difficult,
> of men and women
> who are victims of brutal violence,
> of the elderly and the sick killed
> by indifference or out of misguided mercy.
> Grant that all who believe in your Son
> may *proclaim the Gospel of life*
> with honesty and love
> to the people of our time.
> Obtain for them the grace
> to *accept that Gospel*
> as a gift ever new,
> the joy of *celebrating* it with gratitude
> throughout their lives
> and the courage to *bear witness to it*
> resolutely, in order to build,
> together with all people of good will,

the civilization of truth and love,
to the praise and glory of God,
the Creator and lover of life.

Given in Rome, at Saint Peter's on 25 March, the Solemnity of the Annunciation of the Lord, in the year 1995, the seventeenth of my Pontificate ... Joannes Paulus II.[27]

NOTES

1. Edgar Allan Poe, "Philosophy of Composition" in *Selected Poetry and Prose of Poe*, ed. T. O. Mabbott (New York: The Modern Library, 1951) 364-65.

2. Henry David Thoreau, *Walden and Civil Disobedience*, ed. Owen Thomas (New York: W. W. Norton and Co., 1966) 1.

3. Neil Postman, *Technopoly* (New York: Vintage, 1992) 196.

4. John J. Hunt, "A Tale of Two Countries: German and American Attitudes Toward Abortion Since World War II" in *Life and Learning IV: Proceedings of the Fourth University Faculty for Life Conference*, ed. Joseph W. Koterski, S.J. (Washington, D.C.: University Faculty for Life, 1995) 128.

5. Romans 12[3]: "not to think *of himself* more highly than he ought to think; but to think soberly."

6. *More Conversations with Walker Percy*, ed. Jervis A. Lawson and Victor A. Kramer (Jackson: Univ. Press of Mississippi, 1993) 61.

7. Reprinted with permission from *Anemone* 3/2 (Winter 1987) 16.

8. Pope John Paul II, *The Gospel of Life [Evangelium Vitae]* #12.

9. "The lady doth protest too much, methinks." William Shakespeare, *Hamlet* III, ii, 242.

10. John Paul II, *The Gospel of Life* #4.

11. From an unpublished manuscript of poems entitled *About Women*.

12. *The American Heritage Dictionary* (New York: American Heritage, 1969) 43.

13. Ibid.

14. Ibid.

15. John Paul II, *The Gospel of Life* #2.

16. Quoted in Lawson and Kramer 242.

17. John Paul II, *The Gospel of Life* #17.

18. Reprinted with permission from *Second Glance* 2 (Spring 1994) 9.

19. "That willing suspension of disbelief for the moment, which constitutes poetic faith." Samuel Taylor Coleridge, *Biographia Literaria*, Chapter XIV (London: George Bell and Sons, 1898) 145.

20. Quoted in Lawson and Kramer 183.

21. From an uncompleted manuscript of poems, currently titled *The Collected Poems of Alice Brooks-Smith*, edited by Carl Winderl.

22. See the book of "Judith."

23. John Paul II, *The Gospel of Life*, #18.

24. Ibid. #59.

25. Ibid. #4.

26. Quote in Lawson and Kramer 200.

27. John Paul II, *The Gospel of Life* #105.

> When Judge Joseph W. Moylan of Omaha, Nebraska, was asked to approve a teenager's request to waive the requirement that she seek her parents' approval for abortion, he faced a crisis of conscience. Unable to adhere to the law of the state, the 61-year-old judge with more than two decades on the bench, resigned saying, "I simply cannot enter an order authorizing one human life to put to death another totally innocent human being.... I am reminded of Lincoln's statement: 'No law can give me the right to do what is wrong' (from *Omaha World Herald*, 10/8/94).

NO LAW CAN GIVE ME THE RIGHT TO DO WHAT IS WRONG

Judge Joseph W. Moylan

First of all, I want to thank University Faculty for Life for the honor of being here today to speak about my resignation. Let me begin by repeating a true story told by Charles Rice, a University of Notre Dame law professor:

On October 26, 1991, Alan Hayat, M.D., performed an abortion on twenty-year-old Rosa Rodriguez in his Manhattan clinic. He charged her fifteen hundred dollars. Doctor Hayat had estimated that she was between the twelfth and sixteenth week of pregnancy. In fact, she was between thirty-two and thirty-four weeks. New York law permits abortion after the twenty-fourth week only to preserve the mother's life. When Miss Rodriguez awoke from the anesthetic, Dr. Hayat told her the abortion was incomplete and advised her to go home and return to him the next day. That night, however, she delivered a live baby girl, Ana Rosa Rodriguez, whose right arm had been severed below her shoulder. The New York State Department of Health had been investigating complaints against Dr. Hayat for several years. After the Rodriguez case hit the papers, seven other women came forward to accuse him of botching abortions he had performed on them. The Department then moved to revoke his medical license.

Ana Rosa's severed arm triggered the outcry that cost Dr. Hayat his license. If he had done his job skillfully — if he had killed the child instead of mutilating her — the case never would have come to public notice. The outpouring of indignation and sympathy for Ana Rosa after her birth, however, could not change the reality that, in public opinion as in law, she was regarded before her birth as less than human. She lacked even protections against cruelty afforded by the law to animals. In the usual abortion procedure, as in the attempt on her life, the living child is torn limb from limb, which procedure could mean a jail term if it were inflicted on a dog or cat.

There is a federal law that if you move, damage, or destroy an eagle's egg or nest, you can be subject to a $5000 fine or a year in prison, but there is no penalty for putting to death a human in the womb.

In 1991 Nebraska passed what is called a Parental Notification Abortion Law. By this law, if a pregnant teenager (seventeen or younger) wants to have an abortion, she has to notify a parent. The law also provides that if she does not want to do this, she can file a petition in court to get a hearing. That sounded good when first introduced. In fact, I think judges were quite lax in not keeping up on this bill before it got passed. When this bill, taken from a Minnesota law, did get passed, it stated that at the hearing the pregnant minor is entitled to have an attorney appointed for her, and even a guardian *ad litem*. There is nobody on the other side, unless a judge takes it on himself. Now I know of no other case that is like that, where it is truly one-sided. If after that one-sided hearing, the judge finds that the girl is mature and can give an informed consent, then the judge is *required* to authorize the abortion physician to perform the abortion. That was quite unsettling to a lot of judges. It looks like, and I still believe, that a judge so acting would be a direct material participant, and the only thing that occurred to me is that it is like putting a contract out on somebody. You are just as guilty as if you did the actual killing. The abortion could not be performed unless I signed the order. I thought that was especially ironic for me. In Juvenile Court for twenty-one years I had been assigned to protect young children and infants from abuse and neglect, and now I was being called upon to inflict the ultimate abuse. I knew, of course, that abortion was wrong, but I felt I needed to know more.

Without much effort I found that with *Roe v Wade* the Supreme Court, for the second time in history, had declared a whole class of people not protected by the Constitution. The other time, of course, was 1858 in the *Dred Scott* decision when black people were declared non-persons and thus were not included in the constitutional protection of liberty. I also learned, in regard to the development of the child in the womb, that within three weeks there is a heartbeat, within five weeks there are brain waves, and within eight weeks all the vital organs are in place and functioning. In addition, I found out that the infant can feel pain, which surprised me. Then I read that doctors sometimes perform operations on infants in the womb, and when they do that, they anesthetize that infant because of the pain. And yet, of course, in abortion they don't anesthetize them. They don't want to recognize, I guess, that the child is human, that it can feel pain. My reading led me to realize that the infant is not a part of the mother; oftentimes it has a different blood type, and it has a separate heartbeat and has been destined naturally to live outside of the mother's womb.

Now in regard to the procedures used in abortion, there are approximately seven of those. In the suction aspiration method, the abortionist inserts a plastic hollow tube into the dilated uterus. The tube is connected to a powerful suction apparatus, and the suction tears the baby's body into pieces. The dilation and curettage method is similar to the suction procedure: a tiny hoe-like instrument is inserted into the uterus, and with this the abortionist cuts the baby into pieces and scrapes him or her into a basin. In the dilation and evacuation method, used after twelve weeks, the abortionist inserts an instrument into the uterus, seizes a leg or other body part, and with a twisting motion tears it from the baby's body. Often the skull must be crushed in order to remove it from the womb. All the other methods, of course, are similar. Ultimately I decided that I could not go along with this law.

It was two years before I was assigned one of these cases. The reason was that most pregnant minors do tell their parents, and in fact many of the parents encourage the abortion. Also, some minors use fake ID's and abortion clinic workers don't question them. Another reason is that the judges are picked at random and do not take their turn, so all the judges' names are in a hat, so to speak, and when a case is filed, they pick one out. One judge could get five cases while another judge gets none. I understood that I was the last judge to get one. In our city there are approximately fifteen district judges and two juvenile judges who can handle this type of case. Anyway, I got a call from the clerk of the District Court one day saying I was assigned one of these cases, and I asked her if there were any way out of it. She said she didn't know but would check on it. In the meantime I called my pastor, Father Robert Gass, and told him the problem and my thoughts about it. He totally agreed with me. When the clerk called back saying the case was mine, I said, "Well, I'm going to resign. I can't take this case."

The problem is, I took an oath to uphold the laws of the State of Nebraska. There is also a canon in the Code of Judicial Ethics that you have to take any case assigned to you unless there's an excuse named in it, like personal involvement in the case, financial involvement, a relative, or something similar.

I called my wife. We had talked about this for two

years, and she agreed with me. She said I should wait a day before turning in my resignation. I did that and by the next morning the word has gotten around. Five or six judges called me and really urged me not to do this. The reason most of them gave was that it is really the girl's decision. I answered that they can't have the abortion unless I authorize the physician to perform it. One said he had resolved it morally; I didn't ask him how. Another judge, who had been there as long as I had, said he couldn't afford to resign. All through these two years a scriptural phrase kept coming back to me, "What does it profit a man to gain the whole world...?" I prepared and sent the following letter to the Chief Justice of the Supreme Court of Nebraska:

Dear Justice Hastings,
    I was assigned a matter today concerning a hearing pursuant to Section 71-6903, which I declined. In reviewing the Abortion Parental Notification Law, I noticed that the definition of abortion is "an act, a procedure, producing the premature expulsion, removal, or termination of human life" (that's right in the definition, in the law) "within the womb of the pregnant woman." If, after a hearing, I find that the minor pregnant woman can give an informed consent, and is mature enough to undergo this procedure without notifying a parent, then I must enter an order authorizing the abortion physician to perform the abortion resulting in the death of the human life.
    I simply cannot enter an order authorizing one human life to put to death another totally innocent human life. I am reminded of Lincoln's statement, "No law can give me the right to do what is wrong."
    This is the first law I have encountered in twenty-one years in this position that I am unable to enforce. Since I took an oath to uphold the laws of Nebraska and cannot comply, I am resigning my position as a judge of the Separate Juvenile Court.

I had decided long before that if I did resign, I wanted to make it public and try to do something positive for the pro-life movement. So I was not going to do this quietly. I called a reporter for the *Omaha World Herald*, Mike Kelly, whom I had known years ago. He came up to my office and we spent about an hour together. He took a copy of the law and a copy of my resignation letter with him. I asked him not to have anything printed until the following evening because I wanted the Supreme Court Justice to get my letter before that. The following evening, a Friday evening, I was surprised when I got home to find that my resignation was the front-page headline story. This astonished me because the *Omaha World-Herald* is not pro-life. The next day there were two more articles; one was a discussion of my conversation with Mike Kelly in his regular daily column, and one of the things I said was that I believed that sometime we are going to have to appear before our final Judge and we're going to have to account for what we do. I said that there are a lot of things I wish I didn't have to account for, and I don't really care to add this to the list. He printed everything I said except for one sentence. I had said, "The procedures used in abortion are horrendous." I don't believe he took it out. I believe it was higher up. It occurred to me then, thinking about that, I never see any article in the secular press describing what goes on in abortions. At any rate, that was my resignation.

Many people have wondered what response I received. There are approximately 140 judges in Nebraska who have jurisdiction to hear this type of case. Now I put them on the spot. I knew that, and I didn't like to. A lot of them were friends. I didn't know what to do except this. I heard from two out of 140 judges. They were both out-state. One is not pro-life, I know, and the other one is. He called me and was really strongly supportive, but that was all the response from any judge anywhere. I did get a letter, which surprised me, from Lou McHardy, the Executive Director of the National Council of Juvenile and Family Court Judges in Reno, Nevada:

Dear Judge Moylan,

A colleague of mine, Jim Toner, directed my attention to the article about you in *Our Sunday Visitor*. I understand that you resigned from the bench rather than issue an order permitting a teenager to obtain an abortion. In my estimation you have responded faithfully to a higher call of morality and decency. Truly you fully deserve the salutation of "Your Honor." Most of us do not have the courage you demonstrated. I commend you and admire you and urge you to call upon me whenever you feel I may be of assistance. Trusting that Our Good Lord will bless you in many ways....

I received over a hundred phone calls and more than two hundred letters, all of them positive. Fifteen to twenty priests that I know mentioned my action in their sermons, and several ministers also did so. Reporters from religious magazines and newspapers and five Christian radio stations from different states called and interviewed me. *Our Sunday Visitor* had a full-page article and an editorial. *National Catholic Register*, *Celebrate Life* (American Life League's publication), *First Things*, and the HLI newsletter all published accounts of my resignation. The editor of *Human Life Review* called last year and asked me to write an article, which I did. It was printed in the fall issue. Recently, in May, an article appeared in *Citizen* magazine published by "Focus on the Family." There have been no interviews for secular magazines or for secular newspapers other than the *Omaha World Herald*. Several bishops were also supportive, including my own bishop, Archbishop Eldon Curtiss. The bishop of the Lincoln, Nebraska diocese, Bishop Bruskiewicz, wrote, "I am sure your action in resigning from the bench makes a stronger contribution than all of your other wonderful works and acts over the course of your judicial career." Father Val Peter, Director of BoysTown, sent a strong letter of support comparing me to St. Thomas More. I wrote back and said that I thought that was a little bit overdone. I said, He lost his head; I just lost my job. A Jesuit from Washington, Fr. Brian Van Hove, wrote, "It reminds me of all those Dutch physicians who refused to cooperate with the Nazi imposed sterilization laws during the occupation. Our century has not seen much good, but a few solitary witnesses always encourage the faint-hearted. "

A sampling of responses from lay people includes a note from a young Omaha man who wrote: "You have inspired me to become more active in the pro-life movement." A lady from Lincoln, Nebraska said, "I have a fourth grader who had to do an assignment at school, and he chose the article in *The World Herald* about you. A lady from Blair, Nebraska wrote that she was having a talk with her thirteen year old daughter on values and how important it is to act, knowing what is right. She picked up the evening paper, saw the headline, read the article regarding my resignation, and quoted it to her daughter as an example of what she was talking about. She said she wanted me to know how much it helped her to get her point across and what an impact it had on her child. A nun from Flint, Michigan wrote, "The Gospel is indeed radical, and God must be pleased." A teacher at a Catholic girls' school, and advisor to their Respect Life Club sent a letter, as did many of the students. One of the girl wrote, "I think it's great that a person in your position has some guts." Another interesting letter came from the founder of "International Cops for Christ" in New York City. He wrote, "I read about the courageous stand you took for the life of the innocent unborn. Thank you for doing this. It is an inspiration for all pro-lifers to see such resolve." He sent a booklet entitled "Bloodshed Touching Bloodshed" which he had written from the perspective of a law enforcement officer to educate other law enforcement officers about the pro-life issues. From a high school coach in Wisconsin I read, "I heard your story on WEMI concerning the stand you took. I have been teaching, coaching, and just plain serving in the community for twenty-two years, and I am always looking for role models. As an encouragement and credit to you, I plan to use your example in my senior health class when we get to the point of decision-making by using beliefs. I commend you on your strong stand." Another letter from a young man said, "I was unable to bring myself to commit to praying at one of the abortion mills, but after reading your article I am going to try."

One of the reasons the judges gave in *Roe v Wade* to justify their decision was that these unborn humans have *not yet reached the capability of meaningful life*. It is interesting — or tragic, I suppose, is the right word — that legislation introduced so far to legalize euthanasia states that it may be used when the patient is *no longer capable of meaningful life*. Now the words of the Hippocratic oath, recited by doctors since the fourth century B.C., are: "Thou shalt not give poison, thou shalt not procure abortion." These words, I believe, have now been changed. They had to be. Scientists and biologists agree that the baby in the womb is a human life from the moment of conception. The Declaration of Independence states that we are endowed by our Creator with unalienable rights to life and liberty. As Christians we believe that we are created in the image and likeness of God.

I'd like to close with this comment by Mother Teresa, which was cited in a brief in a case in this country:

America needs no words from me to see how your decision in *Roe v Wade* has deformed a great nation. The so-called right to abortion has pitted mothers against their children, and women against men. It has sown violence and discord at the heart of the most intimate human relationships. It has aggravated the derogation of the father's role in an increasingly fatherless society. It has portrayed the greatest of gifts, a child, as a competitor, an intrusion, and an inconvenience. It has nominally accorded mothers unfettered dominion over the independent lives of the physically dependent lives of their sons and daughters. Human rights are not a privilege conferred by government. They are every human being's entitlement by virtue of his humanity. The right to life does not depend and must not be declared to be contingent on the pleasure of anyone else, not even a parent or a sovereign.

ABORTION MALPRACTICE: EXPLORING THE SAFETY OF LEGAL ABORTION

Teresa Stanton Collett[1]

> "Prolife, your name's a lie,
> you don't care if women die."
> - Chant of Abortion Rights Activists[2]

Implicit in the chant of abortion rights activists is the argument that the legalization of abortion has converted what was once a terrifying dangerous experience at the hands of an unscrupulous amateur into a relatively risk-free medical procedure performed by caring physicians.[3] The success of this argument is evidenced by its inclusion in a dissenting opinion in *Webster v. Reproductive Health Services*.[4] Other commentators have carefully examined the argument that abortions were both numerous and dangerous prior to 1973, when the Supreme Court ruled that the states must permit abortions if necessary to preserve the health of the mother.[5] These commentators discovered that the numbers of pre-1973 deaths most often used by abortion rights activists are not credible, and are not relied upon in serious discussions, even by those who use them in political rhetoric.[6]

Part I of this article explores the second half of the abortion activists' argument; that legal abortions are relatively risk-free medical procedures performed by caring physicians. This contention is brought into question by newspaper accounts of abortion providers allegedly providing substandard medical care to women. The 1978 *Chicago Sun-Times* investigative series entitled "The Abortion Profiteers" is an example of such reports. Reported cases of abortion malpractice provide some evidence of the practices reported in the newspaper accounts.

Abortion is the most common surgical procedure performed in the United States by providers that remain virtually unregulated.[7] Even in the jurisdictions that appear to have laws that would mandate meaningful regulation, regulatory agencies have been slow to intervene. This is due in part to lack of funding and personnel,[8] in part to lack of political will,[9] and in part to the procedural protections afforded anyone determined to have violated the state regulatory scheme.[10]

In attempts to limit abortion providers' ability to profit from the taking of human life (both mother and child), Part II of this article suggests that medical malpractice may provide a meaningful supplement to regulation. Various legal theories that allow women to recover from the injuries received at the hands of the abortionist will be described, as well as the defenses most often employed by abortion providers. Particular litigation strategies and trial tactics of abortionists will be outlined, as well as the effects of these tactics upon women who sue.

Part III of this article will briefly suggest areas where research is needed in order to insure that women who are injured by abortions recover for those injuries. Scholars involved with University Faculty for Life can provide valuable assistance to the efforts of lawyers seeking to protect both mother and child from those who profit from abortions.[11]

I. INJURIES FROM LEGAL ABORTIONS

Sometimes spoken and sometimes not,[12] the initial premise of almost all advocates of abortion rights is that legalization of abortions results in safer medical procedures. Government statistics maintained by federal centers for disease control and prevention seemingly support this assumption.[13] Yet even some government officials question the validity of those statistics in light of the manner in which the information is gathered. The statistics reflecting deaths caused by abortion are compiled from death certificates issued by each state. Because those certificates are based upon the doctor's characterization of the cause of death, it is the individual provider who determines whether a death would be characterized as caused by abortion or some other medical procedure or complication.

The leading factors in death to due [sic] legal abortion include complications of anesthesia, hemorrhaging, infection, and amniotic embolism. Deaths from complications of anesthesia are sometimes deleted from mortality statistics, though common sense would say that the deaths were due to the abortion procedure if, but for undergoing the abortion, the woman would have lived.[14]

Both public officials and private physicians have been accused of deliberately altering medical records in order to avoid evidencing a causal connection between abortion and physical injuries or death.[15] Challenges to the reporting system have motivated a group of women Republican state lawmakers to create a "Contract with American Women" requiring the creation of a new federal abortion surveillance agency.[16]

These challenges often arise after public reports of misconduct or incompetence on the part of abortion providers. The 1978 *Chicago Sun-Times* series of newspaper articles is an example of reports motivating attempts to regulate abortion providers.[17]

1978 INVESTIGATIVE FINDINGS

On November 12, 1978, the *Chicago Sun-Times* began a series of in-depth articles reporting the results of a five-month investigation into what the paper characterized as "Chicago's thriving abortion business."[18] During the investigation, reporters and investigators worked in six clinics. The clinics were selected, in part, because they provided the greatest number of abortions in the area. Collectively the six clinics performed more than half of the

60,000 abortions provided in Illinois the previous year.[19] "In four of those clinics women's reproductive lives — indeed, their very lives — were endangered every day."[20] Abuses reported after the investigation included: 1) abortive procedures performed on women who were not pregnant[21]; 2) abortions performed by incompetent or unqualified individuals[22]; 3) abortions performed without anesthetic, or prior to anesthetic taking effect[23]; and 4) routine postoperative pathology reports ignored or not ordered. These practices resulted in women suffering postoperative infections and complications, including death in at least two cases.[24]

In addition to injuries suffered during abortions, it was reported that at least one abortionist refused to provide postoperative care for injuries suffered during the abortion, absent additional payment. The paper reports that one clinic offered discounts for abortions performed on Wednesdays. Instead of the usual $125.00, the clinic charged $110.00. However, based upon the experience of one patient, if a Wednesday abortion proved to be incomplete, the patient was required to pay an additional $25.00 in order to obtain follow-up treatment. If unable to make the additional payment, the patient would be told to leave the clinic without treatment. If she refused, the police were called to escort the "trespasser" away.[25]

Races to see who could perform the most abortions on a given day were reported. Not only did victory convey "bragging rights" as to speed and surgical prowess, but rapid abortions assured increased compensation since each doctor was paid according to the number of abortions performed.[26]

Other decisions reportedly driven by the economics of abortion practice include actions ranging from the seemingly petty, like the directive that recuperating patients not be allowed to have more than three cookies (in order to reduce clinic "cookie" expenses), to the far more ominous, such as the following statements reported from a staff meeting: "We have to sell abortions. We have to use all of the tactics we can because, just like my other business, we have competition. Now, we have to go by the rules, but rules have to be broken if we are gonna get things done."[27]

RECENT REPORTS OF ABORTION-RELATED INJURIES

In addition to the *Chicago Sun-Times* exposé, several cases of women injured by abortionists have received public attention.[28] In California, Dr. Leo Kenneally was suspended from the practice of medicine in 1995 after a five-year court battle over charges resulting from the death of three patients.[29]

Also in the news were stories about Dr. Thomas Tucker, who was found guilty of 32 counts involving falsified paper work and faulty procedures in his abortion clinics in Jackson, Mississippi.[30] Just the year before, local papers had published articles featuring Dr. Tucker's practice. These stories quoted Dr. Tucker's explanation of his choice to perform abortions. "It started out as a financial thing, but I got heavy into the [abortion rights] movement and realized there was a lot of need for physicians."[31]

More recently the case of Dr. David Benjamin received national attention when New York district attorneys persuaded a jury to convict Dr. Benjamin of second degree murder in the 1993 death of his patient after he attempted to perform a late-term abortion. At the time of the patient's death, Dr. Benjamin's medical license had been revoked, but he was allowed to practice while he appealed the board's decision.[32]

As a final example, Dr. Steven Brigham agreed to provide abortions in Florida after the murder of Dr. Britton. His hero status among abortion rights advocates was tarnished, however, by reports that he was under investigation for medical misconduct in five states.[33] Most recently Florida authorities suspended Dr. Brigham's medical license.[34]

II. MALPRACTICE CLAIMS FOR ABORTION-RELATED INJURIES

In *Roe v. Wade* the United States Supreme Court ruled that the U.S. Constitution limited the ability of states to intervene in the private decision-making of a woman and her doctor in deciding whether to terminate a pregnancy.[35] Until *Planned Parenthood v. Casey,*[36] the Court continually expanded this holding until it seemed that any regulation of abortion was invalid, even when an extensive record of misconduct by abortion providers existed, and the legislation was primarily designed to insure the physical safety of the mother. With *Casey*, the Court upheld Pennsylvania statutes that required abortion providers to give women specific information concerning the procedure at least 24-hours prior to the abortion.[37] This change in the Court's position on regulations governing abortion providers foretells increased regulation of clinics and abortionists.

Yet the mere existence of regulations is not enough. Several actions reported in the *Chicago Sun-Times* violated state and local regulations that were in effect at the time.[38] Yet subsequent events have revealed the inability of regulators to respond swiftly to the deceptive practices and threats to women's health reported in the exposé. In order for regulation to be effective, there have to be both the political will and the necessary government resources to enforce the law. Regulators argue that they rarely receive the support necessary to police this politically volatile industry.[39]

Medical malpractice claims by women who are injured during an abortion provide a mechanism supplementary to regulation. By recognizing and compensating women injured by abortion, courts require those who profit from the argument that abortion is simply another elective surgery to meet the standards that other providers of surgical procedures must meet. Abortion malpractice suits also reveal the economic motivation of many abortion providers, and the duplicity of those who seek to characterize all abortion providers as defenders of women's rights.[40]

CLAIMS THAT MAY ARISE FROM ABORTION MALPRACTICE

Women injured by abortion providers may seek compensation for those injuries through filing malpractice suits. The particular claims that may be asserted in such cases include negligence, failure to obtain informed consent to the abortion, battery, infliction of emotional distress, fraud or negligent misrepresentation, breach of contract, deceptive trade practices, and any statutory claims that may be created by state statutes. Each of these claims (or "causes of action") require the woman to establish specific acts of misconduct by the abortion providers, and that those acts were the legal cause ("proximate cause") of the injuries she seeks compensation for.

Negligence. In order to prevail on a claim of negligence the woman must establish four things: 1) the abortion provider owed her a duty to conform to a certain standard of conduct; 2) the provider failed to conform to the standard of conduct; 3) the failure was both the factual and legal cause of the woman's injuries; and 4) the injuries were of the type and extent that the law requires compensation for.[41] Failure to establish any one of these elements is fatal to the woman's claim.

In seeking to establish the first element, the woman rarely has to worry about whether the doctor owed her a duty. The law has long recognized that doctors owe patients a general duty to treat them in accordance with the standards observed by other doctors in good standing in the medical community.[42] However, when the woman sues the clinic or hospital in addition to the doctor, the existence of a duty can be a hotly disputed point. The clinic or hospital may claim that the doctor is an "independent contractor"[43] and that the clinic or hospital has no responsibility (and thus liability) for any actions of the doctor.

Separate from the question of whether a duty exists is the question of what the scope of that duty is. For example, while the agreement to provide an abortion creates a general duty to use all reasonable means to achieve that end, does it include a requirement that the abortionist forward all fetal tissue to a pathologist or laboratory to determine if the abortion has been successful? Does failure to do so create liability for injuries the woman suffers from the incomplete abortion?[44] This is an example of questions that arise in the context of satisfying the requirement that the woman show that the provider failed to meet the standard of care.

Expert testimony is usually required in order to establish what a reasonable doctor would do in the same or similar circumstances.[45] The expert must be able to discuss what is required in order to perform an abortion which is safe for the woman. While any physician probably could testify as to the textbook requirements of the abortion procedure, book knowledge is rarely sufficient to qualify. Instead most courts require a showing that the expert witness either has done extensive studies concerning the procedures as part of a scholarly endeavor, or that the doctor has actually performed abortions.[46] Absent such qualifications, the court will refuse to allow the doctor to testify on the grounds that he or she is not an expert. Since many prolife physicians have never performed an abortion, these doctors can not act as effective witnesses in abortion malpractice cases.

After the plaintiff has established that the defendants owed her a duty of care of a particular nature and scope, the woman must show that the provider failed to perform the duty. Often this is established through notations in the medical records, or the testimony of the provider or other witnesses to the abortion.

Next the woman must prove that the failure to perform the duty was the legal and factual case of her injuries.[47] Proof of factual cause requires a showing that "but for" the action or inaction of the abortion providers, the woman would not have suffered the injuries. Proof of legal cause (also called "proximate case") requires that the injuries be a foreseeable result of the provider's duty.[48]

Finally, the woman must prove that legally recognizable injuries resulted from the provider's negligence.[49] Thus some courts have refused to recognize claims where the injuries complained of are the birth of a healthy child.[50]

Lack of Informed Consent/Battery. Claims for lack of informed consent are based upon the right of patients to have sufficient information prior to agreeing to medical treatment.[51]

[I]t is generally held that a physician who performs a diagnostic, therapeutic, or surgical procedure has a duty to disclose to a patient of sound mind, in the absence of an emergency that warrants immediate medical treatment, (1) the diagnosis, (2) the general nature of the contemplated procedure, (3) the material risks involved in the procedure, (4) the probability of success associated with the procedure, (5) the prognosis if the procedure is not carried out, and (6) the existence of any alternatives to the procedure.[52]

In cases involving minors or women determined to be legally incapable of consenting, it may be sufficient for the doctor to obtain the consent of the minor's parent or the guardian of the incapacitated woman.[53]

The primary dispute in abortion malpractice cases alleging lack of informed consent is what constitutes "material risks" that the abortion provider must warn of. For example, in *Humes v. Clinton* the court rejected a claim asserting liability for failure to warn about the psychological risks abortion poses to some women.[54] In *Reynier v. Delta Women's Clinic, Inc.* the court suggested that a perforated uterus was a normal risk of an abortion that need not be discussed with the patient prior to performing the abortion.[55]

Establishing that the abortion provider failed to warn of a material risk is not sufficient, in and of itself, to create liability for failure to obtain informed consent. The woman also must establish that she would have foregone the abortion if she had known of the risk that in fact occurred.[56]

If the woman succeeds in establishing that the abortion provider failed to obtain her informed consent, liability may be imposed under either a theory of battery or negligence.[57] Battery is an intentional and unconsented to touching which is harmful or offensive.[58] The older medical malpractice cases involving lack of informed consent treat the failure to inform as negating the consent given by the woman who was ignorant of the risk.[59] More recent cases treat the failure to obtained informed consent as a failure to conform to the standard of care, essentially fulfilling the first two elements of a claim of negligence.[60]

Related to, but distinct from the duty to obtain informed consent, is a claim of negligent counseling.[*] Often this claim is asserted when pre-abortion counseling is provided by someone other than a healthcare professional.[61] Negligent counseling seeks to protect similar interests to those protected by the requirement of informed consent.[62]

Infliction of Emotional Distress.   Claims of emotional distress related to the women's experiences in pregnancy and childbirth have received mixed treatment by the courts.[63]   This is particularly true where a woman seeks compensation for emotional distress suffered from an incomplete abortion.[64]

To be entitled to recovery for the negligent infliction of emotional distress, a plaintiff must prove three elements: (1) the plaintiff must have been in the zone of danger; (2) the plaintiff must have felt contemporaneous fear for his safety; and (3) the plaintiff must show some sign of physical injury or illness as a result of his emotional distress. The physical illness or injury requirement indicates a desire to permit compensation only in cases involving severe or serious emotional distress.[65]

These requirements exist to protect against bogus claims, and limit liability for conduct that is not intended to, yet results in distress suffered by others. In order to establish the first and second elements, a woman must show that she felt distress from a threat to her physical well-being. The third element of physical injury is required where the conduct causing the distress is merely negligent.[66] If the conduct causing the distress is outrageous, a growing number of jurisdictions do not require that the plaintiff show physical illness or injury resulting from the distress.[67]

Fraud, Deceit, or Negligent Misrepresentation. Actions for fraud or deceit require that the plaintiff show that: 1) the defendant made a false representation; 2) the defendant knew it was false at the time the representation was made; 3) the representation was made with the intention that the plaintiff would rely upon it; 4) the plaintiff justifiably relied upon it; and 5) the plaintiff was injured as a result of her reliance.[68] Fraud claims have enjoyed some success when asserted against abortion providers when the providers have made false statements that the woman was pregnant.[69] Liability for misrepresentation may also exist in cases where abortion providers conceal information necessary for women to maintain claims against them.[70]

Breach of Contract. "A breach of contract claim arising out of the rendering of medical services will be held legally sufficient only when it is based on 'an express special promise to effect a cure or to accomplish some definite result.'"[71] Most consent forms used by abortion providers expressly disclaim any promise "to cure."[72] However, where evidence exists that the abortion provider expressly promised that the abortion was or would be successful, women may sue claiming that the abortionist has breached his or her contract.[73]

Deceptive Trade Practices. Many states have enacted statutes that provide extensive protection against business practices designed to deceive consumers. Whether these statutes apply to abortion providers has yet to be determined. At least one commentator has expressed reservations about the propriety of applying deceptive trade practices acts to medical professionals for anything other than intentional misconduct.[74] This limitation would not preclude many claims that could be asserted by women injured by abortions. Clearly the reported practices of misrepresenting the results of pregnancy tests[75] or paying "commissions" to "counselors" for each abortion sold[76] could be maintained under a deceptive trade practice act which limits liability for healthcare providers to intentional acts. Alternatively, there is some ground for arguing that abortion clinics are not medical facilities for purposes of requiring that all claims be submitted to medical compensation funds or protection under special statutes of limitations.[77] The existence of these cases suggests that abortion clinics may not be protected by any exemption limited to medical providers.

The advantage of pursuing a claim under such statutes is the availability of treble damages and attorneys' fees. In cases where the harmful conduct is properly characterized as a "business practice," this type of claim should be serious considered.[78]

Violations of State Statutes. In addition to the claims recognized at common law, states often have statutes that provide for enforcement by private parties. In the alternative criminal statutes may require restitution be made to victims.[79] Any statutory claims should not be overlooked.

DEFENSES AND TACTICS OF ABORTION PROVIDERS

Abortion providers rarely recognize liability for the injuries women suffer. Typically they contest every element of the woman's claim. Additionally providers often assert defenses based upon the statute of limitations, waivers or releases contained within a consent form, and the "bad woman" defense.

Statute of Limitations. Statutes of limitations require plaintiffs to bring suit within a specified period of time. Failure to do so will allow the defendant to have the case dismissed.[80] Statutes of limitations protect potential defendants against false claims, as well as insure that evidence supporting any defense will still be available.[81]

However, depending upon the nature of the injuries suffered due to the abortion, the woman may not even know that she has been injured until several years after the abortion. This is particularly true where the injury is sterility. Courts have recognized this problem in medical malpractice actions and have crafted three rules that allows the statutes of limitations to be suspended ("tolled"). In some jurisdictions, statutes of limitations do not begin to run during the existence of the physician and patient relationship. Others state place an affirmative duty on doctors to reveal any injuries to the patient. The third, and most common way courts avoid overly harsh application of a statute of limitation is to allow women to bring suit anytime within the statutory period after they reasonably should have discovered their injuries.[82]

Waiver and Release. Even when women sue abortion providers within the statute of limitations, the abortionists often assert that the woman signed a document that waives any liability.[83] Blanket waivers and releases are frowned upon by the courts, and therefore a defense based upon too general a document stands little chance of success. However, abortion providers often include detailed descriptions of potential complications in the consent to treatment. These are much more likely to preclude a woman succeeding in her claim.

Bad Woman Defense. While not constituting legal defenses (and often contrary to the rules of procedure and legal ethics), tactics such as wide-ranging inquiry into the woman's personal life and attacks upon her integrity, dissuade women from filing suit, or if a suit is filed, persuade them to settle for small amounts. This makes abortion malpractice cases less attractive to lawyers who often rely upon a contingent fee arrangement to insure payment for their services to clients who otherwise would be unable to afford the expenses of filing and prosecuting a medical malpractice claim.[84]

Separate from illicit attempts to coerce the plaintiff to dismiss or settle her claim through improper discovery are the attempts to introduce into the trial irrelevant information about the plaintiff's sexual habits or past abortions. Although experienced in cases involving issues other than abortion malpractice,[85] commentators suggest that such tactics are common where the claim arises from a failed or unsafe abortion. And, unfortunately, the tactics are all too effective.[86] There is a certain grim irony in "defenders of women's rights" using such tactics, yet until courts or legislatures effectively forbid such conduct, it will probably continue.

III. AREAS NEEDING ADDITIONAL RESEARCH

Several areas of research could be helpful as women and their lawyers seeking to hold abortion providers accountable for the injuries they inflict. Listed below are just a few:

■ Recent reports of research establishing a causal connection between abortion and breast cancer is an example of the sort of information that can be very useful to a woman seeking compensation for abortion-related injuries. Any additional adverse physical effects that can be established must be warned of if abortion providers are to avoid liability for lack of informed consent.

■ Trial lawyers need to know the extent and nature of insurance coverage carried by abortion providers, as well as the incidents of claims on the policies that exist, in order to maximize the settlements women receive.

■ Identification and documentation of common business practices of abortion providers would assist women if they seek to assert claims under their state's deceptive trade practices act.

■ A compilation of state agencies' policies in regulating abortion clinic would provide attorneys a starting point for determining whether the clinic or abortionist have violated any laws in the treatment of the woman injured by abortion.

■ Research defining what counseling techniques should be used if a woman's consent to abortion is to be fully voluntary would assist in establishing negligent counseling claims.

CONCLUSION

Members of University Faculty for Life can play a significant role in the development of the law that will reduce abortions through holding abortion providers liable for the injuries they inflict upon women. Women and their lawyers must rely upon scholars and researchers to develop the empirical evidence that abortion hurts women, that the abortion industry should be highly regulated while abortion remains legal, and ultimately, that there are solid pragmatic reasons legally to limit abortions to cases where the woman's life is at stake.

NOTES

1. This article benefits from the excellent research assistance I received from my student assistants, Christa Kerney and Kathryn Elias.

2. Kim Cobb, "Abortion Demonstrators Swap Insults Outside Buffalo Clinics" in *Houston Chronicle*, Apr. 21, 1992 at 1, 1992 WL 8061039 HOUSTON CHRONICLE A NEWS. See also David Germain (Assoc. Press), "Clinics Open as Groups Begin Siege in Buffalo" in *Orange County (Cal.) Register*, Apr. 21, 1992 at A05, 1992 WL 6347823, and John F. Harris, "Both Sides of Abortion Debate Take Case to Fairfax Hospital" in *Wash. Post (Metro)*, May 14, 1989 at B03, 1989 WL 2055552.

3. See Diane Curtis, "Doctored Rights: Menstrual Extraction, Self-Help Gynecological Care and the Law" in 20 *N.Y.U. Rev. L. & Soc. Change* 427, 428 (1993-1994): "The campaign for legal abortion has always been premised on the still largely unquestioned assumption that only legal abortions are safe abortions because they are performed by physicians, who are licensed (and therefore presumably skilled), rather than by the notorious 'back-alley abortionists' (who are presumably untrained and unskilled). For many people, to imagine abortions performed by nonphysicians is to conjure nightmares of bloody coat hangers, turpentine or lye ingestion, and other 'home remedies' leading to injury and even death." Susan R. Estrich and Kathleen M. Sullivan, "Abortion Politics: Writing for an Audience of One" in 138 *U. Pa. L. Rev.* 119, 154 (1989): "In the years before *Roe*, '[p]oor and minority women were virtually precluded from obtaining safe, legal procedures, the overwhelming majority of which were obtained by white women in the private hospital services on psychiatric indications.' Women without access to safe and legal abortions often had dangerous and illegal ones. According to one study, mishandled criminal abortions were the leading cause of maternal deaths in the 1960s, and mortality rates for African-American women were as much as nine times the rate for white women." Rachael N. Pine and Sylvia A. Law, "Envisioning a Future for Reproductive Liberty: Strategies for Making the Rights Real" in 27 *Harv. C.R.-C.L. Rev.* 407, 463 (Symposium, 1992): "The fact-finding role of the trial court, Fed.R.Civ.P. 52(a), permits litigants to introduce evidence about, inter alia, the medical and psychological realities of pregnancy and childbirth, the psychological and socio-economic consequences of denial of legal abortion, the medical consequences of "back alley" abortions, and the disproportionately harsh impact of laws regulating abortion on low-income, young and rural women."

4. "The result, as we know from experience, see Cates & Rochat, "Illegal Abortions in The United States: 1972-1974" in *Family*

Planning Perspectives 86, 92 (1976), would be that every year hundred of thousands of women, in desperation, would defy the law, and place their health and safety in the unclean and unsympathetic hands of back-alley abortionists, or they would attempt to perform abortions upon themselves, with disastrous results." *Webster v. Reproductive Health Services*, 492 U.S. 490, 558 (1989), J. Blackmun, dissenting.

5. Brian W. Clowes, "The Role of Maternal Deaths in the Abortion Debate" in 13 *St. Louis U. Pub. L. Rev.* 327 (1993) and Clarke D. Forsythe, "The Effective Enforcement of Abortion Law Before Roe v. Wade" in *The Silent Subject: Reflections on the Unborn in American Culture*, ed. Brad Stetson (1996).

6. Ibid.

7. Informal regulation may occur through professional associations. "There is a split among NAF's [National Abortion Federation Legal Clearinghouse] members over what the group has done to ensure the quality of abortion services. CO [Colorado] abortion-provider Dr. Warren Hern, who helped write NAF's abortion-care standards, said that the group has become 'ornamental.' He added that NAF 'has never pursued a serious program of standards, implementation and program evaluation.' Hern explained that the bottom line is money: 'Following good standards costs money and people don't want to do that.' But WA [Washington] abortion-provider Dr. Suzanne Poppema, who heads NAF's clinical guideline committee, said that Hern's charges are 'unfair': 'NAF is an educational membership organization that strives to maintain excellence in care through education.' He added that overall, abortion is 'one of the safest' surgeries in the U.S.: 'We just don't want to be singled out for regulations while other surgeries are not.' (AMN, 2/6)." "National Briefing Abortion Malpractice: Attempts to Put Providers Out of Work?" in 6 *Am. Pol. Network Abortion Rep.*, Feb. 7, 1995.

8. See Pamela Zekman and Karen Koshner, "State to Act on Abortion Clinics" in *Chicago Sun-Times*, Nov. 13, 1978 at 3 and 11.

9. See G. Robert Hillman, "License All Abortion-Clinic Counselors, Daley Asks" in *Chicago Sun-Times*, Nov. 15, 1978 at 60.

10. *See Rucker v. Wilson*, 475 F. Supp. 1164 (E.D. Mich., 1979) (doctor argues that delay in processing complaint requires dismissal of

complaint under due process); *Tampa Bay & State, St. Petersburg Times* (FL.), Feb. 7, 1995, at 4B (abortionist vows to fight Florida suspension of license based upon suspension of license in other states due to medical negligence); and *Shkolnik v. Nyquist*, 59 A.D.2d 954, 399 N.Y.S.2d 482 (N.Y. App. Div. 1977) (physician appeals revocation of medical license despite showing that he fraudulently represented the association of an abortion clinic, which he ran, with Bellevue Hospital; maintained incomplete records; failed to submit accurate records of abortions; aborted patients who were more than 12 weeks pregnant; failed to examine a patient before performing an abortion; diagnosed pregnancy based upon a male's urine specimen, and practiced in inadequate facilities).

11. *Okereke v. State*, 129 A.D.2d 373, 518 N.Y.S.2d 210 (N.Y. App. Div., 1987) (reviewing suspension of doctor based upon finding that he had engaged in (1) the fraudulent practice of medicine for having established the Erie Women's Center so that it might refer abortion patients to him in return for money; (2) unprofessional conduct for, inter alia, failing to timely file fetal death certificates; (3) for splitting fees illegally; and (4) for advertising the Erie Women's Center in a manner not in the public interest); and *Holtzman v. Samuel*, 130 Misc.2d. 976, 495 N.Y.S.2d. 583 (N.Y. Sup. Ct. 1985) (reviewing order permitting forfeiture of bank account containing proceeds from clinic that routinely advised women they were pregnant regardless of the results of urine test for the purpose of inducing the women to agree to abortions). Cf. *Ragsdale v. Turnock*, 841 F.2d 1358 at 1391 (7th Cir. 1988) (Coffey, Circuit Judge, dissenting) (criticizing majority for disregarding the possibility that Dr. Ragsdale's motivation for challenging regulation of abortion clinics might be protection of his $875,000 income from performing abortions). See also text accompanying nn. 56-57.

12. E.g., "Keep Abortion Out of the Back Alley" (Editorial) in *St. Louis Post Dispatch*, Aug. 17, 1992 at 2B.

13. Joyce Price, "Statistics May be Misleading on Deaths Caused by Abortion" in *Washington Times* (D.C.), June 4, 1994 at A5.

14. Forsythe (see note 5 above).

15. "Maryland's D.H.M.H. Secretary Sabitini's Credibility Questioned by Human Life International" in *P.R. Newswire*, Oct. 30, 1992

(challenging report indicating no deaths related to abortion in 1989; challengers pointed to the deaths of three women recorded in the press during the period covered by the government report) and *Hachamovitch v. State Bd. for Professional Medical Conduct*, 206 A.D.2d 637, 614 N.Y.S.2d 608 (N.Y. App. Div., 1994) (doctor disciplined for practicing medicine fraudulently by making entry in patient's office record that patient did not have bleeding following abortion procedure performed by physician).

16. "'Contract' Unveiled" in *Tulsa World*, Jan. 23, 1996 at D6 (Oklahoma State Representative Joan Greenwood identified the need for such contracts as "The Centers for Disease Control, which is presently charged with that task [abortion surveillance], makes biased reports that minimize the health risks of abortion").

17. *Thornburg v. Am. College of Obstetrics & Gynecologists*, 476 U.S. 747 (1986) and *City of Akron v. Akron Ctr. for Reprod. Health*, 462 U.S. 416 (1983). After the *Chicago Sun-Times* series, the Illinois legislature passed several statutes aimed at eliminating the abuses identified in the articles. Even with these reports, the legislation was overturned by the federal courts. *Charles v. Daley*, 749 F.2d 452 at 462-63 (7th Cir., 1984).

18. Pamela Zekman and Pamela Warrick, "The Abortion Profiteers: Making a Killing in Michigan Ave. Clinics" in *Chicago Sun-Times*, Nov. 12, 1978 at 1.

19. Ibid.

20. Ibid.

21. "Men Who Profit from Women's Pain" in *Chicago Sun-Times*, Nov. 13, 1978. Subsequent reports of similar conduct include Beth Holland, "Abortion Doc Nailed: Unlicensed MD Arrested in Police Sting" in *Newsday*, Jan. 14, 1992 at 7. Use of undercover agents to determine abortion as compliance with state requirements is not unprecedented. See *Penn Cas. Co. v. Simopoulos, M.D., Ltd.*, 235 Va. 460, 369 S.E.2d 166 (1988). (Physician arrested while preparing to perform an abortion on policewoman who was not pregnant.)

22. "Men Who Profit from Women's Pain" in *Chicago Sun-Times*, Nov. 13, 1978 and "Women Take Chances with 'Tryout' Doctors" in

Chicago Sun-Times, Nov. 14, 1978.

23. Pamela Zekman and Pamela Warrick, "Dr. Ming Kow Hah: Physician of Pain" in *Chicago Sun-Times*, Nov. 15, 1978 at 1.

24. Ibid. See also "Infamous Doctor is Detroit Connection" in *Chicago Sun-Times*, Nov. 21, 1978; Pamela Zekman and Karen Koshner, "Probe Michigan Ave. Abortion Clinic Death" in *Chicago Sun-Times*, Nov. 17, 1978 at 1 (reporting that the family of Sherry Emry had filed a $5 million medical malpractice suit against Water Tower Reproductive Center); UPI Feb. 17, 1987 (reporting that Illinois state officials had charged one abortionist with gross malpractice as a result of Sylvia Moore's death from complications related to an abortion performed December 31, 1986); and Pamela Zekman and Pamela Warrick, "12 Dead After Abortions in State's Walk-In Clinics" in *Chicago Sun-Times*, Nov. 17, 1978 at 19 (reporting 11 deaths of patients other than Sherry Emry and Sylvia Moore). Subsequent claims against doctors included in the article include *Fowler v. Bickham*, 550 F.Supp. 71 (N.D. Ill., 1982) (case settled for $15,000) and *Chicago Tribune*, Sept. 14, 1989 at 5 (sued for $10 million by patient alleging a botched abortion).

25. Pamela Zekman and Pamela Warrick, "The Abortion Profiteers: Making a Killing in Michigan Ave. Clinics" in *Chicago Sun-Times*, Nov. 12, 1978 at 6. There are other reports of the practice of demanding additional payment prior to performing a second abortion when the original operation was incomplete. See *Showery v. State*, 678 S.W.2d 103, 105 (Tex. Ct. App., 1984): ("The [still pregnant] complainant returned to Dr. Showery to complain of the results of his surgery. After indicating that he was not 'Sears' and didn't guarantee his work, he offered several explanations for her condition. He agreed to perform a second abortion and accepted $300.00 in cash. The operation was performed on April 20.").

26. Pamela Zekman and Pamela Warrick, "The Abortion Profiteers: Making a Killing in Michigan Ave. Clinics" in *Chicago Sun-Times*, Nov. 12, 1978 at 5, and Pamela Zekman and Pamela Warrick, "Dr. Ming Kow Hah: Physician of Pain" in *Chicago Sun-Times*, Nov. 15, 1978 at 1. It has been reported that Dr. Hah is no longer practicing medicine. Beth Holland, "Abortion Doc Nailed: Unlicensed MD Arrested in Police Sting" in *Newsday*, Jan. 14, 1992 at 7.

27. Pamela Zekman and Pamela Warrick, "The Abortion Profiteers: Making a Killing in Michigan Ave. Clinics" in *Chicago Sun-Times*, Nov. 12, 1978 at 5.

28. *Hachamovitch v. State Bd. Prof. Med. Conduct*, 206 A.D.2d 637, 614 N.Y.S.2d 608 (N.Y. App. Div., 1994) *leave to appeal denied*, 84 N.Y.2d 809, 645 N.E.2d 1218, 621 N.Y.S.2d 518 (1994) (doctor's license suspended for fraudulent entry upon medical chart relating to post-abortion bleeding); *Holtzman v. Samuel*, 130 Misc.2d 976, 495 N.Y.S.2d 583 (N.Y. Sup. Ct., 1985) (reviewing order permitting forfeiture of bank account containing proceeds from clinic that routinely advised women they were pregnant regardless of the results of urine test for the purpose of inducing women to agree to abortions); *Showrey v. State*, 678 S.W.2d 103 (Tex. Ct. App., 1984) ("[d]uring her testimony, the complainant testified that following the second abortion procedure she began to eject fetal parts, causing nightmares and extreme emotional distress. She testified that she reported this incident to her physician Dr. Turner Sharp, who eventually hospitalized her for one week for suicidal depression. Dr. Sharp testified that he referred the complainant for psychiatric counseling due to suicidal depression but she never reported any discharge of fetal parts.")

29. Such charges are described in Virginia Ellis, "State Panel Accuses MD of Negligence in 3 Deaths" in *L.A. Times*, May 5, 1990 at 1. On May 25, 1995, the *L.A. Times* reported that Dr. Kenneally's license was revoked. (Douglas P. Shuit, "Doctor Tied to 2 Deaths Loses License" in *L.A. Times*, May 25, 1995 at 3).

30. "Mississippi Loses Abortion Clinics; Just One Left in State as Doctors Suspended" in *Cincinnati Post*, May 9, 1994 at 2A, 1994 WL 6837478.

31. Jim Yardley, "Abortion Doctor Says It's the Cause, and the Cash, That Keeps Him Driving" in *Atlantic J. & Const.*, May 16, 1993 at A1. *See also* Steve Pokin, "At the Eye of the Abortion Storm Dr. Edward Allred Has Made a Fortune in Abortions" in *Press-Enterprise*, Nov. 8, 1992 at A01. ("In Allred's own eyes, he is simply a shrewd businessman who happened 25 years ago to start a medical practice just as abortion was made legal in California and as a better way of doing abortions became available.")

32. Abraham Abramovsky, "Depraved Indifference in the Incompetent Doctor" in *N.Y.L.J.*, Nov. 8, 1995 at 3 (Col.1).

33. Ronald Smothers, "Abortion Doctor is Linked to Complaints in 5 States" in *N.Y.Times*, Sept. 30, 1994 at A-19 (reporting suspension of Dr. Brigham's license in New York and Georgia, as well as investigations in other states) and *Tampa Bay & State*, *St. Petersburg Times* (FL.), Feb. 7, 1995 at 4B (abortionist vows to fight Florida suspension of license based upon suspension of license in other states due to medical negligence).

34. Regional Reports, "Florida Abort Doc's License Lifted" in *The National L.J.*, Feb. 20, 1995 at A8 (col. 1).

35. 410 U.S. 113 (1973).

36. 112 S. Ct. 2791 (1992).

37. 112 S. Ct. 2791 (1992).

38. G. Robert Hillman, "License All Counselors, Daley Asks" in *Chicago Sun-Times*, Nov. 15, 1978 at 5.

39. Pamela Zekman and Karen Koshner, "State to Act on Abortion Clinics" in *Chicago Sun-Times*, Nov. 13, 1978.

40. See n. 21. It is interesting to note that almost every Supreme Court case after *Roe* has been brought by abortion providers rather than women seeking abortions.

41. W. Page Keeton, Dan B. Dobbs, Robert E. Keeton, & David G. Owen, *Prosser & Keeton on the Law of Torts*, Sec. 30 (5th Ed., 1984).

42. Ibid. at Sec. 32: "But by undertaking to render medical services, even though gratuitously, a doctor will ordinarily be understood to hold himself out as having a standard professional skill and knowledge."

43. Cf. *Cole v. Delaware League for Planned Parenthood, Inc.*, 530 A.2d 1119 (Del. Super. Ct. 1987) (found that local Planned Parenthood affiliate was not entitled to shortened statute of limitations

available to "health care providers").

44. See *Williams v. Robinson*, 512 So.2d 58 (Ala. 1987) and *Stills v. Gratton*, 55 Cal. App. 3d 698, 127 Cal. Rptr. 652 (Cal. Ct. App., 1976). Compare *Dunmore v. Babaoff*, 149 Mich. App. 140, 386 N.W.2d 154 (1985).

45. *S.A. v. Thomasville Hosp.*, 636 So.2d 1 (Ala. 1993) (claiming that physician breached the standard of care in a second-trimester abortion not supported by testimony of plaintiff's expert); *Koehler v. Schwartz*, 67 A.D.2d 963, 413 N.Y.S.2d 462 (N.Y. App. Div. 1979), order affirmed by *Koehler v. Schwartz*, 48 N.Y.2d 807, 399 N.E.2d 1140, 424 N.Y.S.2d 119 (1979) and *Senesac v. Assoc. in Obstetrics & Gynecology*, 449 A.2d 900 (Vt., 1982) (statements by defendant physician that she had "made a mistake," were not sufficient evidence of negligence in the absence of expert testimony that the care failed to meet the standard of care observed by abortions).

46. Cases discussing the various requirements for expert testimony in medical malpractice cases were collected and analyzed in Jay M. Zitter, J.D., Annotation, "Standard of Care Owed to Patients by Medical Specialist as Determined by Local, 'Like Community,' State, National, or Other Standards" in 18 A.L.R.4th 603; James O. Pearson, J.D., Annotation, "Modern Status of 'Locality Rule' in Malpractice Action Against Physician Who is not a Specialist" in 99 A.L.R.3d 1133; A.S Klein, Annotation, "Competency of General Practitioner to Testify as Expert Witness in Action Against Specialist for Medical Malpractice" in 31 A.L.R.3d 1163; and H.H. Henry, Annotation, "Necessity of Expert Evidence to Support an Action for Malpractice Against a Physician or Surgeon" in 81 A.L.R.2d 597.

47. *Edison v. Reproductive Health Services*, 863 S.W.2d 621 (Mo. Ct. App., 1993) (parents of minor who committed suicide after abortion failed to establish that the abortion provider's negligence was the proximate cause of the suicide) and *Holmquest v. Hanson*, 1992 WL 196213 (Minn. App., 1992) (plaintiff failed to establish that doctor's failure to advise her of abnormal PAP smear results caused emotional distress).

48. See *Coleman v. Atlantic Obstetrics & Gynecology Group, P.A.*, 390 S.E.2d 856, *superseded* 398 S.E.2d 16 (Ga. App. Ct., 1990).

49. *Speck v. Feingold*, 497 Pa. 77, 439 A.2d 110 (1981) (holding that the parents of a genetically defective child, born due to the negligence of physicians performing in performing vasectomy and abortion procedures, had a cause of action in tort against the physician for the recovery of expenses attributable to the birth and raising of the child, and for the mental stress and physical inconvenience attributable to the birth of the child).

50. *Zapata v. Rosenfield*, 811 S.W.2d 182 (Tex. Ct. App., 1991), *error denied* (1991); *Nanke v. Napier*, 346 N.W.2d 520 (Iowa, 1984); and *Delaney v. Krafte*, 98 A.D.2d 128, 470 N.Y.S.2d 936 (N.Y. App. Div., 1984). *Contra Stills v. Gratton*, 55 Cal. App.3d 698, 707-709, 127 Cal. Rptr. 652 (1976) (mother of child born after negligently performed abortion entitled to full compensation under established tort principles); *Miller v. Johnson*, 231 Va. 177, 343 S.E.2d 301 (1986) (permitting recovery for damages, if proven, for medical expenses, pain and suffering, and lost wages for a reasonable period, directly resulting from the negligently performed abortion, the continuing pregnancy, and the ensuing childbirth, as well as damages, if proven, for emotional distress causally resulting from the tortiously caused physical injury). Some courts have distinguished the cases involving the birth of a handicapped child, *see Speck v. Finegold*, 268 Pa. Super. 342, 408 A.2d 496 (Pa. Super. Ct., 1979), *modified* 439 A.2d 110 (Pa., 1981). See generally "Note: Wrongful Birth in the Abortion Context" in 53 *Denver L. J.* 501 (1976).

51. This cause of action is explored extensively in Thomas R. Eller, "Informed Consent Civil Actions for Post Abortion Psychological Trauma" in 71 *Notre Dame L. Rev.* (forthcoming May, 1996) and Joseph W. Stuart, "Abortion and Informed Consent: A Cause of Action" in 14 *Ohio N. U. L. Rev.* 1 (1987).

52. *Tisdale v. Pruitt*, 302 S.C. 238, 241, 394 S.E.2d 857, 859 (1990) (doctor examines and performs an abortion on patient only seeking second opinion concerning the medical necessity of terminating a pregnancy she wished to continue) and *Collins v. Thakkar*, 552 N.E.2d 507 (Ind. Ct. App., 1990) (doctor sued for performing abortion on lover who only agreed to submit to a pelvic exam).

53. *Powers v. Floyd*, 904 S.W.2d 713 (Tex. Ct. App., 1995), rehearing overruled (1995), error denied (1995), pet. cert. filed (1995) (rejecting claim that consent of mother was ineffective for abortion

performed upon 16 year old girl in 1974). Cf. *Northern Ins. Co. of New York v. Superior Court in and for City and County of San Francisco*, 91 Cal. App.3d 541, 154 Cal. Rptr 198 (1979) (insurer refused to defend physician from claim arising from "administrative" error in that tortious conduct was that of a clerical employee who mistook patient for another and directed patient to a treatment room where an abortion was mistakenly performed).

54. 246 Kan. 590, 790 P.2d 1032 (1990).

55. 359 So.2d 733 (La. Ct. App, 1978) (the court opined that, based upon the plaintiff's testimony, she would not have been dissuaded from having the abortion if the risk had been disclosed, and therefore her claim failed).

56. Ibid. See also *Prosser & Keeton on Torts*, Sec. 32.

57. *Prosser & Keeton on Torts*, Sec. 32.

58. Ibid. at Sec. 9.

59. Ibid. at Sec. 32.

60. "If treatment is completely unauthorized and performed without any consent at all, there has been a battery. However, if a physician obtains a patient's consent but has breached his duty to inform, the patient has a cause of action sounding in negligence." *Scott v. Bradford*, 606 P.2d 554, 557 (Okla., 1979).

61. *Cole v. Delaware League for Planned Parenthood, Inc.*, 530 A.2d 1119, 1122 (Del. Super. Ct., 1987) (court finds that negligent counseling claim is defined by Section 323 of the Restatement (Second) of Torts which provides: "Negligent Performance of Undertaking to Render Services: One who undertakes, gratuitously or for consideration, to render services to another which he should recognize as necessary for the protection of the other's person or things, is subject to liability to the other for physical harm resulting from his failure to exercise reasonable care to perform his undertaking, if (a) his failure to exercise such care increases the risk of such harm, or (b) the harm is suffered because of the other's reliance upon the undertaking."

62. See *Eidson v. Reproductive Health Services*, 863 S.W.2d 621 (Mo. Ct. App., 1993) (unsuccessful claim by parents of daughter who committed suicide after abortion).

63. Carolyn A. Goodzeit, Note, "Rethinking Emotional Distress Law: Prenatal Malpractice and Feminist Theory" in 63 *Fordham L. Rev.* 175, 178-9 (1994).

64. *Sabot v. Fargo Women's Health Organization*, 500 N.W.2d 889 (N.D., 1993). See also *Ferrara v. Bernstein*, 81 N.Y.2d 895, 613 N.E.2d 542, 597 N.Y.S.2d 636 (1993) (affirming judgment against abortion providers for damages where "[a]s a result of the experience [miscarriage following failed abortion], plaintiff claimed she required psychiatric care; suffered posttraumatic depression, nightmares and sleeplessness; became withdrawn; and was reluctant for a substantial period of time to resume intimate relations with men"); *Humes v. Clinton*, 246 Kan. 590, 792 P.2d 1032 (1990) (denying recovery for emotional distress caused by physician's failure to warn about possible physical and psychological consequences of obtaining abortion where no physical injury occurs); *Abbey v. Jackson*, 483 A.2d 330 (D.C., 1984) (plaintiff underwent an abortion at a clinic and was later treated for complications at a hospital. She sued the owners/operators of the clinic alleging negligence in two counts: 10 negligent nondisclosure of information pertinent to appellant's consent to the procedure, and 2) negligent infliction of emotional distress). *Cf. Maguire v. State*, 254 Mont. 178, 835 P.2d 755 (1992) (rejecting mother's claim for emotional distress suffered in deciding whether to direct continuation of retarded daughter's pregnancy that was the result of rape) and *Przbyla v. Przbyla*, 87 Wis.2d 441, 275 N.W.2d 112 (1978) (rejecting claim against ex-wife for emotional distress suffered by husband due to wife's obtaining abortion).

65. *Shirk v. Kelsey*, 246 Ill. App. 3d 1054, 1068, 617 N.E.2d 152, 161, 186 Ill. Dec. 913, 922 (1993), *appeal denied Shirk v. Kelsey*, 152 Ill.2d 580, 622 N.E.2d 1228, 190 Ill.Dec. 911 (1993): "Around September, plaintiff noticed a knot in her stomach, and that she was gaining weight. Plaintiff and her mother both thought that she might still be pregnant because of her appearance. On September 27, plaintiff began experiencing severe stomach cramps and passed a lot of blood clotting. Plaintiff's mother thought she might be having a baby, so she instructed plaintiff's brother to take her to St. Francis Hospital in Peoria. Plaintiff received a pelvic examination upon

arriving at the hospital and was told that there was a foot protruding into her vaginal area, and that she was going to have a baby. After two to three hours of labor, plaintiff delivered a baby boy who lived for approximately 90 minutes. She remained in the hospital for a few days, and was discharged with some restrictions as to work and leisure activities.

"Plaintiff stated that as a result of this incident, she has experienced emotional problems. As explained by the plaintiff: 'I've had a lot of nightmares. I wake up nights reliving the baby's birth, the baby's death. I relive having the abortion. I go through a terrible morning [sic] periods a month before the baby's death. I'm detached from my husband and my kids for at least a month before and weeks afterward. It puts a lot of strain on my marriage because I'm not really fit to be around.' According to the plaintiff, she still mourns her son's death every year. What happened to her was her 'worst nightmare' and she felt as though she was 'being repaid' for the two abortions she had undergone." 246 Ill.App.3d 1054, 1058, 617 N.E.2d 152, 155, 186 Ill. Dec. 913, 916 (Ill. App. Ct., 1993).

66. *Prosser & Keeton on Torts*, Sec. 54.

67. Ibid. at Sec. 12. Compare *Martinez v. Long Island Jewish Hillside Medical Center*, 70 N.Y.2d 697, 699, 512 N.E.2d 538, 539, 518 N.Y.S.2d 955, 956 (1978) (plaintiff allowed to recover on claim of negligent infliction of emotional distress absent showing of physical injury where the medical care providers knew that plaintiff's religious beliefs forbade abortion except under exceptional circumstances, and the providers negligently gave plaintiff-mother incorrect information concerning her unborn child, as a result of which she decided on an abortion). *Cf. Boykin v. Magnolia Bay, Inc.*, 570 So.2d 639 (Ala., 1990) (rejecting parents' claim for emotional distress based upon outrageous conduct, where conduct complained of is providing abortion to minor who misrepresented her age in order to avoid parental requirement).

68. *Prosser & Keeton on Torts*, Sec. 105.

69. *Clair v. Reproductive Health Services*, 720 S.W.2d 793 (Mo. Ct. App., 1986) (abortion procedures performed on non-pregnant women). *Cf. Perry v. Atkinson*, 195 Cal.App.3d 14, 19-20, 240 Cal. Rptr. 402, 405-406 (1987) (affirming dismissal of women's fraud and deceit cause of action for pain caused by abortion done in reliance on defendant's

promise he would impregnate plaintiff later).

70. Cf. *Henry v. Deen*, 310 S.E.2d 326 (N.C., 1984) (doctor could be held liable for altering medical records).

71. *Delaney v. Krafte*, 98 A.D.2d 128, 130, 470 N.Y.S.2d 936, 938 (N.Y. App. Div., 1984) (quoting *Mitchell v. Spataro*, 89 A.D.2d 599, 452 N.Y.S.2d 646 (N.Y. App. Div., 1982). Other abortion malpractice cases alleging breach of contract include *Walsh v. Women's Health Center, Inc.*, 376 So.2d 250 (Fla. Dist. Ct. App., 1979); *Wilczynski v. Goodman*, 73 Ill.App.3d 51, 391 N.E.2d 479, 29 Ill.Dec. 216 (1979); and *Ladies Center of Clearwater, Inc. v. Reno*, 341 So.2d 543 (Fla. Dist. Ct. App., 1977).

72. *Zapata v. Rosenfeld*, 811 S.W.2d 182 (Tex. Ct. App., 1991) (disclaimer in abortion consent form effective to preclude finding of breach of contract).

73. "There are some justifications for excluding medical professionals from 'the good and workmanlike manner implied warranty [under the Texas Deceptive Trade Practices Act].' Application of this warranty to medical professionals may be unnecessary. Medical professionals can be sued on tort theories, including negligence, misrepresentation, infliction of mental anguish, assault, battery, and under the DTPA for non-negligence causes of action. Thus, one may question why another cause of action against medical professionals is necessary. Generally, in medical malpractice cases, damages are sufficient to warrant bringing a suit. Generally, a plaintiff injured by a negligent health care provider can recover sufficient damages, so that the DTPA's incentives of attorney's fees and treble damages are not necessary to encourage attorneys to take the case.

"In contrast, in the application of 'the good and workmanlike manner implied warranty' as originally created in *Melody Home*, the repair costs may be negligible, and the DTPA's additional recovery is necessary to discourage shoddy workmanship and encourage plaintiffs to file suit although damages may be minimal. Other considerations indicate that another cause of action against medical professionals is unnecessary. Although a medical professional may be sued under a negligence theory, it may be extremely difficult to prove causation. Also, even though a plaintiff may recover punitive damages in a tort cause of action, under a DTPA cause of action a successful plaintiff may recover attorney's fees, court costs, and punitive damages in the form of treble damages. Because it is unlikely that a plaintiff will fit under the laundry list of deceptive practices, only the breach of a *Melody Home* type warranty will allow a plaintiff to recover under the DTPA against a medical professional. Just because consumers of medical services have other causes of action does not automatically preclude application of 'the good and workmanlike manner implied warranty.'" Lisa L. Havens-Corte, Comment, "Melody Home, DTPA, and the Medical Profession" in 45 *Baylor L. Rev.* 985, 1002 (1993).

74. See cases cited in note 11 above.

75. *Holtzman v. Samuel*, 130 Misc.2d 976, 495 N.Y.S.2d 583 (N.Y. Sup. Ct., 1985).

76. *Cole v. Delaware League for Planned Parenthood, Inc*, 530 A.2d 1119 (Del. Super. Ct., 1987).

77. For an excellent discussion of the general applicability of deceptive trade practices acts to health care providers, see Lee Ann Bundren, Commentary, "State Consumer Fraud Legislation Applied to the Health Care Industry" in 16 *J. Legal Med*. 133 (1995).

78. Cf. *Holzman v. Samuel*, supra; *Showery v. State*, 678 S.W.2d 103 (Tex. Ct. App., 1984) (criminal conviction of abortionist for misapplication of fiduciary property over $200 in value [proceeds from health insurance policy] resulting in four years imprisonment) and *People v. Franklin*, 683 P.2d 775 (Colo., 1984) (upholding manslaughter and criminal abortion conviction of osteopath who caused the death of a patient through performing an illegal abortion).

79. *Bryan v. Conn. Dept. of Public Health & Addictive Services*, 1995 WL 780932 (Conn. Super. Ct., 1995) (rejecting plaintiff's claim that fraudulent concealment tolled statute of limitations for period equal to time necessary to obtain evidence of every element of claim); *Bryant v. Crider*, 209 Ga. App. 623, 434 S.E.2d 161 (Ga. Ct. App., 1993) (2 year statute of limitations began to run when plaintiff became aware of significant physical symptoms immediately after abortion and not when plaintiff received diagnosis of "probable Ashermann's Syndrome"); *Vitner v. Miller*, 208 Ga. App. 306, 430 S.E.2d 671 (Ga. Ct. App., 1993), *cert. dismissed* (1993); *Kirby v. Jarrett*, 190 Ill.App.3d 8, 545 N.E.2d 965, 137 Ill.Dec. 204 (1989) (statute of limitations begins to run from date that plaintiff knew or should have known of

her injuries); *Schafer v. Lehrer*, 476 So.2d (Fla. Dist. Ct. App., 1985) (statute of limitations tolled by physician's concealment of injury); and *Cole v. Delaware League for Planned Parenthood, Inc.*, 530 A.2d 1119 (Del. Super. Ct., 1987).

80. *Prosser & Keeton on Torts*, Sec. 30.

81. Ibid.

82. *Abbey v. Jackson*, 483 A.2d 330 (D.C., 1984).

83. Lawsuits seeking compensation for injuries suffered as a result of abortion malpractice have been listed as the second most undesirable type of case to file. Lewis L. Laska, "Medical Malpractice Cases Not to File" in 20 *Mem. St. L. U. Rev.* 27 (1989). However, injured women (or their surviving family members) who persevere may reap significant rewards. See *Estate of Ruckman v. Barrett*, 1991 WL 444085 (Green Cty., Mo. Cir. Ct., 1991) ($25,000,000 verdict for abortion death) and *Redding v. Bramwell*, 1990 WL 468158 (Cobb Cty., Ga. Sup. Ct., 1991) ($500,000 verdict for abortion death).

84. *Green v. Aberle*, 150 Misc.2d 306, 568 N.Y.S.2d 300 (N.Y. Sup. Ct., 1991) (striking interrogatories requesting past history of abortions in male college student's action for defamation, negligence and intentional infliction of emotional distress against female college student who accused him of rape) and *Garcia v. Providence Medical Center*, 60 Wash.App.635, 806 P.2d 766 (1991) (improper to introduce evidence of past abortions in case where plaintiff's claim is for emotional damages caused by infant son's death which allegedly resulted from negligent care before and during labor and delivery).

85. Lewis L. Laska, "Medical Malpractice Cases Not to File" in 20 *Mem. St. L. U. Rev.* 27 (1989).

86. Ibid.

THE CRITICAL NEED FOR SOCIAL SCIENCE RESEARCH FOR THE PUBLIC POLICY BATTLE FOR LIFE

Clark D. Forsythe, Esq.

INTRODUCTION

There is a critical need for social science research for the public policy battle on the life issues. There is a need for original social science research, for critical analysis of pro-abortion and pro-euthanasia claims, and for greater coordination and cooperative sharing of such research among pro-life legal, public policy, educational and scholarly organizations in order to promote pro-life strategies in litigation, legislation, and public education. The question is not *whether* social science will be used for such ends, but rather whether the social science being done is good science and whether it is being used fairly in the public policy debate. The issue is the thoroughness, fairness, and the credibility of the social science that is being published and publicized.

SOCIAL SCIENCE AND LITIGATION

Social science research is used and desperately needed for purposes of litigation. The Supreme Court's decisions in *Roe v. Wade* and *Planned Parenthood v. Casey* heavily relied on social science assumptions. Despite the *Casey* decision, *Roe v. Wade* will be overturned one way or another. It has no basis in American history, law or culture; in fact, it is at war with the American tradition, stretches back to the English common law. Twenty-two years after <u>Roe</u>, public opinion polls show that the American people — when informed — still reject the extreme regime of abortion on demand imposed by *Roe*. *Roe* will be swamped by the growing tide of protection for the unborn child in other areas of the law. Fully informed consent will be the undoing of *Casey*. Growing cultural and political trends point to an American society where communal values are taking precedence over individual autonomy and an America where greater political authority is being returned to the states. Look at the growing support for federalism and for welfare reform. No matter what one's view on welfare reform, it cannot be denied that there is a growing consensus that the system is broken and needs fixing.

Yet, whether these cultural and political trends reach a climax with greater support for the sanctity of human life, or dissipate, may be significantly determined by our ability to conduct, popularize, and disseminate social science research on the life issues.

SOCIAL SCIENCE AND PUBLIC POLICY

It is well-known that the Supreme Court's 1954 decision in *Brown v. Board of Education* inaugurated the modern use of social science data in constitutional litigation. Social science claims have driven the abortion issue in American society since the 1960^s and, in recent years, they have been critical in Supreme Court cases such as *Webster* and *Casey*. *Roe* and *Casey* are probably the purest examples of sociological jurisprudence in American history.

In the abortion area, two myths that were used to great effect to drive the abortion rights movement of the 1960's were the claims that there were 1-2 million illegal abortions annually in the United States and that 5-10,000 maternal deaths from abortion annually. These myths are still perpetuated today in popular and scholarly books and articles.

Public policy is constructed of sound bites, and slogans, and labels. The labels that the public sees often have their origin in social science data. Most social science research that affects the public debate on the life issues is disseminated in newspapers and journals, distributed to journalists, or used by pro-abortion activists in public policy campaigns.

For example, in state legislatures all over the country, it is regularly claimed that "abortion is safer than childbirth" or that "abortion is safer than a shot of penicillin." Where do these claims come from? If you can trace these claims — and often you can't — you'll find their basis in various articles or briefs that are put together by Planned Parenthood, or the ACLU, or the Alan Guttmacher Institute (AGI). These are ostensibly based on national maternal mortality statistics comparing maternal mortality from childbirth with maternal mortality from abortion.

The fact of the matter is that the public debate about abortion today — this year, this month — is completely dominated by social science research compiled and disseminated by the Alan Guttmacher Institute of New York — or AGI. AGI was formerly the formal research arm of Planned Parenthood and is still intimately connected with Planned Parenthood. Look at nearly any newspaper article published on the abortion issue, and, if it cites data, the source that is almost invariably cited is AGI. AGI publishes its own bi-monthly journal, *Family Planning Perspectives*, by which it disseminates its own in-house writings, which is usually cited as though it was a neutral, objective publication. The Pro-life Movement is not going to make much progress in changing American law and culture until that domination by AGI ends.

USE OF RESEARCH

Social science research on abortion can be used in a number of ways to promote the sanctity of human life in American law and culture. Popular mass education, advertising, media strategies, litigation, and legislative campaigns must be grounded in scholarly and scientific research and publications. Scholarship needs to be retailed or popularized to be effective in this arena.

Ideally, this research should be published in peer review journals. After such reputable publication, it can be revised and published in popular periodicals. Then, it can also be used in litigation, supported by expert testimony, or in briefs in appellate courts. In addition, such research can provide a compelling basis for state or federal legislation. Finally, mass education, advertizing, and media strategies should be based on impeccable social science research.

EXAMPLES OF PAST RESEARCH AND ITS IMPACT

Frankly, there is too little social science research being conducted and published to support the sanctity of human life. But there are some excellent examples of past research that has had a significant impact on the abortion debate in American society.

In 1990, Americans United for Life (AUL) commissioned the Gallup Organization to conduct the most indepth and comprehensive survey ever conducted of American attitudes toward abortion. The survey instrument was designed by a team headed by Professor James Davison Hunter of the University of Virginia. The resulting data will serve as a fertile source of research and analysis for years to come. In 1994, Hunter published much of this research in his book, *Before the Shooting Begins*, and a number of recent, proabortion books — such as those by Roger Rosenblatt and Ronald Dworkin — have cited the survey as authoritative and have had to deal with the findings.

Second, in 1991, James Rogers, a Professor of Psychology from Wheaton College in Illinois, analyzed official demographic data from the MN Dept of Public Health concerning adolescent abortion, birth and pregnancy rates during the 4 1/2 years that the MN parental notice of abortion law was in effect between 1981 and 1986. That data showed significant decreases in abortion and pregnancy rates and a continuing decline in birth rates, and the data was published in the April, 1991 issue of the American Journal of Public Health. It continues to dominate the public policy debate over parental notice and consent legislation in the states.

Finally, we are all familiar with claims about the impact on unwanted children from denied abortion. One of the primary proabortion books of this genre is Henry David's *Born Unwanted: Development Effects of Denied Abortion*, published in 1988. It is a prominent source cited in proabortion articles, briefs and books. A careful analysis of this book demonstrates that assumptions that denied abortion predictably results in women abusing their children or in children suffering severe social or psychological dysfunction are erroneous. In fact, David's book and other research show that a high percentage of women and children has positive outcomes and that denied abortion imposes no long-term or severely negative outcome on any significant percentage of women or children.

SPECIFIC EXAMPLES OF NEEDED RESEARCH

There are numerous examples of research that needs to be done. The Rogers' research on adolescent birth, abortion and pregnancy rates in Minnesota needs to be replicated in other states. Data needs to be collected and analyzed to determine the impact of the Mississippi parental consent and informed consent for abortion (or women's right to know) laws on adult and adolescent pregnancy, birth and abortion rates. (Mississippi recently became the first state with both types of laws enforced simultaneously.) In 1981, Surgeon General C. Everett Koop issued a letter to President Reagan in 1988 decrying the absence of longitudinal studies on psychological sequelae from abortion. Since then, no longitudinal studies have been completed. The abortion-breast cancer (ABC) link — which has received publicity in the past year — needs to be studied further.

COORDINATION AND COLLABORATION

There is also a great need for coordination and collaboration with research. There is a need for prioritization, collaboration between different disciplines, distribution on a wide scale throughout the country, and popularization of scholarly research.

CONCLUSION

Commentators have suggested in recent years that the American abortion debate is at a "stalemate." In a similar vein, it is often said that Americans are "pro-choice" but "anti-abortion." Although these commentators often suggest that this is a contradiction that cannot be explained, there is public opinion data — primarily from the 1991 Gallup Poll — which does explain this. And it suggests a public education strategy that might dramatically change American attitudes toward abortion in the next few years.

Considerable evidence from public opinion polls and media articles and reports shows that we can identify the essential obstacle to progress in the abortion fight: *public belief that legalized abortion is a "necessary evil" to avert back alley abortions.* If we could change public opinion on this score, we would see significant change on the issue.

Let me explain. The Pro-life Movement has essentially won the intellectual battle. Most Americans consider abortion to be the taking of human life if not murder itself. The 1990 Gallup Poll confirms this. Most Americans oppose abortion on demand and support it only for "hard cases" early in pregnancy.

This is also supported by the growing evidence that state legislators are willing to increase protection for the unborn child *in the non-abortion context*, prosecutors are willing to aggressively use those laws, juries are willing to convict, and judges are willing to enforce the laws.

As a result, many commentators (including House Speaker Newt Gingrich most recently) have observed that Americans are anti-abortion but pro-choice. Many say that this is contradictory and they can't explain it, but there is an explanation, and that is that Americans see legalized abortion as a "necessary evil." But "necessary" for what? I suggest that Americans see abortion as necessary to avert the "back alley." ("Yeah, abortion is the taking of human life, but if it wasn't legal, millions of women would go to the "back alley.") Americans have fully bought the myths spouted by pro-abortion advocates for 30 years about the horrors of the "back alley." This is demonstrated most recently by Newt Gingrich's statements on "Meet the Press."

Accordingly, a critical need of the Pro-life Movement is a national, educational strategy directed to overcoming the myth that legalized abortion is a "necessary evil." There are several components of this notion that need to be individually addressed through nationwide advertising and media strategies:

- the myth that legalized abortion services today are done by caring, competent doctors;
- the myth that legal abortions are significantly safer than illegal abortions (the legal-illegal myth);
- the myth that there were millions of illegal abortions before legalized abortion;
- the myth that thousands of women died from back alley abortions before legalization;
- the myth that there are no realistic alternatives to abortion.

A national educational campaign that addresses these five myths is a critical need. It would aid all our other efforts in public policy. It would bring us significantly closer to a time when our law and culture truly protects the sanctity of human life.

ABORTION MALPRACTICE:
WHEN PATIENT NEEDS
AND ABORTION PRACTICE COLLIDE

Vincent M. Rue

In contemporary American life, legal remedy for harm or injury resulting from substandard or negligent medical care is commonplace. Too often the only arbiter between the needs and rights of the patient and the adequacy and standards of the health care services provided is medical malpractice litigation.

Because litigation mirrors contemporary social conflict, it provides an intense arena in which to scrutinize highly volatile issues. Nowhere is this more evident than in the fierce political controversy surrounding reproductive rights and induced abortion: "the heat of the conflict tends to melt the boundaries between demonstrated fact and personal belief."[1] Resistance to the reality that some women and men are psychologically harmed post-abortion is considerable, both in the courtroom and out.

Not all women who elect abortion have a traumatic response. Nor, however, is abortion such a benign psychological experience that women should be misinformed about its significant emotional risks for some individuals. The fact is, insufficient scientific data is available in this country to determine conclusively how many women and men are negatively impacted by abortion and which types of individuals are at risk compared to other possible alternatives. Though existing research has identifiable methodological weaknesses, in the aggregate, these studies suggest a *direction of harm* and a significant percent of individuals likely to be negatively impacted. Politics aside, some women experience serious psychological harm post-abortion.

Recent publications in peer-reviewed professional journals have also documented the psychological risks of induced abortion, including the studies by Rue (1986), Hittner (1987), Zakus and Wilday (1987), Campbell, Franco and Jurs (1988), Ney and Wickett (1989), Rogers, Stoms and Phifer (1989), DeVeber, Ajzenstat and Chisholm (1991), Rogers (1991), El-Mallakh and Tasman (1991), Rue and Speckhard (1991), Angelo (1992), Speckhard and Rue (1992), Rosenfeld (1992), Franz and Reardon (1992), Speckhard and Rue (1993), Congelton and Calhoun (1993), Bagarozzi (1993), Bagarozzi (1994) and Ney (1994).[2]

With increased recognition of the psychological harm abortion can cause some women, it is not surprising that more and more women are filing abortion malpractice suits in the U.S.[3] This article will address the underlying reasons for these cases, provide a profile of a "typical plaintiff," and will offer recommendations that might better protect women from harm if they are considering an abortion.

THE NATURE OF THE ABORTION DECISION

The abortion decision is a unique one, complex in nature, necessitating due deliberation and the evaluation of considerable information, some of which may be emotionally trying. The U.S. Supreme Court has ruled: (1) that "abortion is inherently different from other medical procedures, because no other procedure involves the purposeful termination of potential life" (*Harris v. McRae* 448 U.S. 297, 325 (1980); (2) that the decision whether or not to abort should be made "in light of all circumstances — psychological and emotional as well as physical — that might be relevant to the well being of the patient" (*Planned Parenthood v. Danforth* 428 U.S. 52, 66 (1976); and (3) that the "medical, emotional and psychological consequences of an abortion are serious and can be lasting..." (*H. L. v. Matheson* 450 U.S. 411 (1981). Because of the medical, moral, societal and psychological controversies surrounding abortion, some states are now insisting that reasoned and deliberate abortion decision-making be legally mandated. In particular, women's "right to know" laws have been enacted that precisely determine the content of information and the timing as to when information should be made available before an abortion may be performed.[4]

In the United States today, the following elements of informed consent have been mandated in a number of states: (1) the medical risks associated with pregnancy determination; (2) the probable gestational age of the unborn child; (3) the alternative risks associated with carrying to term; (4) the medical assistance benefits if childbirth were elected; (5) the father's liability for financial assistance; (6) the opportunity to review printed information descriptive of fetal development; and (7) some waiting period for deliberation, usually 24-48 hours. Additionally, a number of states now have parental consultation statutes requiring minors seeking abortions to involve their parents in their decision-making. This is to protect the adolescent from making a secret and hasty abortion-decision and to insure that her decision is truly informed and voluntary.

These informed consent requirements are additive in nature, insuring that the woman has more rather than less information. These requirements do not appear to restrict the patient's decision-making capacity — they enhance it. How is it possible for a woman to weigh the benefits and risks of electing an abortion if information regarding abortion alternatives are conspicuously absent in the "counseling process"? Indeed, if informed consent is not obtained prior to an abortion, then grounds for medical malpractice litigation are warranted based on personal injury.[5]

Because the doctrine of informed consent is well established, courts and legislatures have consistently required physicians to provide a minimum of information to the patient prior to making a decision regarding treatment. This information is generally composed of a determined diagnosis, reasonable prognosis, the risks and benefits of proposed treatment and non-treatment, all of which should be provided in terms that the patient can comprehend. The practice of abortion has been an exception to this standard of care.

THE "TYPICAL" PLAINTIFF

In numerous cases in which we have either evaluated the patient, testified as expert witnesses, or consulted generally on a case, it is apparent to us that most plaintiffs have a number of factors in common.

1. Most were between 22 and 35 years of age, unmarried and had experienced both physical and emotional injuries post-abortion.
2. Most did not receive pre-abortion counseling, or if they did, it was so deficient as to be meaningless to the plaintiff at the time of the abortion.
3. Most of these women remembered signing "informed consent forms" but did not read or understand them.
4. Most were not given "options" counseling, nor the opportunity to ask questions privately.
5. Most had four to eight predisposing risk factors to post-abortion trauma that were unacknowledged or unexplored at the abortion clinic or minimized by either the abortion counselor or the physician.
6. Most experienced the staff and abortion-provider as insensitive to their special circumstances or emotional state.
7. Most felt ill-prepared for the emotional traumatization post-abortion and deceived by the abortion counselor regarding the developmental characteristics and humanity of the fetus.
8. Most plaintiffs have suffered serious and significant emotional injury that has negatively impacted their primary relationships, subsequent parent-child interactions, and resulted in lowered self-esteem, the use of dysfunctional coping mechanisms (drinking, drugs, food, avoidance behaviors, emotional numbing) and experienced post-traumatic decline in

overall functioning.

9. Most of these women all had first trimester abortions.

10. Most of these women had some pre-existing psy-chosocial stressors, most were competent and functioning individuals in society prior to their abortion traumatization.

The following cases are presented here by way of example of the degree and variance of post-abortion emotional injury.

CASE ONE

D. had a first trimester abortion to hide the fact that she was having sex with someone other than her mate.   She felt she had no other choice.   She did not receive any pre-abortion counseling.   After the procedure she found herself thinking about the abortion hundreds of times during the day.   When she had her menstrual period, she would save whatever blood clots that had passed into the toilet and place them in glass bottles every month.   Every week since the abortion, this woman has had oral sex with her mate twice a week.   Unknown to her sexual partner, she collects his semen in her mouth and goes to the bathroom immediately afterwards.   There she spits it into a turkey baster and then inserts the semen into her vagina, hoping to become pregnant.   In addition, she has nightmares and suffers from depression and unrelenting guilt.

CASE TWO

M. had a first trimester abortion.   She had approximately five minutes of pre-abortion counseling.   After the abortion she returned to the abortion clinic for her follow-up visit.   She reported that she was continuing to bleed and that the pain was severe.   In her own words: "they wouldn't listen to me.   They told me there was nothing wrong except rectum strain.   I told them that I couldn't sleep and they gave me Halcium.   I think they just wanted me to die in my sleep."   For the next three months this woman was traumatized by her incomplete abortion. She had unrelenting pain, diarrhea, and kept smelling something rotten coming from her vagina. She continued bleeding. She felt she was going crazy because the smell was intermittent and the pain was overwhelming. Her mate discounted her feelings and called her names. The experience finally culminated in an emergency D&E abortion, at which time a fetal corpse was identified in her cervix and was removed.

CASE THREE

G. had a first trimester abortion. During pre-abortion counseling she asked if this was a baby and her counselor assured her "it is just a clump of tissue." Shortly afterwards she went home and took a shower. Afterwards she felt something strange and looked down at the bathroom floor: "I looked down and it had two eyes, the formation of a nose and a mouth; the rib cage was sticking out. It was all broken up. You could even see an arm. You could just see what it was." In her shock and panic, she quickly picked it up and took it into the kitchen and put it in the cupboard. Then she just started to shake and cry.

KNOWN DEFICIENCIES OF ABORTION COUNSELING

The two most common causes of action in abortion malpractice are: (1) negligence in evaluating/screening a patient pre-abortion; and (2) lack of informed consent, which constitutes battery. Because abortion is a medical procedure, legally it is the physician's duty to evaluate, counsel and assess the patient beforehand.

Current abortion practice, though, severely limits physician-patient contact, and instead pre-abortion counseling is most typically delegated to the physician's agent, i.e., the abortion counselor. Nevertheless, it is the physician who actually performs the abortion, and it is always his/her ultimate responsibility to (a) protect the patient's health; (b) to see to it that the patient's decision is firm, freely made, and duly thoughtful; and (c) that her consent is truly informed.

THE ABORTION COUNSELOR

Abortion counseling in most countries suffers from obvious and serious conflicts of interest and procedural inadequacies. Abortion counseling between physician and patient is largely non-existent. Instead, the patient is "counseled" by someone other than a physician, i.e., his agent, who most typically is not professionally trained and who receives "on the job training." In the U.S. abortion counselors as a "profession" are unlicensed and are unregulated in 95% of the States. "Professional background is considered less important than such personal attributes as warmth, caring, empathy and *a commitment to the pro-choice cause.*"[6]

Counselor-bias can clearly be a negative force in the counseling process, particularly if the situation is compounded by a conflict of interest, e.g., pecuniary benefit in the outcome, namely, abortion.

All too often the abortion counselor has only a high school diploma, has herself had one or two abortions, and feels compelled to assist others by affirming the abortion decision. She thereby affirms her own decision, unknown to her and her client. Because she may be in denial about the emotional aftereffects of her own abortion, she is either unaware of post-abortion emotional trauma because she needs to be, or is simply uninformed.

One abortion counselor worked two days at the clinic and the remainder of her work-week as a bartender at a "biker's bar." Another abortion counselor, when asked at her deposition when human life began, responded: "it begins at birth." Sadly, this kind of counselor and counseling may be more the rule than the exception.

DURATION OF PRE-ABORTION COUNSELING

Contemporary abortion counseling is so time-limited and volume-oriented as to make it impossible to be tailored to the unique needs and circumstances of the individual patient. Indeed, thorough, thoughtful and deliberative pregnancy-outcome decision-making is handicapped by existing abortion counseling procedures.

Several empirical studies in the U.S. have indicated the deficiencies of current abortion counseling practices with the majority of respondents reporting insufficient information provided by the abortion counselor, insensitive, unhelpful abortion clinic personnel with respect to providing assistance in decision-making, and the provision of misinformation, thereby contributing to increased anxiety, confusion, and levels of post-abortion depression and hostility.[7]

Clearly, effective counseling that is empathic, durational and substantive in content benefits women considering abortion as a solution to an undesired pregnancy. On the other hand, biased "counseling" which is of 5-15 minutes duration, outcome-oriented, deficient of sufficient information and not allowing for multiple visits or time to deliberate is harmful to women considering abortion.

NATURE OF PRE-ABORTION COUNSELING

Current standards of care for abortion counseling have appropriately been criticized in the U.S. on at least three counts: (1) the health profession inadequately fulfills women's needs for abortion counseling; (2) current laws, by not mandating or regulating the practice of abortion counseling, thus undermines maternal health; and (3) abortion counseling must of necessity expand and include assistance in remediating post-procedural problems.[8]

The value of nondirective crisis pregnancy counseling was underscored by Cook. She reported: "When women may act only within a short span of gestation, they may be denied the opportunity to consider their options fully and take necessary steps for continuation or termination. Women could thereby be denied the choice to continue a pregnancy and give birth. The agendas of both antichoice and prochoice activists may be served by affording women opportunities for nondirective counseling and planning, and not obliging them to make their decisions in haste."[9]

INFORMATION DEFICIENCIES

It is a tragic reality that abortion clinics go to great lengths to disguise, minimize, deny, disavow or dissuade their patients' concerns about the humanity of the fetal child.

Not offering a woman the opportunity to receive fetal information is also not following good counseling procedures, for in the absence of such procedures a directive counseling environment is created. In the absence of an opportunity to receive fetal information, the woman's attention is focused on the limited information which the counselor chooses to disclose, and her decision is thereby directed by the limited information she receives. In such a directive counseling situation, the woman is denied the opportunity to consider thoroughly all her options, as information that would allow such has been withheld by the counselor.

In addition, many women are not familiar with the facts of fetal development but would consider information on fetal development to be important in making their abortion-decision because they would not wish to have an abortion if their unborn child were sufficiently developed to have readily identifiable arms, legs, a beating heart, etc.

The provision of information on fetal development further insures that, in deciding whether or not to have an abortion, a woman has an opportunity to use her own personal values, including her view of the time at which human life begins. If she is informed about fetal development and concludes that the unborn child is indeed a human life, then given her legal options, she can act accordingly in light of her own values. If she concludes that either the product of conception or the aborted material is not human, and decides to abort it, then she will have minimized the risk of future potential psychological harm arising from post-operative reflection prompted by obtaining fetal information not made available to her before it took place.

If information causes discomfort or dissonance, this does not mean it is antithetical to the doctrine of informed consent. According to U.S. Supreme Court Chief Just Rehnquist and Justice White: "It is in the very nature of informed consent provisions that they may produce some anxiety in the patient and influence her in her choice. This is in fact their reason for existence, and — provided that the information required is accurate and non-misleading — it is an entirely salutary reason."[10]

DECISION-MAKING AND NON-EVALUATING

One of the most important roles of the abortion counselor is to ascertain whether or not a woman's decision is indeed her own, made with sufficient information and reflection, made voluntarily, and without undue pressure or coercion. In addition the counselor should obtain a psychosocial as well as a medical history, and accordingly assess the risk for any post-abortion negative emotional adjustment.

The current nature of pre-abortion counseling virtually insures the impossibility of achieving its objectives. This is so because of: (a) the lack of professional education and training on the part of the counselor; (b) the severe time-constraints placed upon the session (5-15 minutes); (c) often the reliance upon group versus individual counseling; (d) the absence of objective information; (e) the non-exploration of alternatives; (f) the absence of information on fetal development; (g) the conflict of interest for the abortion counselor; and (h) the counselor's biases.

PREDISPOSING RISK FACTORS FOR POST-ABORTION TRAUMA

Research evidence is clear that certain women are predisposed to significant negative post-abortion adjustment. Existing biased abortion counseling places maternal health of these women at risk. These women are in need of *more* counseling, *more* information, exploration, and deliberation-time, and *more* assistance than others.

Abortion traumatization may in many cases be prevented or remediated if women who give evidence of documented risk factors receive adequate counsel to make a decision that fits their unique psychological and social needs.

In the current marketplace of abortion practice, nowhere is the disparity between the patient's best interests and the reality of care provided more evident than in the abortion "counseling" provided. Sadly, in this examiner's opinion, it is normative today for *all* women seeking abortions to be treated *identically*. Women that need special attention and time are treated the same way as everyone else. Individual evaluation of patient needs tends to be more the ideal than the reality of contemporary abortion practice.

Empirical evidence suggests emotional harm from abortion is probable when the following risk factors are present:

1. prior history of mental illness
2. immature interpersonal relationships
3. unstable, conflicted relationships with one's partner
4. history of a negative relationship with one's mother
5. ambivalence regarding abortion
6. religious or cultural background hostile to abortion
7. single status, especially if one has not borne children
8. age, particularly adolescents versus adult women
9. second-trimester versus first-trimester abortions
10. abortion for genetic reasons, i.e., fetal anomaly
11. pressure or coercion to abort
12. prior abortion
13. prior children
14. maternal orientation
15. biased pre-abortion counseling

An example of inadequate abortion counseling is illustrated by Donna M., who came to the Institute for emotional and behavioral evaluation pending a medical malpractice suit against her abortion-provider. Because information about gestation and fetal characteristics was not made available, her traumatization was worsened post-abortion. She recalls: "... I guess I was a little bit naive. You know, three months, you look at yourself and say, 'I don't look any bigger,' and I hadn't gained any weight, and I felt, you know, what could be really inside of you?" Prior to her abortion she failed to keep two appointments at the clinic, expressed considerable ambivalence and moral conflict with the decision, felt pressure to abort by her social worker, and possessed ten of fifteen risk factors for post-abortion traumatization, none of which were considered in her pre-abortion counseling. Clinical evaluation of this patient's functioning supported the impact of Post-Abortion Syndrome (PAS),[11] a type of Post-traumatic Stress Disorder, in her life and the painful reality of post-traumatic decline since her pregnancy termination.

Women who are emotionally traumatized by their abortions, and perhaps physically traumatized as well, are frequently overwhelmed by the depths of emotions that the abortion experience evokes. The factors of being surprised and overwhelmed by the intensity of the emotional and physical response to the abortion experience frequently act upon the post-abortive woman in a manner which causes her to resort to the defenses of repression and denial.

Women who repress or deny their emotional responses to the abortion trauma are more likely to re-experience that trauma in memory at a later time.[12] When denial breaks and painful symptoms cause significant suffering, it is far more likely at this point that a woman will consider bringing a lawsuit against her abortion provider.

In the case of PAS, re-experience of the abortion event can occur in nightmares or any events during the day associated with childbearing or with abortion. One woman reported a recurring nightmare in which she dreams that her aborted baby is pointing a gun at her and she wakes up in a sweat just before the trigger is pulled.

Re-experience also occurs in PAS women in the form of preoccupation in their waking and sleeping moments with thoughts about pregnancy in general, and the aborted child in specific. Such preoccupation frequently becomes most intense on subsequent anniversary dates of the abortion or on anniversaries of the projected due-date of the aborted child.

PAS re-experience also occurs in the form of flashbacks to the abortion experience. As one woman described her flashbacks, "Every time my period comes around and I see blood, I just start shaking. There it all is again in front of me."

It has been the author's experience in counseling hundreds of women that many encounter guilt, anxiety, loss, and depression now associated with Post-Abortion Syndrome. This condition was worsened because they received inadequate and misleading information prior to their abortion. All too often we have heard: "If I knew then what I know now, I would never have allowed myself to get into this mess."

VICTIMS NO LONGER
While some find their lives filled with daily emotional torture from their abortions, others may be living marginally and unconnected to their abortion feelings. For these women it may be too difficult or threatening to face the unacknowledged pain of their abortion experience. These women believe feelings buried by design are best left buried.

For this reason, denial is common among women who have elected abortion. In particular, some women may minimize or deny: (a) that they have experienced an emotional injury, especially when they "chose" to have the procedure; (b) that they feel grief and/or were traumatized; (c) the extent of their emotional suffering from the abortion, particularly when this is minimized by society, friends, and family; (d) that they have had multiple abortions because of the shame and guilt attached to these experiences and because of unmastered unconscious repetition compulsions; (e) the extent of psychological disruption the abortion caused in their psyches and lives because they "deserved" it as warranted punishment; and (f) the need for treatment because the media and many professionals minimize the painful reality of post-abortion trauma.

Consequently, the story of the after-effects of abortion is largely untold and unknown. While appearing "invisible" at the societal level, the story is very visible at the personal level where rhetoric collides with reality and where women live out the consequences of their decisions.

It is recommended that the following necessary changes be instituted to enable enhanced informed consent and remediate deficient standards of abortion counseling:

- Counseling for women considering abortion should only be undertaken by professionals who are trained and who possess a minimum of a master's degree in the mental health field.
- Counseling for women considering abortion should include complete, full and factual information regarding fetal development, all possible pregnancy outcome alternatives and appropriate referral sources, risks and benefits of each alternative, and risks of non-treatment.
- All women seeking abortion should be required to attend a minimum of three individual counseling sessions of one-hour duration before being able to provide their informed consent for the procedure.
- There should be a minimum waiting period of at least

one week before being able to provide their assent to abortion.

- All psychological risks of abortion should be explained and carefully evaluated according to each person's individual background and emotional status.
- Adolescents should be required to obtain the consent of their parents in order to obtain an abortion, or in the event of severe family dysfunction and/or abuse, an alternative method of evaluation may be substituted, e.g., a juvenile court may appoint an independent social worker to provide a psychosocial assessment of the individual and her circumstances.
- All women seeking an abortion should be fully appraised of their legal rights to carry to term and their right to obtain financial assistance from the child's father.
- All women seeking an abortion should have the right to unbiased professional counseling and a full opportunity to discuss any and all information concerning their crisis pregnancy and possible outcome, as well as be afforded the opportunity to ask questions freely and privately.
- All women considering an abortion should be provided with the opportunity to view a video-presentation that is scientifically accurate that depicts human fetal development. In addition, all women should be afforded the opportunity to view a video-presentation that depicts both sides of the scientific controversy over Post-Abortion Syndrome.
- Abortion counseling should *not* be undertaken by any provider who has any financial interest in the outcome of the pregnancy decision-making process.
- Each State should be required by law to compile health statistics on abortion, including morbidity and mortality, and these statistics should be annually forwarded according to federal regulations to the Centers for Disease Control.

NOTES

1. N. Stotland, "The Myth of the Abortion Trauma Syndrome" in *Journal of the American Medical Association* 268 (1992) 2078.

2. V. Rue, "Abortion in Relationship Context" in *International Review of Natural Family Planning* 19/2 (1986) 95-121; A. Hittner, "Feelings of Well-Being Before and After an Abortion" in *American Mental Health Counselors Association Journal* 9/2 (1987) 98-104; G. Zakus and S. Wilday, "Adolescent Abortion Option" in *Social Work in Health Care* 12/4 (1987) 77-91; N. Campbell, K. Franco and S. Jurs, "Abortion in Adolescence" in *Adolescence* 23/92 (1988) 813-23; P. Ney and A. Wickett, "Mental Health and Abortion: Review and Analysis" in *Psychiatric Journal of the University of Ottawa* 14 (1989) 506-16; J. Rogers, G. Stoms, and J. Phifer, "Psychological Impact of Abortion" in *Health Care for Women International* 10 (1989) 347-76; L. DeVeber, J. Ajzenstat, and D. Chisholm, "Postabortion Grief: Psychological Sequelae of Induced Abortion" in *Humane Medicine* 7 (1991) 203-09; J. Rogers, "Utilization of Data in the Ongoing Public Debate Over Abortion" in *Family Perspective* 25/3 (1991) 179-99; R. El-Mallakh and A. Tasman, "Recurrent Abortions in a Bulimic: Implications Regarding Pathogenesis" in *International Journal of Eating Disorders* 10/2 (1991) 215-19; V. Rue and A. Speckhard, "Postabortion Trauma: Incidence and Diagnostic Considerations" in *Medicine and Mind* 6/1 (1991) 57-74; E. J. Angelo, "Psychiatric Sequelae of Abortion: the Many Faces of Post-Abortion Grief" in *Linacre Quarterly* 59/2 (1992) 69-80; A. Speckhard and V. Rue, "Postabortion Syndrome: an Emerging Public Health Concern" in *Journal of Social Issues* 42/3 (1992) 95-119; J. Rosenfeld, "Emotional Responses to Therapeutic Abortion" in *American Family Physician* 45/1 (1992) 137-40; W. Franz and D. Reardon, "Differential Impact of Abortions on Adolescents and Adults" in *Adolescence* 27/105 (1992) 162-72; A. Speckhard and V. Rue, "Complicated Mourning and Abortion" in *Journal of Pre- and Peri-Natal Psychology* 8/1 (1993) 5-32; G. Congleton and L. Calhoun, "Post-Abortion Perceptions: a Comparison on Self-Identified Distressed and Non-Distressed Populations" in *International Journal of Social Psychiatry* 39/4 (1993) 255-65; D. Bagarozzi, "Post-traumatic Stress Disorders in Women Following Abortion: Some Considerations and Implications for Marital/Couple Therapy" in *International Journal of Family and Marriage* 1 (1993) 51-68; D. Bagarozzi, "Identification, Assessment, and Treatment of Women Suffering from Post-traumatic Stress After

Abortion" in *Journal of Family Psychotherapy* 5/3 (1994) 25-54; P. Ney et al., "The Effects of Pregnancy Loss on Women's Health" in *Social Science Medicine* 38/9 (1994) 1193-1200.

3. See D. Reardon, *Abortion Malpractice* (Dallas: Life Dynamics 1994).

4. In the U.S., the States of Ohio, Pennsylvania, North Dakota, South Dakota, Utah, Montana, Mississippi and Indiana have enacted statutes that expressly proscribe the nature and content of informed consent in pre-abortion counseling and decision-making.

5. J. Stuart, "Abortion and Informed Consent: a Cause of Action" in *Ohio Northern University Law Review* 14/1 (1987) 1-20.

6. U. Landy, "Abortion Counseling — A New Component of Medical Care" in *Clinics in Obstetrics and Gynecology* 33 (1986) 37.

7. C. Barnard, *The Long Term Psychological Effects of Abortion* (Portsmouth: Institute for Abortion Recovery and Research 1990); and H. Vaughan, *Canonical Variates of Post Abortion Syndrome* (Portsmouth: Institute for Abortion Recovery and Research 1990).

8. T. Steinberg, "Abortion Counseling: To Benefit Maternal Health" in *American Journal of Law and Medicine* 15 (1989) 483.

9. R. Cook, "Abortion Laws and Policies: Challenges and Opportunities" in *International Journal of Gynecology and Obstetrics* (1989, supplement 3) 61-87 at 74.

10. B. White and R. Rehnquist, Dissenting Opinion in *Thornburgh v. American College of Obstetrics and Gynecologists* 84-495 (1985) 16.

11. For a more detailed exposition of PAS see V. Rue, "Postabortion Syndrome: a Variant of Posttraumatic Stress Disorder" in P. Doherty, ed., *Post-Abortion Syndrome* (Dublin: Four Courts Press 1995) 15-28; and V. Rue, "The Psychological Aftermath of Induced Abortion" in M. Mannion, ed., *Post-abortion Aftermath* (Kansas City: Sheed and Ward 1994) 5-43.

12. A. Speckhard, *Psycho-Social Stress Following Abortion* (Kansas City: Sheed and Ward 1987).

EFFECTS OF HOSPICE INTERVENTIONS ON BEHAVIORS, DISCOMFORT, AND PHYSICAL COMPLICATIONS OF END-STAGE DEMENTIA NURSING HOME RESIDENTS

Christine R. Kovach
Sarah A. Wilson
Patricia E. Noonan

INTRODUCTION[1]

In recent years an increasing number of articles have focused on the type of care that should be provided to older adults with dementia in the nursing home.[2] A plethora of activity has ensued in developing special care units for people with mid-stage dementia.[3] Research is scant and at times contradictory regarding the efficacy of these units.[4] The qualities that make a unit "special" are ill-defined, and there is evidence that some of these units do nothing more than segregate residents with a similar diagnosis on the same unit.[5]

The resident with advanced or end-stage dementia often does not qualify for admission to these special care units or is discharged when physical needs increase and the ability to engage in group programming activities deteriorates.[6] In addition, residents with end-stage dementia may reside in the nursing home for ten years or more.[7] Currently, the literature is equivocal when discussing the therapeutic obligation of nursing homes when treating residents with end-stage dementia. Even though the hospice movement has provided many strategies for treating the person who is no longer a candidate for curative or rehabilitative services, implementation of these interventions has been fragmented and cursory. Health care workers in long-term care need to increase the armamentarium of interventions that are used to assist residents at the end-stage of a dementing illness in maintaining quality of life and dignity. The purpose of this study was to test the effect of delivering case-managed hospice care to residents in long-term care on discomfort, behaviors associated with dementia, and common physical complications. It was expected that this more individualized delivery model with a strong focus on comfort and quality of life would decrease discomfort, behavioral problems, and commonly occurring physical complications.

BACKGROUND LITERATURE

Luchins and Hanrahan[8] surveyed 819 physicians, 1,000 randomly selected non-physician members of the Gerontological Society of America and 500 families of relatives with dementia. The majority of physicians (61%), gerontologists from other professions (55%), and families (71%) chose "palliative care only" as appropriate for end-stage dementia residents. Increased age of the respondent and experience with terminal care choices were associated with the choice of palliative care. The majority preferred hospice care for end-stage dementia. Interestingly, 69% of the professionals in this study favored home hospice, while 56% of family members favored institution-based hospice care.

Hospice is commonly thought of as a delivery model for people with terminal cancer. Only recently have health care professionals begun to examine the application of hospice concepts to the care of people with end-stage dementia. There are, however, disturbing subtexts in some of these discussions. Implicit in some public policy debates is the notion that people have an obligation to "die on time" in order to relieve an economic burden on their family and society.[9]

Hospice care provides an alternative that is based on compassion and competent care, but there is a lack of consensus in defining the essential concepts that relate to hospice care for people with end-stage dementia. Volicer[10] defines hospice care as "palliative care that is aimed toward maximal comfort and not maximal survival of the patient" (p. 656). More holistic approaches include interventions that address palliative symptom control, psychosocial needs of the patient and family, amelioration of the negative effects of the disease process that impair the patient's quality of life, dignity, safety, respect for personhood, emphasis on use of intact patient abilities, and manipulation of the environment.[11] "Dying is viewed not as a medical problem, but rather as a significant event in life's journey that involves the patient, the family, and the community."[12] End-stage dementia care differs from care of end-stage cancer patients because end-stage dementia residents generally cannot communicate their needs or wishes, use much less narcotic analgesia, and have a more unpredictable course of illness.

There is also a difference of opinion regarding treatment of physical complications in hospice literature. For example, one hospice program for end-stage dementia does not treat infections with antibiotics, but residents are kept as comfortable as possible with antipyretics and analgesics.[13] It is suggested that this "antidysthanasia" approach merely allows death to proceed from the underlying dementing disease which was responsible for the infection. However, in considering the needs of both the resident and the family, Levy[14] maintains that families that watch a loved one die of a treatable condition may suffer feelings of guilt and remorse. Frequently, families of patients with Alzheimer's disease (AD) have feelings of self-doubt and guilt when faced with negative choices.[15]

Rango[16] provides a comprehensive discussion of the treatment needed that avoids both minimalist care and active euthanasia. Rango states, "Because failure to provide effective palliation constitutes nothing less than neglect of the dying person, the decision to forego medical treatment must always be accompanied by an intensification of palliative efforts, both in terms of pharmacologic intervention and human agency" (p. 838).

The primary emphasis of hospice care is on living life to the fullest — with comfort, dignity, and a sense of connectedness. While the goal of hospice is not necessarily to prolong life, hospice also is not associated with efforts to end life more quickly than natural. Even though there is no hope that the person with end-stage dementia will recover memory, people do not consist of memory alone. Human beings have physical, psychosocial and spiritual dimensions that are inherently individual, complex, interrelated and meaningful. Hospice workers, by focusing on the whole person, on comfort, and quality of life, may find ways to touch, ameliorate, and transcend the human condition of end-stage dementia.

With these assumptions regarding hospice care, a study was undertaken to determine if the application of hospice concepts to the care of a sample of residents with end-stage dementia would improve the resident's quality of life. Specifically, this study was guided by the following research question: What is the effect of hospice-oriented care on comfort, physical complications, and behaviors associated with dementia for residents of long-term care with an end-stage dementing illness?

METHODS: SAMPLE

Three long-term care facilities were chosen by convenience as sites for the study. The facilities were all close geographically which facilitated interagency meetings, and, coincidentally, all had the same religious affiliation. The goal of the project was to have 16 subjects in each facility serve as study subjects, and 16 serve as control subjects. In order to be considered in the end-stages of a dementing illness and to be considered for inclusion in the study, subjects had to meet the following criteria: a) be diagnosed with irreversible dementia; b) have a score on the Short Portable Mental Status Questionnaire (SPMSQ) which indicates severe cognitive impairment[17]; c) be identified by the staff as usually unable to engage in group programming designed for residents with dementia; d) have at least two of the following symptoms: aphasia (disorder of language due to brain dysfunction); apraxia (inability to carry out purposive activities despite intact sensory and motor function); agnosia (failure to recognize or identify common objects despite intact sensory function); and constructional difficulty (inability to copy three-dimensional figures); and e) have advanced directives that request no cardiopulmonary resuscitation (CPR) be initiated. It was felt that requesting more restrictions on care such as no further hospitalizations or no tube feedings would have been unethical because family members may have to choose between enhanced palliative care and feeding/hydrating the resident or treating an acute illness. By only accepting subjects who had previously had an advanced directive of no CPR, it was felt that we would at least be consistent in our primary emphasis on comfort rather than rehabilitation or cure.

One hundred eighteen residents at the three facilities met eligibility criteria. Consent was obtained from 92 of the subjects' guardians. Seventeen subjects died in the five month period between the time consent was obtained and the interventions were implemented. Two subjects in the experimental group refused to make necessary room changes as a part of the intervention, and were dropped from the study. One subject in the control group moved to another city. When the households opened, 35 subjects were in the treatment group and 37 subjects served as a control group. Two months after the unit opened post-testing was done. There were five more deaths in the treatment group and five more deaths in the control group over this two month time period yielding a sample size of 62 for post-testing.

Table 1 provides data which supports that random assignment to groups was effective in yielding equivalent groups. Subjects in the treatment and control group were not significantly different in age, sex, length of stay, or marital status. All subjects were Caucasian.

TABLE 1: DESCRIPTION OF SAMPLE

Variable	Treatment Group	Control Group	Test Statistic	p
Age	X = 88.06	X = 87.78	t = .181	.857
Sex	Female = 30 Male = 5	Female = 28 Male = 9	χ^2 = 1.56	.210
Length of stay	X = 40 months	X = 36 months	t = .419	.677
Marital status	Widowed=26 Married=7 Single=1 Divorced=1	Widowed=22 Married=12 Single=2 Divorced=1	χ^2 = 4.33	.228

DESIGN

A pre-test—post-test experimental design was used. Subjects who met eligibility criteria and for whom consent from a guardian was obtained, were randomly assigned to the treatment or control group. Two months before the households were opened, measurements of comfort, behavior, and physical complications were obtained. Subjects in the treatment group received the hospice household intervention and the control group received the traditional care provided by the facility. Two months after the interventions were implemented the outcome variables were measured again. The relatively short timing of the assessments was chosen because of the high mortality rate of this group. Individual interviews with a convenience sample of 15 staff and 13 family members were also conducted before and after the interventions were implemented to assess satisfaction and identification of changes. The complete analysis of these interviews will be reported elsewhere but findings are briefly summarized in the results section. Measurements and interviews were done by two graduate nursing students with experience in gerontology.

MEASUREMENT

Cognitive impairment. Presence and degree of cognitive impairment was assessed using the SPMSQ. This 10-item instrument compares with results of a clinical psychiatric diagnosis of organic brain syndrome with 92% agreement when the SPMSQ indicates definite impairment and 88% when the SPMSQ indicated either no impairment or mild impairment.[18]

Behaviors associated with dementia. The BEHAVE-AD scale was specifically designed to assess commonly occurring and potentially remediable behavioral symptoms associated with Alzheimer's disease and related dementias.[19] Sclan[20] found agreement between a rater and the BEHAVE-AD tool total score was .96. Patterson[21] found that for 20 of the 25 items, kappas were .619-1.00 and agreement was fair on the five remaining items.

Comfort. The Discomfort Scale for Dementia of the Alzheimer's Type (DS-DAT) is an objective scale for measuring discomfort in people with advanced dementia who have lost communication abilities. Discomfort was operationally defined as, "the presence of behaviors considered to express a negative emotional and/or physical state that are capable of being observed by a trained rater unfamiliar with the usual behavior pattern of the patient."[22] Ratings on the nine-item scale were made by assessing magnitude of its defining characteristics on a 100mm horizontal line visual analogue scale from absent (0) to extreme (100). The rater waited for 15 minutes after any event that might induce discomfort (such as a position change) and observed the subject for five minutes. The possible range of scores was 0-900. The tool has a content validity index of 1.0 and an internal consistency reliability of .86-.89.[23]

Physical complications. Physical problems commonly experienced in end-stages of a dementing illness were determined through consultation with three nurse administrators in long-terms care and through a review of the literature. Based on this compilation, a data collection form was constructed that was used during a chart review. Major categories of problems in the tool were: Nutrition, elimination, sleep, mobility, and infection.

DESCRIPTION OF THE HOSPICE HOUSEHOLD INTERVENTION

The intervention was implemented through a four-pronged approach: a) interdisciplinary development of the intervention strategies for the new households; b) development of the households; c) use of a hospice nurse as a case manager; and d) education of staff.

Development of Interventions. An interdisciplinary task force from the three facilities was formed and included two nurse consultants from the university. Hallmarks of this program were to provide comfort, quality of life, and dignity. The task force operationalized these hallmarks into a set of practice guidelines that became, in essence, the contract the staff made with the researchers regarding the enhanced care that would be provided. The residents day became much busier with the addition of a full schedule of therapeutic activities, but, an effort was made to balance sensory stimulating and sensory calming activities. Examples of common activities were: quilting, rummage boxes, one-on-one friendly visiting, massage, music therapy, afternoon social hour with non-alcoholic wine, baking, and a variety of other sensory stimulating activities. Providing meaningful human interaction every day for every resident was paramount.

Development of Households. Rather than being isolated on a distant unit, residents were clustered in 6-8 bed areas on units that were 22-44 beds. Efforts were made to make these households as homelike as possible through the following interventions: using colorful afghans, pillows, and furniture from home; letting in as much natural light as possible; displaying pictures and biographical sketches of each resident whose guardian consented; providing plants in each room. Each facility provided a lounge for the project. Residents were able to eat meals in this room and it also became the hub for many of the individual and group therapeutic activities.

Case Management. Case managers were chosen by the Director of Nursing from each facility. It had been intended that nurses would be randomly chosen to serve as case manager, but, because there were few RN's at the facilities who were available for the project, randomization was not possible. Two of the case managers had a bachelor's degree, and one had a master's degree in nursing. Case managers received formal classes in hospice, care planning, assessment techniques, and case management from the researchers as well as much informal support and instruction. The case manager led a smaller interdisciplinary team at her facility in the development of individualized care plans that were consistent with the ideology of treating the whole patient, maintaining comfort, and quality of life. The case manager assisted in implementing the care plan, served as a role model, direct caregiver, coordinator of services, and as an advocate for the resident, family and staff.

The staff. An all-day conference was held at the university for all staff involved in the project. There were over 80 people in attendance. Classes focused on hospice concepts, dementia, treatment of behaviors associated with dementia, activity programming, and family and spiritual care. In addition, the nurses received a class that focused on improving recognition and early treatment of commonly occurring physical conditions. Lung assessment was presented with an emphasis on early intervention to treat pneumonia and pulmonary edema. Nurses were taught to use an LE dipstick to assess for potential urinary tract infection (UTI) when the resident displayed common signs of UTI in the elderly (e.g. changed behavior, change in appearance of urine). Common signs and symptoms of skin and soft tissue infections were reviewed. A "give when needed" Tylenol prescription was obtained for all residents in the treatment group and nurses were instructed to try administering Tylenol rather than a chemical restraint if the patient displayed behavior such as agitation or perseverance, and behavioral interventions and/or assessment were ineffective in calming the behavior or identifying the meaning behind the behavior. These physical assessments and interventions were designed to provide comfort and keep these residents out of the acute care setting if possible.

RESULTS

At pre-test there were no significant differences between the groups in discomfort ($t = .477$, $p = .635$), behaviors associated with dementia ($t = .317$, $p = .752$), or physical iatrogenic problems ($t = .404$, $p = .688$). These findings support that the two groups were very similar on the outcome variables of interest and that random assignment was effective in yielding equivalent groups. Because the groups were this similar at pre-test, there was not a need to covary out pre-test differences. A between group independent t-test was therefore used to analyze results rather than analysis of covariance (ANCOVA).

Scatterplots and frequency distributions were obtained for all of the variables and associations tested. There was no evidence of nonlinearity or marked skew in these graphs. Also, the variances for each set of variables tested were not significantly different.

As seen in Table 2, at post-test, there was a statistically significant difference in discomfort levels between the treatment and control groups (t=3.88, p<.001). Table 3 shows the frequency of specific behaviors associated with dementia and physical complications. Social interaction difficulties, diurnal rhythm disturbances, activity disturbances, and aggression were the most prevalent problems experienced by this sample. At post-testing, the treatment group had decreased the frequency of all behavior problems except delusions and hallucinations. The most striking improvements in behavior problems were decreased aggression and improved ability to interact in a group. The control group also showed a more moderate decreased frequency of many behavior problems, but had an increased incidence of delusions, hallucinations, and phobias. Even though the treatment group showed lower scores on the tool that assessed behavior problems, the differences were not large enough to be statistically significant (t=1.44, p=.155).

TABLE 2: DIFFERENCES BETWEEN TREATMENT AND CONTROL GROUPS AT POST-TESTING

Condition/ Variable	Treatment Group		Control Group		t	p
	M	SD	M	SD		
Behaviors	4.52	5.2	6.58	6.0	1.44	.155
Discomfort	218.10	142.1	368.88	168.3	3.88	<.001*
Physical	1.68	1.74	1.66	1.3	.054	.957

* Statistically significant result

TABLE 3: FREQUENCY OF BEHAVIORS ASSOCIATED WITH
DEMENTIA AND PHYSICAL COMPLICATIONS FOR TREATMENT
AND CONTROL GROUPS AT PRE AND POST-TESTING

Variable	Pre-testing		Post-testing	
	Treatment Group N=35	Control Group N=37	Treatment Group N=30	Control Group N=32
Behaviors				
Activity Disturbances	18	21	12	16
Aggression	22	22	10	17
Diurnal Rhythm Disturbances	20	22	12	16
Affective Disturbances	14	11	8	6
Phobias	14	13	8	16
Delusions	4	5	4	6
Hallucinations	2	2	2	6
Social Interaction Difficulties	29	24	16	23
Physical Complications				
Nutrition	11	15	9	4
Elimination	17	20	9	13
Skin	15	16	14	11
Mobility	13	19	7	9
Infections	10	12	4	15

This sample had a high frequency of physical complications. There was not a difference in the number of physical complications experienced by the treatment and control groups (t = .054, p = .957). Examination of frequency of physical complications does reveal that at post-testing the treatment group had fewer iatrogenic infections (N = 4) than the control group (N = 15).

Interviews with staff revealed improved job satisfaction,

increased sense of empathy and caring, and recognition that there was an observable improvement in some residents. The comment "they have woken up," and "they maintain eye contact," and "they're alive again," reflect the staff's perceptions of improvement in residents. Several residents who had been nonverbal began speaking and were able to call the staff person by name. Some residents began participating more in their self-care. For example, one resident who had to be fed was able to feed herself with cues from the staff.

One nurse commented, "It changed how I look at those with dementia. They are not those poor unfortunates. There is lots we can do and they can laugh and have their quality of life and not just be stuck in a wheelchair looking out a window." A certified nursing assistant (CNA) said, "It helped me to understand the resident more. You learn to be a little more friendly, be assertive instead of aggressive..." Another CNA said, "I learned a lot and she (resident) learned too. It helps. It's working here. Every home should have this program."

Compared to the nursing staff, family members noted fewer changes in the residents. Several family members indicated that it was difficult for them to visit the nursing home when the resident shows little or no recognition of them and cannot participate in a conversation. One family member noted that a resident was able to sleep better at night, and several commented that there were periods when the resident was more alert.

DISCUSSION

The results supported that application of hospice concepts to care of nursing home residents with end-stage dementia is associated with decreased discomfort levels. This is a critical finding, because comfort is fundamental to a focus on palliation rather than cure or rehabilitation. Additionally, there exists a prevalent view that there is little that the health care system has to offer people in the latter stages of a dementing illness. This controlled study supports that palliation can have positive influences on quality of life. Even though the differences between the treatment and control group BEHAVE-AD scores were not statistically significant, the means suggest that the treatment group was experiencing fewer behavior problems. These interventions were implemented without additional staff and with minimal cost for the purchase of appropriate therapeutic activity materials and some environmental modifications.

Comfort and behavior "problems" in the end-stages of dementia are perplexing problems because of the communication difficulties during the latter stages of dementia, difficulties sorting out the meaning behind certain behaviors, and difficulties measuring variables of interest in this population. Although it does appear that some effect of the interventions used were captured by the discomfort scale, the need remains for better measurements in researching outcome variables of interest. Further studies on behaviors associated with dementia and comfort levels of people with end-stage dementia are needed to advance understanding of these complex, intertwined problems. The differential impact of specific interventions used in this study on reliable, valid, and clinically meaningful outcome measures must be confirmed and explored further.

The results failed to confirm that the application of hospice concepts reduces physical complications experienced by residents of long-term care with end-stage dementia. Physical complications may not be highly amenable to intervention at this stage of the illness, and this may explain the lack of difference in physical complications. Before any conclusions can be made about the differences between the treatment and control group infection rates, these results would need to be replicated. Because the interventions implemented in this study were fairly global and multifaceted, there is a need to design a study that focuses entirely on physical problems, and the prevention and early diagnosis of common physical problems. Because this is a group that generally fairs poorly when admitted to acute care facilities, there is a need to study ways in which improved assessment, early recognition, and early treatment in nursing homes can possibly reduce the need for acute care admissions.

The differences in the observations of family members and staff may reflect that staff were able to notice more changes as a result of day-to-day interactions with residents. Family members may have expected more dramatic improvements, even though all family members expressed satisfaction with care in the nursing home and with participation in the project. The differences between perceptions of staff and family members may also reflect differences in the sense of loss, grief, and observed change from the residents' pre-demented state.

The line that separates palliative care from curative care is often blurred. The danger in this lack of clarity results in the potential for some practitioners to interpret that palliative care means little or no intervention. This study did not address these important issues beyond using as eligibility criteria for admission to the study that there be an advanced directive of no cardiopulmonary resuscitation. The difficulty in deciding when to forego medical treatment is complicated by the high degree of prognostic uncertainty associated with dementing illnesses.[24] Empirical studies are needed that address the treatment decisions made for people with end-stage dementia. There is a need for greater understanding of the course of the dementing illnesses, and the influence of various physical, pharmacological, social, cognitive, nutritional, and psychological interventions on the rate and decline of life expectancy.

Since much of the research on special care units for dementia is inconclusive, future research should focus less on identifying if the units are effective than on differentiating which specific interventions are associated with improved comfort, health status, or quality of life. There is a need to move beyond the noble notions of improved care to better understood and moré firmly established principles and interventions for care of persons with early to end-stage dementia.

NOTES

1. This study was funded by a grant from the Helen Bader Foundation.

2. L. Berg, K. C. Buckwalter, P. K. Chafetz, L. P. Gwyther, and D. Holmes, "Special Care Units for People with Dementia" in *Journal of the American Geriatric Society* 39 (1991) 1229-1236. G. R. Hall and K. C. Buckwalter, "From Almshouse to Dedicated Unit: Care of Institutionalized Elderly with Behavior Problems" in *Archives of Psychiatric Nursing* 4 (1990) 3-11. T. H. Koff, "Nursing Home Management of Alzheimer's Disease: A Plea for Standards" in *Am. J. Alzheimer Care and Related Disorders Research* 1 (1986) 12-15.

3. D. Holmes, J. Teresi and C. Monaco, "Special Care Units in Nursing Homes: Prevalence in Five States" in *The Gerontologist* 32 (1992) 191-196.

4. J. Green, J. Asp and N. Crane, "Specialized Management of the Alzheimer's Patient: Does It Make a Difference? A Preliminary Progress Report" in *J. Tenn Medical Association* 78 (1985) 58-63. G. Hall, M. V. Kirschling and S. Todd, "Sheltered Freedom: An Alzheimer's Unit in an ICF" in *Geriatric Nursing* 32 (1986) 191-196. L. Volicer, Y. Rheaume, J. Brown, K. Fabiszewski and R. Brady, "Hospice Approach to the Treatment of Patients with Advanced Dementia of the Alzheimer's Type" in *JAMA* 256 (1986) 2210-2213. C. R. Kovach and S. A. Stearns, "Dementia Specific Care Units: A Study of Behavior Before and After Residence" in *Journal of Gerontological Nursing* 20 /2 (1994) 33-39. P. K. Chafetz and H. C. West, "Longitudinal Control Group Evaluation of a Special Care Unit for Dementia Patients: Initial Findings" presented at the 40th annual scientific meeting of the Gerontological Society of America, Washington, D.C., November 22, 1987.

5. M. M. Carley, "Regulating Alzheimer's Special Care Units" in *Contemporary Long Term Care* 16 (1993) 76-88.

6. R. N. Riter and B. E. Fries, "Predictors of the Placement of Cognitively Impaired Residents on Special Care Units" in *The Gerontologist* 32 (1992) 184-190.

7. B. Reisberg, "Clinical Presentation, Diagnosis, and Symptomatology of Age-Associated Cognitive Decline and Alzheimer's Disease" in *Alzheimer's Disease*, ed. B. Reichberg (New York: The Free Press, 1983) 173-188.

8. D. J. Luchins and P. Hanrahan, "What Is Appropriate Health Care for End-stage Dementia?" in *Journal of the American Geriatrics Society* 41 (1993) 25-50.

9. H. Caplan, "We Can't Afford to Prolong So Many Hopeless Lives" in *Medical Economics for Surgeons* (Dec. 1982) 62-66. J. C. d'Oronzio, "Good Ethics, Good Health Economics" in *New York Times* (June 1993) A25. E. J. Emanuel and L. L. Emanuel, "The Economics of Dying — the Illusion of Cost Savings at the End of Life" in *New England Journal of Medicine* 330 (1994) 540-44. R. W. Evans, "Health Care Technology and the Inevitability of Resource Allocation and Rationing Decisions" in *JAMA* 249 (1983) 2047-53. J. F. Fries, C. E. Koop, C. E. Beadle, P. P. Cooper, M. J. England, R. F. Greaves, J. J. Sokolov, and D. Wright, "The Health Project Consortium: Reducing Health Care Costs by Reducing the Need and Demand for Medical Services" in *New England Journal of Medicine* 329 (1993) 321-24. M. R. Gillick, "Is the Care of the Chronically Ill a Medical Prerogative?" in *New England Journal of Medicine* 310 (1984) 190-93. G. D. Lundberg, "National Health Care Reform: The Aura of Inevitability Intensifies" in *JAMA* 267 (1992) 2521-24. G. D. Lundberg, "American Health Care System Management Objectives: The Aura of Inevitability Becomes Incarnate" in *JAMA* 269 (1993) 2554-56.

10. L. Volicer, "Need for Hospice Approach to Treatment of Patients with Advanced Progressive Dementia" in *Journal of the American Geriatrics Society* 34 (1986) 655-58.

11. B. Austin and P. Melbourne, "Hospice Services for the Terminal Alzheimer's Patient" in *Caring* 9/11 (1990) 60-62. K. J. Fabiszewski,

M. E. Riley, D. Berkley, J. Karner and S. Shea, "Management of Advanced Alzheimer Dementia" in *Clinical Management of Alzheimer's Disease*, eds. L. Volicer, K. J. Fabiszewski, Y. L. Rheaume and K. E. Lasch (Rockville, Md.: Aspen, 1988) 87-109. P. Heacock, C. Walton, C. Beck and S. Mercer, "Caring for the Cognitively Impaired: Reconceptualizing Disability and Rehabilitation" in *Journal of Gerontological Nursing* 17/3 (1991) 22-26. V. Mor and S. Masterson-Allen, *Hospice Care Systems: Structure, Process, Costs, and Outcome* (New York: Springer, 1987).

12. B. G. Brechling, J. D. Heyworth, D. Kuhn and M. F. Peranteau, "Extending Hospice Care to End-stage Dementia Patients and Families" in *The American Journal of Alzheimer's Care and Related Disorders & Research* 4 (1989) 21-29 at 22.

13. See Volicer (cited in n. 4 above) at 658.

14. J. A. Levy, "The Hospice in the Context of an Aging Society" in *Journal of Aging Studies* 3 (1989) 385-99.

15. H. S. Wilson, "Family Caregiving for a Relative with Alzheimer's Dementia: Coping with Negative Choices" in *Nursing Research* 38 (1989) 94-98.

16. N. Rango, "The Nursing Home Resident with Dementia" in *Annals of Internal Medicine* 102 (1985) 835-41.

17. E. Pfeiffer, "A Short Portable Mental Status Questionnaire for the Assessment of Organic Brain Deficits in Elderly Patients" in *Journal of the American Geriatrics Society* 23 (1975) 433-41.

18. Ibid.

19. B. Reisberg, J. Borenstein, S. P. Slaob, S. H. Ferris, E. Franssen and A. Gergotas, "Behavioral Symptoms in Alzheimer's Disease: Phenomenology and Treatment" in *Journal of Clinical Psychiatry* 48 (1987) 9-15.

20. S. G. Sclan, B. Reisberg, E. Franssen, C. Torossian and S. H. Ferris, "Remediable Behavioral Symptoms of Alzheimer's Disease: A Cognitive Independent Syndrome" at the American College of Neuropsychopharmacology 29th Annual Meeting, Abstract (1990) 150.

21. M. B. Patterson, A. H. Schnell, R. J. Martin, M. F. Mendez, K. A. Smyth and P. J. Whitehouse, "Assessment of Behavioral and Affective Symptoms in Alzheimer's Disease" in *Journal of Geriatric Psychiatry and Neurology* 3 (1990) 21-30.

22. A. C. Hurley, B. J. Volicer, P. A. Hanrahan, S. Houde and L. Volicer, "Assessment of Discomfort in Advanced Alzheimer's Patients" in *Research in Nursing & Health* 15 (1992) 369-77 at 370.

23. Ibid.

24. Rango (cited in n. 16 above) and Reisberg (cited in n. 7 above).

NEW DIMENSIONS TO EUTHANASIA

Eugene F. Diamond, M.D.

The New England Journal of Medicine has been the launching pad for numerous bioethical trial balloons over the years. Death as the treatment of choice for handicapped newborns was first suggested in print in the pages of this prestigious journal by Duff and Campbell in 1973, and as late as 1984 the imprimatur of publication was accorded to apologists for *third trimester* abortion. The publication of "The Physician's Responsibility toward Hopelessly Ill Patients"[1] must be scrutinized with this record as a background. There are ten different authors from ten different institutions and, not unexpectedly, much of the article is based on an apparent consensus of different backgrounds and widely separated geographical locations. As such, the article is largely platitudinous and exhorts the profession toward a level of care and informed consent already in place and accepted without controversy in most places.

The placid landscape of pious pronouncements, however, is disturbed toward the end of the article by a somewhat muted explosion. After a slight nod to assisted suicide, the authors state that it is "ethically permissible" to withhold "nutrition administered by... gastric tube" from "severely and irreversibly demented patients" as well as those who are "pleasantly senile."

It is obvious that the issue of the ethical permissibility of removing feeding-tubes is highly controverted in medical as well as legal circles. The *Claire Conroy* case in New Jersey resulted in a decision that to remove the tube would be unacceptable in that it would result in death from "a new and independent condition: dehydration and starvation." The Supreme Court of New Jersey overruled the lower Court and said that feeding could be discontinued if

a) a living will so directed, b) the patient verbally directed the doctor to do so, or c) the physician determined that the burden of continuing feeding outweighed its benefits. The last point is fraught with danger in that it allows the attending physician to determine when it was in the patient's interest to be dead.

In the widely publicized Herbert Case in California, two physicians were acquitted of a charge of murder after having taken a patient off of a respirator and having removed his feeding-tube. The basis for the murder charge, however, was the allegation that the removal of respirator-support and tube-feeding had been carried out in an inappropriately hasty manner on a patient whose coma had resulted from possible medical malpractice. The survival of such a patient could result in the award of a judgment far in excess of that resulting from his early death. The Herbert case, then, does not clearly support the removal of any and all feeding-tubes on terminal patients in California. The crux of the matter is whether the tube-feeding constitutes ordinary or extra-ordinary care. Wanzer and his co-authors apparently base their position on the dubious notion that the insertion of a feeding-tube is more uncomfortable than death by starvation for the "severely and irreversibly demented" patient or the "pleasantly senile" patient.

This category of patient is, of course, quite separate from the terminally ill, persistently vegetative, or brain-dead patients (even in the authors' classification in this article). "Dementia" is in no way synonymous with "dying" even if it happens most often to senile patients of advanced age.

Health care planners with a cost-benefit orientation would be delighted with a national policy allowing the removal of feeding-tubes and the withholding of antibiotics from the *entire class* of demented, senile patients in institutions. Savings in the billions could probably be achieved annually. The cost in human terms would be much greater. The American system would slide further down the slippery slope of death worship.

The New England Journal is America's most illustrious medical publication. It does not, of course, establish standards of care and none of its authors can claim to speak *ex cathedra*. It would be ingenuous, however, not to expect that the principles enunciated in this article would have heavy impact on the national conscience.

Those who deplore "slippery slope" type of argumentation will have to concede that there is a progression in permissiveness from the recommendation that feeding be withheld from a) "brain-dead" patients, b) patients in a "chronic vegetative state," c) "irreversibly demented" patients, and finally d) "pleasantly senile" patients. There is also demonstrated here the tendency of a principle to expand to cover a multitude of sins. The principle employed in various contexts is the "right to privacy."[2] This principle, unexpressed in the Constitution but alleged by the Burger Court to be implied in the fifth and fourteenth amendments, was enunciated as the pregnant woman's "right to privacy" in reproductive decision-making which allowed her to abort her child without the interference of law.[3] In the Baby Doe case in Bloomington, Judge Premo in the Indiana lower court enunciated a parental privacy right to choose one form of therapy over another. This right was said to extend to the private right to choose the option of death by starvation for Baby Doe over the option of life-saving corrective surgery.[4] The right to privacy now being invoked is the private right to refuse medical treatment. The principles underlying this right can be summarized as follows:

1. A competent patient has the right to refuse care even if refusal means certain death.
2. The wishes of a once-competent patient, as expressed in writing or verbally to friends or relatives, must be accorded great weight after he has become incompetent.

3. When the patient is a child, parents' decisions should be respected except when they are not in the child's best interest.
4. A physician will be protected if his concurrence in a decision to withhold treatment is a good faith judgment in conformity with generally accepted medical practice.
5. Where a once-competent patient never expressed a preference, if a treatment is excessively burdensome or does not offer a reasonable hope of benefit, it may be eliminated.

This latter balancing of burdens versus benefits is sometimes referred to as the principle of proportionality. The principle of proportionality was enunciated frequently by the President's Commission for the Study of Ethical Problems in Medicine in various contexts.[5] It was also adopted by the California Appellate Court in the Barber Case[6] and is employed by various authors[7] in the medical literature. It is frequently cited as a calculus to be preferred over the more traditional "ordinary" versus "extraordinary" means of prolonging life. It would seem, however, that the differences are more semantic than substantive. A therapy imposing more burdens than benefits would be "extraordinary" and a therapy offering more benefits than burdens would be "ordinary." In fact, Pius XII, in his epoch-making address to the anesthesiologists alludes to burdens and benefits while defining the distinction between ordinary and extraordinary means.[8]

It is obvious that the benefit/burden equation is relevant to the decision to withdraw nutritional support and that the application of the principle of proportionality will be contingent on the medical condition of the patient:

1. If the patient is *brain-dead* there is obviously no benefit to be derived from continuing nutrition except in those instances where it might be maintained briefly for the benefit of harvesting organs for transplantation.

2. If death is imminent, in the sense that it will occur with or without treatment, in a short time, the provision of nutrition would be ineffective and therefore could be

withheld in those instances where it could only be provided with great difficulty.[9] Connery has suggested that "imminent" in this context means two weeks or less.

3. If the patient is in a *persistent vegetative state* the discontinuation of hydration and nutrition would be highly questionable. A patient in a persistent vegetative state is not presumed to be dying. The prognosis for the regaining of consciousness and cognitive function is generally presumed to be hopeless. However, in one highly publicized case, Sgt. David Mack of Minneapolis[10] regained consciousness after 22 months of coma to testify that he had been aware of happenings around him for six months. Najenson,[11] in his studies of Israeli servicemen in coma as a result of injuries suffered in combat, concluded that the prognosis could be improved by doubling the dose of calories usually provided. He concluded that the cause of death was likely to be either aspiration or starvation. By increasing feedings and keeping patients upright, he achieved a 70% rate of recovery.

Whatever the prognosis, however, the duty to prolong life is not abrogated by a hopeless prognosis. As Connery has pointed out, "A patient may live a long time with a hopeless disease. One cannot simply argue that the disease is incurable and thus no obligation exists to preserve life." Brodeur,[12] on the other hand, argues against perceiving quality of life and sanctity of life as polar opposites: "If life has a spiritual value to which temporal ends are subordinated, how does the permanent comatose patient pursue these ends? If a pure physiological existence ensues, which is what happens to a person in a persistent vegetative state, does a moral obligation to continue life-sustaining treatment still exists?" The inference may be drawn that a person not in pursuit of spiritual values may be leading a less than meaningful life. To paraphrase, "Let him who is leading a full spiritual life pull the first plug."

The problem in deciding about nutritional support for the

chronically comatose patient may derive from the classification of food and drink as modalities of medical treatment. As Meilander[13] has pointed out, "the care involved in feeding is not, in any strict sense, medical treatment, even if provided in a hospital. It is ordinary human care and is not given as treatment for any life-threatening disease." Viewed in this light, feeding is neither useless nor excessively burdensome. As strategies for providing nutritional support have become more complicated, there has been a tendency to evaluate them along with other invasive technologies such as respirators and dialysis-machines. It is probably more valid to view self-feeding, assisted feeding, nasogastric tube-feeding, hyperalimentation, and gastrostomy-feedings as strategies for providing basic support for persons capable of varying degrees of cooperation. (The decision to use one or the other may be related as much as to staff-convenience as patient-competence. It may be a lot quicker to feed by tube rather than by teaspoon.) The benefit of feeding for the permanently comatose patient is the preservation of his life even if he has no capacity for life with the quality of consciousness. If anything, the burden of providing nutrition is reduced by the advancement of technology (such as the technology of introducing flexible gastronomy-tubes by way of endoscopy).[14]

4. *Irreversibly demented* patients and those *pleasantly senile*. We mention these categories only to condemn the rationale of using such categories as an excuse for withholding food and water. Neither category justifies the withholding of nutritional support, the tortured rationale of the Wanzer group notwithstanding.

THE PROBLEM OF PAIN

Justification for the removal of nutritional support is often included under the rubric of shortening a painful existence. The British Medical Research Council[15] has reported in a long study that pain can be relieved without shortening life. An adequate number of drugs has been shown to be available for control of pain of varying severity[16] but these are apparently underutilized[17] and withholding food and drink leads to death by starvation and dehydration. Dehydration leads to death through hemoconcentration, hyperosmolarity, azotemia and hyperatremia.[18] Thirst and hunger to the extreme will be experienced to the degree that the patient is conscious and aware of these sensations. In summary, death by starvation is painful. Pain resulting from terminal illness can be controlled without shortening life. As Ramsey[19] has pointed out, relief of discomfort is a primary objective of the physician caring for the terminally ill.

LEGAL ASPECTS

Myers[20] has summarized the legal arguments for continuing patient nourishment, as follows:

1. Nourishment is included within that minimum level of care that anyone has a right to expect to be continued.
2. The expectation of certain minimal care, including nutrition, is essential to the maintenance of trust and confidence in the physician-patient relationship.
3. The dignity of the patient requires that hydration and nutrition continue even when other care is withdrawn.
4. Artificial nourishment can be provided in a simple non-invasive manner.
5. Nourishment is not medical treatment but a basic necessity of life.
6. To withdraw nourishment causes death by means independent of the underlying illness.
7. Nourishment allows life to continue while the illness runs its course.
8. Withdrawal of nourishment is beyond the powers of the surrogate decision-maker.
9. Few, if any, patients express, in advance, a desire not to be fed.
10. To withdraw food and water is to cause a painful, agonized death.

Most of the above arguments are subject to refutation in a court of law. The death of Karen Quinlan in June of 1985 reminded the nation of her remarkable survival for over nine years after she was removed from a respirator and provided comfort care only, including tube-feedings. Karen had originally lapsed into coma following an ingestion of an unknown combination of drugs. The etiology of the coma was unknown and the prognosis, therefore unsure. In November 1975 Judge Muir refused the Quinlan family permission to remove the respirator. In March 1976 the New Jersey Supreme Court overruled Judge Muir, stating that an individual's right to privacy is "broad enough to encompass a patient's decision to decline medical treatment under certain circumstances."[21] Although the Quinlan family never petitioned the court to remove her feeding-tube, many of the subsequent decisions can be considered Karen Quinlan case law progeny. The three principal feeding-tube cases are those of Clarence Herbert, Claire Conroy, and Paul Brophy.

Since the Wanzer article is unquestionably the watershed publication on the issue of discontinuing feeding for certain classes of patients, we must examine the contents carefully for what seems to be a pro-euthanasia bias. On the issue of assisted suicide, for example, the paper seems to be on both sides of the issue. They say, "Although a rare patient may contemplate suicide, the physician cannot participate by assisting in the act for this is contrary to the law." The subliminal message is that there is regret about the law. The next sentence states, for example, "On the other hand, the physician is not obligated to assume that every wish (for suicide) is irrational and requires coercive intervention." From an ethical standpoint, the fact that suicide is against the law is the least important reason why it should not occur. The authors of the Wanzer article imply that while we regretfully cannot assist suicide, we should not work too hard to prevent it. The article then walks a fine line between an endorsement of euthanasia and the responsible choice to refuse therapy when its burden far outweighs its benefit. It is important to note, for example, that the conferences upon which the paper is based were held under the auspices of the *Society for the Right to Die*. This is the latest name for the group which was known from 1938 to 1967 as the *Euthanasia Society of America* and from 1967 to 1975 as the *Euthanasia Educational Council*. The important distinction in this instance is between *what* is done and why it is done. The Vatican Declaration on Euthanasia of 1980[22] states: "By euthanasia is understood an action or omission which of itself or by intention causes death." The terms of reference for euthanasia then are to be found both in the intention of the will and in the methods used.

The authors state that "financial ruin of the patient's family as well as the drain on resources for other patients who are not hopelessly ill should be weighed in the decision-making process." Cost-containment is thus given a prominent place in the evaluation of therapy. Some Catholic authors boldly assert the propriety of including cost-containment in the hierarchy of values even in our society where no need to triage patients has been demonstrable.

The danger of this emphasis is twofold. First, there is no such thing as inexpensive medical care. The attempt to delineate the difference between ordinary and extraordinary care on the basis of cost alone in an affluent society is almost impossible. (I recently spent a few short days in the hospital for a relatively minor surgical procedure and used up the entire annual salary of a person who would be considered to be above the poverty level.)

The second danger is, of course, the new categories for therapeutic restriction created by the Wanzer group. They go beyond those with terminal illnesses, beyond those in a persistent vegetative state, to address a group known as the "pleasantly senile." They define this group as those with "a permanent mild impairment of competence, somewhat limited in their ability to initiate activities and communicate but who appear to be enjoying their moderately restricted lives." Members of this group are also described as "biologically tenacious," meaning apparently that they are not able to accept Governor Lamm's suggestion that they drop dead. All that is recommended for this group is "freedom from discomfort." If emergency resuscitation and intensive care are required, "they should be provided sparingly," based on, among other things, "the wishes of the patient's family and the prospects for improvement." They recommend that routine monitoring of vital signs should be stopped. Then the clincher. "Food and water given *naturally or artificially*" (emphasis added) may be provided or not "depending on the patient's comfort." When we see how the "pleasantly senile" category is defined, it is obvious that feeding anybody above a certain age becomes an option rather than an obligation under the principles of the Wanzer group and the Right to Die Society. Deciding not to treat the elderly whose competence is only mildly impaired is a quantum leap away from not resuscitating the terminally ill or not prolonging the dying process. It is an ugly, unconscionable step down that slipper slope to active euthanasia.

The society has identified two goals for the care of the chronically and terminally ill: a) cost-containment and b) death with dignity. The medical control of nutrition has been held out as a way of accomplishing both of these goals simultaneously. Daniel Callahan, director of the Hastings Institute, has noted, "Given the increasingly large pool of superannuated chronically ill, physically marginal elderly, denial of nutrition could well become the non-treatment of choice."[23]

Medical spending increased seven-fold from 1970 to 1982. It now costs taxpayers $55 billion and we may go broke by 1996. In that context these proposals could be viewed as a particularly nasty kind of cost-cutting. The elderly have enough worries without wondering whether their attending physician is about to label them pleasantly senile and write them off. Should "health care planners" have anything to do with decisions to withhold treatment? Even to suggest that they do reflects a monumental change in the nature of medical practice in the U.S. The medical profession must resist the tendency for their allegiance to drift from the patient to the paymaster.

As recently as three years ago, the idea that fluids and nourishment might be withdrawn with legal and moral impunity would have been repudiated and condemned by most health professionals. The underlying philosophy is as follows:

1. That for a growing population of patients, the costs and burdens of continued life are perceived as being too great to justify the continuation of life-support.
2. Death is accepted as the outcome to be desired for such patients.
3. The physician is to be the agent bringing the desired outcome about.

The countervailing philosophy would be as follows:

The discontinuation of fluids and foods should be forbidden except in the rare instances where it can be incontrovertibly demonstrated that the problems of maintaining nutrition clearly outweigh the acceptance of death by starvation. This philosophy should prevail until there is much more certainty that denying nutrition will not lead to inevitable calamities for the society.

The benefits of adhering to this alternative philosophy would be as follows:

1. Patients will be protected. Prognosis for term of survival is one of the least accurate and least scientific medical skills, even where the diagnosis is clear and accurate.
2. Society will be protected. The fabric of society is threatened by a drift toward the unscrupulous restriction of care out of cost-benefit consideration.

3. Physicians will be protected. There is evidence that physicians are much more inclined to provide fluids and nutrition in terminal situations than so-called professional ethicists. Three out of four physicians polled by Micetich et al.[24] expressed a desire to provide nutrition even to terminal, unconscious patients.
4. The Hippocratic tradition against direct euthanasia will be preserved for the medical profession.
5. The role of the physician as patient-advocate in quality of life debates will be maintained.
6. The goals of medical therapy can be prioritized to include provision of comfort and amelioration of severity as well as complete recovery.

Most physicians would identify the care of the elderly and the terminally ill as a largely unsatisfactory part of the total picture of American medical care. The U.S. wins the lion's share of Nobel Prizes for medical research and American medicine is on the cutting edge of advances in high technology diagnostic and therapeutic achievement. The hospice movement has represented a welcome development toward the humanization of the care of the terminally ill. In all candor, however, it must be admitted that the level of care in American nursing homes and extended care facilities is more an occasion for scandal than for satisfaction. The quality of life for the elderly in these institutions provides, in the eye of the beholder, an inspiration for short-term, Draconian solutions. The society which groans under the burden of providing acute care under Medicare has been unwilling to accept the reality that personal and financial disaster are still a part of the system for those whose terminal illness escapes the time-frame of acute care. As the make-up of the society changes toward the inverted pyramid of an aging population, the need for the medical profession to address the deficiencies of chronic care will increase. As Mark Siegler[25] has said, "If care is to be withheld, it should be withheld from those who are strongest and most powerful, for they are the ones who can make the best case for themselves. The aged and incompetent cannot speak for themselves and should, therefore, not have to bear the burden of justifying their continued medical treatment."

One person in nine is now over 65. By the 21st century it will be one in five. There have been suggestions that everyone on Medicare be required to have a living will. The National Conference of Commissioners of Uniform State Laws has approved a Model Living Will statute which includes the provision of food and water under "medical treatment."[26] During their deliberations in Minneapolis, the Conference defeated an attempt to restrict the definition to *artificially* administered nutrition and to exclude nutrition provided *naturally*.

Dr. Andre Wynen[27] of Belgium, the Secretary General of the World Health Organization, expressed the following well-grounded fear: "Now that cost containment in health care is an everyday threat to the basis interest of the patient, the conflict calls for the presence of his natural defender, the doctor, to help him against the self-interest of the majority. Just as the lawyer defends an accused in society, so must the doctor defend the patient against his own family when the welfare of the elderly or handicapped is at stake."

NOTES

1. S. Wanzer, "The Physician's Responsibility toward Hopelessly Ill Patients" in *N. Eng. J. Med.* 310 (1984) 955.

2. *Griswold v. Connecticut* 381 U.S. 479, 1965.

3. *Roe v. Wade* 410 U.S. 113, 1972.

4. J. Pless, "The Story of Baby Doe" in *N. Eng. J. Med.* 309 (1983) 664.

5. President's Commission for the Study of Ethical Problems in Medicine, *Deciding to Forego Life Sustaining Treatment* (Washington:

Government Printing Office), pp. 123-70.

6. *Barber v. Los Angeles County*, Cal. Rptr. 195.484, 1983.

7. R. Resser and E. Boisaubin, "Ethics, Law and Nutritional Support" in *Arch. Int. Med.* 145 (1985) 122; D. W. Myers, "Legal Aspects of Withdrawing Nourishment from an Incurably Ill Patient" in *Arch. Int. Med.* 145 (1985) 125.

8. Pope Pius XII, Address to the International Congress of Anesthesiologists, Nov. 24, 1957, in *The Pope Speaks* 4 (1958) 395.

9. J. Connery, "The Clarence Herbert Case: Was Withdrawal of Treatment Justified?" in *Hospital Progress* 70 (1984) 32.

10. "'Rip Van Winkle' Mack" in *Minn. Tribune*, April 25, 1982 at 1.

11. T. Najenson, "Laverstein Rehabilitation Hospital Ra'anana, Israel" (unpublished data).

12. D. Brodeur, "Feeding Policy Protects Patients' Rights, Decisions" in *Hospital Progress* 71 (1985) 38.

13. G. Meilander, "On Removing Food and Water, Against the Stream" in *Hastings Center Report* 14 (1984) 6.

14. J. L. Ponsky et. al., "Percutaneous Endoscopic Gastroscopy" in *Arch. Surg.* 118 (1983) 913.

15. Report of the Board of Science and Education, British Medical Research Council in *Medical Tribune*, Dec. 19, 1973 at 5.

16. W. McGivney and G. Crooks, "The Care of Patients with Severe Chronic Pain" in *JAMA* 251 (1984) 1182.

17. M. Argell, "The Quality of Mercy" in *N. Eng. J. Med.* 306 (1982) 98.

18. J. V. Zerwekh, "The Dehydration Issue" in *Nursing* 13 (1983) 47.

19. P. Ramsey, *The Patient as a Person* (New Haven: Yale Univ. Press 1970) 161-62.

20. See note 7 above.

21. In re: *Quinlan* 429 U.S. 922, 1976.

22. *Declaration on Euthanasia*. Sacred Congregation for the Doctrine of the Faith, May 5, 1980.

23. D. Callahan, "On Feeding and Dying" in *Hastings Center Report* 13 (1983) 22.

24. Micetich et al., "Are Intravenous Fluids Morally Required for a Dying Patient?" in *Arch. Int. Med.* 143 (1983) 975.

25. M. Siegler and A. Weisbard, "Against the Emerging Stream" in *Arch. Int. Med.* 145 (1985) 129.

26. "Uniform Rights of the Terminally Ill Act," National Conference of Commissioners of Uniform State Laws, August 9, 1985.

27. A. Wynen, "Euthanasia Feared as a Solution to Rising Health Costs" in *AMA News*, October 6, 1985, p. 36.

SHIFTING THE FOCUS
IN THE ABORTION DEBATE

Francis J. Beckwith

I believe there is a shift occurring in the way abortion is debated in the legal literature. It is a shift that I believe the pro-life movement, at least in popular political debate, is not prepared to challenge. I hope that my comments can help contribute to preparing us for this challenge.

The judicial and ethical debate over abortion in the United States has for the most part focused on the moral status of the fetus, whether or not the fetus is a human person. Typically the pro-life advocate (and the abortion-rights advocate) has argued in this way:

1. The fetus is a person if and only if abortion in almost every case is unjustified homicide.
2. The fetus is (or is not) a person, therefore,
3. Abortion is (or is not) in almost every case unjustified homicide.

Supreme Court Justice Harry Blackmun, who wrote the majority opinion in *Roe v. Wade* (1973), reasons this way as well when he writes, "If the suggestion of personhood [of the unborn] is established, the appellant's case, of course, collapses, for the fetus' right to life is then guaranteed specifically by the [Fourteenth Amendment]."[1]

As we shall see, this assumption is being challenged by the employment of an argument which is nearly 25 years old. Unfortunately, the popular pro-life movement does not appear prepared for this shift. Also, there seems to be a subtle shift in pro-life thinking, which downplays the humanity of the unborn. I will briefly discuss this pro-life shift at the end of this essay.

331

THE SHIFTING IN PRO-ABORTION LEGAL THINKING

In an article, which by 1986 was "the most widely reprinted essay in all of contemporary philosophy,"[2] Professor Judith Jarvis Thomson argues that even if the fetus is fully a human person with a right to life, this does mean that a woman must be forced to use her bodily organs to sustain its life, just as one does not have a right to use another's kidney if one's kidney has failed. Consequently, a pregnant woman's removal of her fetus from her body, even though it will probably result in its death, is no more immoral than an ordinary person's refusal to donate his kidney to another in need of one, even though this refusal will probably result in the death of the prospective recipient. Thomson uses the following story in order to illustrate her position:

> You wake up in the morning and find yourself back to back in bed with an unconscious violinist. A famous unconscious violinist. He has been found to have a fatal kidney ailment, and the Society of Music Lovers has canvassed all the available medical records and found that you alone have the right blood type to help. They have therefore kidnapped you, and last night the violinist's circulatory system was plugged into yours, so that your kidneys can be used to extract poisons from his blood as well as your own. The director of the hospital now tells you, "Look we're sorry the Society of Music Lovers did this to you — we would never have permitted it if we had known. But still, they did it, and the violinist now is plugged into you. To unplug you would be to kill him. But never mind, it's only for nine months. By then he will have recovered from his ailment, and can safely be unplugged from you." Is it morally incumbent on you to accede to this situation? No doubt it would be very nice of you if you did, a great kindness. But do you *have* to accede to it? What if it were not nine months, but nine years? Or still longer? What if the director of the hospital says, "Tough luck, I agree, but you've now got to stay in bed, with the violinist plugged into you, for the rest of your life. Because remember this. All persons have a right to life, and violinists are persons. Granted you have a right to decide what happens in and to your body, but a person's right to life outweighs your right to decide what happens in and to your body. So you cannot ever be unplugged from him." I imagine that you would regard this as outrageous...[3]

It should not be ignored by the pro-life advocate that Thomson's argument makes some very important observations which have gone virtually unnoticed. For Thomson is asking "what happens if, for the sake of argument, we allow the premise [that the unborn are fully human or persons]. How, precisely, are we supposed to get from there to the conclusion that abortion is morally impermissible?"[4] That is to say, from the fact that a certain living organism is fully a human person how does it logically follow that it is *never* permissible to kill that person? Although a near unanimous number of ethicists maintain that it is *prima facie* wrong to kill an innocent human person, a vast majority agree that there may be some circumstances in which taking a human life or letting a human being die is justified, such as in the event of a just war, capital punishment, self-defense, or withdrawing medical treatment. Thomson's argument, however, includes abortion as one of these justified circumstances, for she maintains that since pregnancy constitutes an infringement by the fetus on the pregnant woman's personal bodily autonomy, the ordinary abortion, although it results in the death of an innocent human person, is not *prima facie* wrong.

One can immediately appreciate the appeal of this argument, especially in light of what is arguably the most quoted passage from *Roe*: "We need not resolve the difficult question of when life begins. When those trained in the respective disciplines of medicine, philosophy, and theology are unable to arrive at any consensus, the judiciary, at this point in the development of man's knowledge, is not in a position to speculate."[5] The Court, however, did not choose to employ Thomson's argument, though there is little doubt that it was brought to its attention. Consequently, the *Roe* Court assumed the major premise of the pro-life position: if and only if the fetus is a person, abortion in almost every case is unjustified homicide. This, according to a growing number of scholars, was a fatal mistake, a mistake which energized the right to life movement.

It appears that the first leading legal scholar to recommend Thomson's argument to the judiciary is Michigan Law School professor, Donald Regan, in a law review article which appeared in 1979.[6] More recently, however, Professor Laurence Tribe of Harvard Law School, whose influence on the Court's liberal wing is well-known, suggests in a 1990 book on abortion that the Court should have seriously considered Thomson's argument. Tribe writes: "...[P]erhaps the Supreme Court's opinion in *Roe*, by gratuitously insisting that the fetus *cannot* be deemed a 'person,' needlessly insulted and alienated those for whom the view that the fetus is a person represents a fundamental article of faith or a bedrock personal commitment... The Court could instead have said: Even if the fetus *is* a person, our Constitution forbids compelling a woman to carry it for nine months and become a mother."[7]

In his highly-acclaimed book, *The Culture of Disbelief*, Stephen Carter of Yale Law School has also recommended Thomson's argument. Carter writes:

...[A]s many theorists have recognized, the right to choose abortion, if indeed it survives, must be based on an approach that allows abortion *even if the fetus is human* — instead of an approach that denies that humanity under cover of the pretense that the definition is none of the state's business. The conclusion of fetal humanity by no means ends the argument; it simply forces the striking of a balance.... My point is that the only fair way around a successful legislative effort to define the fetus as human — the only option that does not deride religiously based moral judgments as inferior to secular ones — is to argue for a right to abortion despite it. And an argument of that kind does not require an attack on the religious motivations of any abortion opponents.[8]

In addition to what has already been mentioned, there seems to have occurred a subtle philosophical shift on the

Supreme Court as well as society at large, which would indicate an openness to Thomson's argument.

First, recent Clinton appointee to the Supreme Court, Justice Ruth Bader Ginsburg, in a 1985 article, chides the Court for appealing to the right to privacy rather than the equal protection clause in its grounding of abortion rights. She argues that since women are unique in their ability to be burdened by pregnancy, giving men a distinct advantage in social and political advancement, women should have the right to abortion based on the constitutional principle that all people, regardless of gender, deserve equal protection under the law. Thus, by permitting women to undergo abortions on the basis of the equal protection clause, the Court would have made a clear stand for gender equity on firm constitutional grounds rather than basing its decision on the controversial and constitutionally vague right to privacy.[9]

Second, the recent physician-assisted suicide cases in Washington state and Michigan, in which a judge in the first case and a jury in the latter acquitted physicians, who had killed consenting patients, by appealing to an almost absolute principle of personal autonomy. The judge in Washington claims she can find it in the 14th amendment, the same place Justice Blackmun found the right to privacy in order to constitutionally ground *Roe*.

Third, in the 1992 case which upheld *Roe* as precedent, *Casey v. Planned Parenthood*, the Court asserted the following about the meaning of the 14th amendment:

Our law affords constitutional protection to personal decisions relating to marriage, procreation, family relationships, child rearing, and education.... These matters, involving the most intimate and personal choices a person may make in a lifetime, choices central to personal dignity and autonomy, are central to the liberty protected by the Fourteenth Amendment. At the heart of liberty is the right to define one's own concept of existence, of meaning, of the universe, and of the mystery of human life. Beliefs about these matters could not define the attributes of personhood were they formed under compulsion by the State.[10]

There is little doubt that a shift is occurring in the abortion debate, which should be addressed by those who oppose abortion as well as those who may not favor legal restrictions on abortion but who see Thomson's argument as a threat to the moral force of parental obligations. Let us, therefore, take a critical look at Professor Thomson's argument.

A CRITIQUE OF THOMSON'S ARGUMENT

Although there are a number of problems with Thomson's argument, six of the following problems are sufficient for the judiciary to reject it for consideration. The seventh problem concerns the conflict between Thomson's argument and the Christian worldview.

1. Thomson assumes ethical voluntarism.

By using the violinist story as a paradigm for all relationships, thus implying that moral obligations must be voluntarily accepted in order to have moral force, Thomson mistakenly infers that all true moral obligations to one's offspring are voluntary. But consider the following story. Suppose a couple has a sexual encounter which is fully protected by several forms of birth-control short of abortion (condom, the Pill, IUD, etc.), but nevertheless results in conception. Instead of getting an abortion, the mother of the conceptus decides to bring it to term although the father is unaware of this decision. After the birth of the child the mother pleads with the father for child support. Because he refuses, she seeks legal action and takes him to court. Although he took every precaution to avoid fatherhood, and thus showing that he did not wish to accept such a status, according to nearly all child support laws in the United States he would still be obligated to pay support *precisely*

because of his relationship to this child.[11] As Michael
Levin points out, "All child-support laws make the parental
body an indirect resource for the child. If the father is a
construction worker, the state will intervene unless some of
his calories he extends lifting equipment go to providing
food for his children."[12] For this reason, Keith Pavlischek,
argues that "given the logic [of Thomson's argument], the
most reasonable course to follow would be to surrender the
defense of paternal support laws for those children whose
fathers would rather have had their children aborted,"
which "will lend some credence not only to the pro-life
insistence on the corollary — that an intimate connection
exists between the way we collectively relate to the unborn
and the way we relate to our children after birth — but also
to the claim made by pro-life feminists that the abortion
mentality simply reaffirms the worst historical failings,
neglect, and chauvinism of males."[13]

2. *A case can be made that the unborn does have a* prima
facie *right to her mother's body.*
     Assuming that there is such a thing as a special filial obli-
gation which does *not* have to be voluntarily accepted in
order to have moral force, it is not obvious that the unborn
entity in ordinary circumstances (that is, with the exception
of when the mother's life is in significant danger) *does not*
have a natural *prima facie* claim to her mother's body.
There are several reasons to suppose that the unborn entity
does have such a natural claim.
     (1) Unlike Thomson's violinist who is artificially attached
to another person in order save his life and is therefore not
naturally dependent on any particular human being, the
unborn entity is a human being who is by her very nature
dependent on her mother, for this is how human beings
are at this stage of their development.
     (2) This period of a human being's *natural* development
occurs in the womb. This is the journey which *we all* must

take and is a necessary condition for *any* human being's post-uterine existence. And this fact alone brings out the most glaring disanalogy between the violinist and the unborn: the womb is the unborn's natural environment whereas being artificially hooked-up to a stranger is not the natural environment for the violinist. It would seem, then, that the unborn has a *prima facie* natural claim upon its mother's body. This brings us the third point.

(3) This same entity, when it becomes a newborn, has a natural claim upon her parents to care for her, regardless of whether her parents "wanted" her (see the above story of the irresponsible father). This is why we prosecute child-abusers, people who throw their babies in trash cans, and parents who abandon their children. Although it should not be ignored that pregnancy and childbirth entail certain emotional, physical, and financial sacrifices on the part of the pregnant woman, these sacrifices are also endemic of *parenthood* in general (which ordinarily lasts much longer than nine months), and do not seem to justify the execution of troublesome infants and younger children whose existence entails a natural claim to certain financial and bodily goods which are under the ownership of their parents. If the unborn entity is fully human, as Thomson is willing to grant, why should the unborn's natural *prima facie* claim to her parents' goods differ before birth? Of course, a court will not force a parent to donate a kidney to her dying offspring, but this sort of dependence on the parent's body is highly unusual and is not part of the ordinary obligations associated with the *natural* process of human development, just as in the case of the violinist's artificial dependency on the reluctant music lover.

As Professor Stephen Schwarz points out: "So, the very thing that makes it plausible to say that the person in bed with the violinist has no duty to sustain him; namely, that he is a stranger unnaturally hooked up to him, is precisely what is absent in the case of the mother and her child."

That is to say, the mother "does have an obligation to take care of her child, to sustain her, to protect her, and especially, to let her live in the only place where she can now be protected, nourished, and allowed to grow, namely the womb."[14]

Now if Thomson responds to this by saying that birth is the threshold at which parents become fully responsible, then she has begged the question, for her violinist argument was supposed to show us *why* there is no parental responsibility before birth. That is to say, Thomson can not appeal to birth as the decisive moment at which parents become responsible in order to prove that birth is the time at which parents become responsible.

It is evident that Thomson's violinist illustration undermines the deep *natural bond* between mother and child by making it seem no different than two strangers artificially hooked-up to each other so that one can "steal" the service of the other's kidneys. Never has something so human, so natural, so beautiful, and so wonderfully demanding of our human creativity and love been reduced to such a brutal caricature.

This is not to say that the unborn entity has an *absolute* natural claim to her mother's body, but simply that she has a *prima facie* natural claim. For one can easily imagine a situation in which this natural claim is outweighed by other important *prima facie* values, such as when a pregnancy significantly endangers the mother's life.

3. Thomson ignores the fact that abortion is indeed killing and not merely the withholding of treatment.

Thomson makes an excellent point in her use of the violinist story; namely, there are times when withholding and/or withdrawing of medical treatment is morally justified. For instance, you are not morally obligated to donate your kidney to Fred, your next door neighbor, simply because he needs a kidney in order to live. In other words, you are not obligated to risk your life so that Fred may live a few years longer. Fred should not expect that of you. If, however, you donate one of your kidneys to Fred, you will have acted above and beyond the call of duty, since you will have performed a supererogatory moral act. But this case is not analogous to pregnancy and abortion.

Levin argues that there is an essential disanalogy between abortion and the unplugging of the violinist. In the case of the violinist (as well as your relationship to Fred's welfare), "the person who withdraws [or withholds] his assistance is not completely responsible for the dependency on him of the person who is about to die, while the mother *is* completely responsible for the dependency of her fetus on her. When one is completely responsible for dependence, refusal to continue to aid is indeed killing." For example, "if a woman brings a newborn home from the hospital, puts it in its crib and refuses to feed it until it has starved to death, it would be absurd to say that she simply refused to assist it and had done nothing for which she should be criminally liable."[15] In other words, just as the withholding of food kills the child after birth, in the case of abortion, it is the *abortion* which kills the child. In neither case is there any ailment from which the child suffers and which highly invasive medical treatment, with the cooperation of another's bodily organs, is necessary in order to cure this ailment and save the child's life.

Or consider the case of a person who returns home after work to find a baby at his doorstep (like in the film with Tom Selleck, Ted Danson, and Steve Guttenberg, *Three Men and a Baby*). Suppose that no one else is able to take care of the child, but this person only has to take care of the child for nine months (after that time a couple will adopt the child). If we assume with Thomson that the fetus is as much a person as you or me, would "withholding treatment" from this child and its subsequent death be justified on the basis that the homeowner was only "withholding treatment" from a child he did not *ask* for in order to benefit himself? Is any person, born or unborn, obligated to sacrifice his life because his death would benefit another person? Consequently, there is no doubt that such "withholding" of treatment (and it seems totally false to call ordinary shelter and sustenance "treatment") is indeed unjustified homicide.

But is it even accurate to refer to abortion as the "withholding of support or treatment"? Professors Schwarz and R. K. Tacelli make the important point that although "a woman who has an abortion is indeed 'withholding support' from her unborn child.... abortion is far more than that. It is the active killing of a human person — by burning him, by crushing him, by dismembering him."[16] Euphemistically calling abortion the "withholding of support or treatment" makes about as much sense as calling suffocating someone with a pillow the withdrawing of oxygen.

4. Thomson's argument ignores family law.

Thomson's argument is inconsistent with the body of well-established family law, which presupposes parental responsibility of a child's welfare. And, of course, assuming as Thomson does that the unborn are fully human, this body of law would also apply to parents' responsibility for their unborn children. According to legal scholars Dennis J. Horan and Burke J. Balche, "All 50 states, the District of Columbia, American Samoa, Guam, and the U.S. Virgin Islands have child abuse and neglect statutes which provide for the protection of a child who does not receive needed medical care." They further state that "a review of cases makes it clear that these statutes are properly applied to secure emergency medical treatment and sustenance (food or water, whether given orally or through intravenous or nasogastric tube) for children when parents, with or without the acquiescence of physicians, refuse to provide it."[17] Evidently, "pulling the plug" on a perfectly healthy fetus, assuming that it is a human person, would clearly violate these statutes.

For example, in a case in New York, the court ruled that the parents' actions constituted neglect when they failed to provide medical care to a child with leukemia: "The parent... may not deprive a child of lifesaving treatment, however well-intentioned. Even when the parents' decision to decline necessary treatment is based on constitutional grounds, such as religious beliefs, it must yield to the State's interests, as parens patriae, in protecting the health and welfare of the child."[18] The fact of the matter is that the "courts have uniformly held that a parent has the legal responsibility of furnishing his dependent child with adequate food and medical care."[19]

It is evident then that child-protection laws reflect our deepest moral intuitions about parental and community responsibility and the utter helplessness of infants and small children. And without these moral scruples — which are undoubtedly undermined by "brave new notions" of a socially contracted "voluntaristic" family (Thomson's view) — the protection of children and the natural bonds and filial obligations that are an integral part of ordinary family life will become a thing of the past. This seems too a high a price for "bodily autonomy."

5. Thomson's argument implies a "macho" view of bodily control, which is inconsistent with true feminism.

Some pro-life feminists have pointed out that Thomson's argument and/or the reasoning behind it, which is supposed to be consistent with feminism, is actually quite anti-feminist.[20] In response to a similar argument from a woman's right to control her own body, one feminist publication asks the question, "What kind of control are we talking about? A control that allows for violence against another human being is a macho, oppressive kind of control. Women rightly object when others try to have that kind of control over them, and the movement for women's rights asserts the moral right of women to be free from the control of others." After all, "abortion involves violence against a small, weak and dependent child. It is macho control, the very kind the feminist movement most eloquently opposes in other contexts."[21]

Professor Celia Wolf-Devine makes the observation that "abortion has something... in common with the behavior ecofeminists and pacifist feminist take to be characteristically masculine; it shows a willingness to use violence in order to take control. The fetus is destroyed by being pulled apart by suction, cut in pieces, or poisoned." Wolf-Devine goes on to point out that "in terms of social thought... it is the masculine models which are most frequently employed in thinking about abortion. If masculine thought is naturally hierarchical and oriented toward power and control, then the interests of the fetus (who has no power) would naturally be suppressed in favor of the interests of the mother. But to the extent that feminist social thought is egalitarian, the question must be raised of why the mother's interests should prevail over the child's.... Feminist thought about abortion has... been deeply pervaded by the individualism which they so ardently criticize."[22]

6. Thomson's argument assumes that no one has or had a right to be born.

One of the unusual consequences that results from Thomson's argument is that in principle nobody has or had a right to be born. Remember that for Thomson childbirth is a supererogatory act, an act that if performed is above and beyond the call of duty, but it is not an act that one is obligated to perform. In fact, if one chooses not to give birth, one has not acted immorally at all. Therefore, each of us has a right to be here, according to Thomson, only because someone else chose not to abort us. That is to say, there is no fundamental right to post-uterine existence. But this seems absurd, since it would mean that the entire human race has no right to be here, because each post-uterine member of the human race has no right be here.

7. *Thomson's argument and the Christian worldview.*

From a distinctively Christian point of view, the "rights" talk in Thomson's argument wrongly construes the relationship between unborn child and mother in adversarial terms, fetal rights vs. mother's rights, when the relationship is instead one of love. Neither the child nor the mother are seen as individuals competing to achieve autonomously independent existence, but as members of the Christian community, which is itself called to express love by protecting both child, a gift from God, and mother.

The Christian ethic from earliest times opposed abortion as a part of its special concern for widows, orphans, the poor, and the unborn.[23] Scripture proclaims God to be the author of life and witnesses to its high value even before birth (Ps. 139; Luke 1:42). Together Scripture and Christian tradition value children and the ethic of love and self-sacrifice highly, and thus conflict fundamentally with Thomson's justification for abortion rights.

THE SHIFTING FOCUS IN PRO-LIFE THINKING

One of the primary accusations leveled against the pro-life movement is that its members do not care about the needs of women who are in crisis pregnancies. The abortion opponent is depicted as caring only for the woman's fetus but only while it remains a fetus. We are told that the pro-lifer has no post-uterine compassion. This apocryphal accusation is raised so often that the press and the general public seem to accept it as if it were as obvious as gravity. Of course, the accusation is false as well as irrelevant to whether elective abortion is unjustified homicide.

In her book, *Real Choices*,[24] Frederica Matthews-Green confronts this accusation head on. A pro-life advocate, she maintains that both opponents and proponents of abortion agree on at least one goal: there should be fewer abortions. (I'm not sure whether the multi-million dollar abortion industry would agree). In order to achieve this goal Matthews-Green developed the Real Choices Project, the results of which are the focus of her book. The purpose of the project was to discover the practical reasons why women have abortions. And based on those findings we can then try to meet the needs of women in crisis pregnancies in order to reduce the number of abortions.

Although much can be said about Matthews-Green's book in terms of its scientific accuracy and data collection methods, what I find disturbing about it, from a moral perspective, is its author's willingness to downplay the humanity of the unborn as fundamentally important in resolving the abortion debate: "Pro-lifers will not be able to break through this deadlock by stressing the humanity of the unborn; as noted above, that is a question nobody is asking. But there is a question they are asking, It is, 'How could we live without it?' The problem is not moral but practical: in this wrecked, off-center world, where women are expected simultaneously to be sexually available and to maintain careers, unplanned pregnancies seem both inevitable and catastrophic."[25]

If anything, what Matthews-Green has shown us is that Americans who are pro-choice and yet concede the humanity of the unborn are either morally untutored or sociopaths. This is about as far away from a practical problem as a moral philosopher can imagine. A practical problem is something like this: how can we make ends meet on only one paycheck. A practical problem is *not*: if only society's expectations were modified, I would not have to commit unjustified homicide. *This* is a deeply moral problem. What it shows is that the pro-life movement has not carefully explained the logic of conceding the humanity of the unborn, for it is evident that simply announcing and arguing for the unborn's humanity has not worked.

The fact that people can say the unborn are human persons and yet permit the termination of 1.5 million of these persons every year means that pro-life Americans have not carefully explained to a large number of its pro-choice fellow citizens the irrationality of maintaining both beliefs simultaneously. Matthews-Green is correct that we should do more than stress the humanity of the unborn. But her remedy is flawed. We must vigorously point out to people that just as one cannot be pro-choice on slavery and say that slaves are human persons one cannot be pro-choice on abortion and maintain that fetuses are fully human. If people are not persuaded by such reasoning, raising their self-esteem is not going to help. It may reduce the number of abortions, but it may have the unfortunate consequence of increasing the number of people who think that unless their needs are pacified they are perfectly justified in performing homicide on the most vulnerable of our population.

Please understand that I have great respect and admiration for the work Matthews-Green is doing. It is important and should be continued. However, not emphasizing the humanity of the unborn, I believe, dooms the pro-life movement, reducing it to just another moralistic cause.

CONCLUDING REMARKS

I would like to thank each and every one of you for the wonderful work you are doing. It is because of your important contributions, in both the academy and the marketplace, that I am confident that the pro-life movement will continue to turn the tide in this country. Let me conclude with the words of one of my heroes, the late Evangelical Protestant theologian, Francis Schaeffer:

Cultures can be judged in many ways, but eventually every nation in every age must be judged by this test: How did it treat people? Each generation, each wave of humanity, evaluates its predecessors on this basis. The final measure of mankind's humanity is how humanely people treat one another.... That there is any respite from evil is due to some courageous people who, on the basis of personal philosophies, have led campaigns against the ill-treatment and use of individuals. Each era faces its own unique blend of problems. Our own is no exception. Those who regard individuals as expendable raw material — to be molded, exploited, and then discarded — do battle on many fronts with those who see each person as unique and special, worthwhile, and irreplaceable.[26]

Thank you for being part of this generation's courageous few.

NOTES

1. Justice Harry Blackmun, "Excerpts from Opinion in Roe v Wade" in *The Problem of Abortion*, 2nd ed., ed. Joel Feinberg (Belmont: Wadsworth, 1984) 195.

2. According to her editor, William Parent, in Judith Jarvis Thomson, *Rights, Restitution, and Risk* (Cambridge: Harvard Univ. Pr. 1986) vii.

3. Judith Jarvis Thomson, "A Defense of Abortion" in *The Problem of Abortion*, 2nd ed., ed. Joel Feinberg (Belmont: Wadsworth, 1984) 174-175. This article was originally published in *Philosophy and Public Affairs* 1 (1971) 47-66. All references to Thomson's article in this paper are from the Feinberg book.

4. Ibid., p. 174.

5. Blackmun, "The 1973 Supreme Court Decisions" p. 195.

6. Donald Regan, "Rewriting *Roe v Wade*" in *Michigan Law Review* 77 (1979).

7. Laurence Tribe, *Abortion: The Clash of Absolutes* (New York: W.W. Norton, 1990) 135.

8. Stephen L. Carter, *The Culture of Disbelief: How American Law and Politics Trivialize Religious Devotion* (New York: Harper Collins, 1993) 257-258.

9. Ruth Bader Ginsburg, "Some Thoughts on Autonomy and Equality in Relation to *Roe v Wade*" in *University of North Carolina Law Review* (1985).

10. Justice O'Connor, Justice Kennedy, and Justice Souter in "*Planned Parenthood v. Casey* (1992)" in *The Abortion Controversy: A Reader*, eds. Louis P. Pojman and Francis J. Beckwith (Boston: Jones & Bartlett, 1994) 54.

11. See *In the Best Interest of the Child: A Guide to State Child Support and Paternity Laws*, eds. Carolyn Royce Kastner and Lawrence R. Young (n.p.: Child Support Enforcement Beneficial Laws Project, National Conference of State Legislatures, 1981).

12. Michael Levin, review of *Life in the Balance* by Robert Wennberg, *Constitutional Commentary* 3 (Summer 1986) 511.

13. Keith J. Pavlischek, "Abortion Logic and Paternal Responsibilities: One More Look at Judith Thomson's 'A Defense of Abortion'" in *Public Affairs Quarterly* 7 (October 1993) 343.

14. Stephen D. Schwarz, *The Moral Question of Abortion* (Chicago: Loyola Univ. Press, 1990) 118.

15. Michael Levin, *Feminism and Freedom* (New Brunswick: Transaction Books, 1987) 288-289.

16. Stephen D. Schwarz and R. K. Tacelli, "Abortion and Some Philosophers: A Critical Examination" in *Public Affairs Quarterly* 3 (April 1989) 85.

17. Dennis J. Horan and Burke J. J. Balch, *Infant Doe and Baby Jane Doe: Medical Treatment of the Handicapped Newborn*, Studies in Law & Medicine Series (Chicago: Americans United for Life, 1985) 2.

18. *In re Storar*, 53 N.Y. 2d 363, 380-381, 420 N.E. 2d 64, 73, 438 N.Y.S. 2d 266, 275 (1981), as quoted in Ibid., 2-3.

19. Horan and Balch, *Infant Doe* 3-4.

20. Although not dealing exclusively with Thomson's argument, Celia Wolf-Devine's article is quite helpful: "Abortion and the 'Feminine Voice'" in *Public Affairs Quarterly* 3 (July 1989). See also Sidney Callahan, "Abortion and the Sexual Agenda" in *Commonweal* 113 (April 25, 1986) and Janet Smith, "Abortion as a Feminist Concern" in *The Zero People*, ed. Jeff Lane Hensley (Ann Arbor: Servant, 1983).

21. *Sound Advice for All Prolife Activists and Candidates Who Wish to Include a Concern for Women's Rights in Their Prolife Advocacy: Feminists for Life Debate Handbook* (Kansas City: Feminists for Life of American, n.d.) 15-16.

22. Wolf-Devine, "Abortion" 86, 87.

23. See *Didache* 2.2.

24. Frederica Matthews-Green, *Real Choices: Offering Practical, Life-Affirming Alternatives to Abortion* (Sisters, Oregon: Multnomah, 1994).

25. Ibid., 32.

26. Francis A. Schaeffer and C. Everett Koop, *Whatever Happened to the Human Race?* (Old Tappan: Fleming H. Revell, 1979), 15-16.

THE HISTORICAL ROOTS
OF THE PRO-LIFE MOVEMENT:
ASSESSING THE PRO-CHOICE ACCOUNT

Keith Cassidy

History is a crucial arena for many social movements which attempt to use the past to legitimize themselves to cast their opponents into disrepute and to give an air of inevitability to the victory of their cause. They can do this by fraud, whether by a deliberate misstatement of the record or by a consciously selective reading of events. But while professional historians often share the convictions and goals of these movements, they are by training less likely to distort the historical record by baldly lying or suppressing contrary testimony. Nonetheless, they do frame questions in a fashion congenial to their interests and presuppositions — usually without being conscious of doing so — and the road to historical insight is often found not in new "facts" but in the clash of different sets of questions and concerns. In the words of a recent book which attempts to assess the nature of historical knowledge in the light of the challenges presented by postmodernism,

Criticism fosters objectivity and thereby enhances reasoned inquiry. Objectivity is not a stance arrived at by sheer willpower, nor is it the way most people, most of the time, make their daily inquiries. Instead it is the result of the clash of social interests, ideologies, and social conventions within the framework of object-oriented and disciplined knowledge-seeking.[1]

The abortion battle is a particularly interesting case of clashing ideologies producing sharply different accounts of the historical record. But we do not need in despair to conclude with the cynic that "history is a pack of tricks the living play upon the dead" and that historical truth is a

350

chimera. It is possible to answer questions about the topic in a fashion which respects scholarly standards, provided that these are framed in a fashion which encourages clarity rather than confusion.

The pro-life movement has always claimed to be the heir to a solid and long-standing tradition of opposition to the practice of abortion, an opposition based on respect for the sanctity of human life, and thus to have been in the mainstream, if not of contemporary societal attitudes, then of the deeper currents of our civilization. Is this true? Pro-lifers have long believed that they represent the continued defense, in John Noonan's famous phrase, of "an almost absolute value in history."[2] But pro-lifers should be aware that a substantial body of material, both popular and scholarly, asserts the contrary. Is the pro-life claim valid? Through an examination of the counter-claims of the movement's opponents we can arrive at some estimate of the accuracy of the pro-life assertions. We should be careful, however, to make clear just exactly what is being asked. It is *not whether abortion was almost unknown before the 20th century*, or *whether abortion was always opposed from the start of pregnancy only or primarily because of the defense of human life*, or *whether exceptions were ever made for abortion where another life was in danger*. Rather, the point in question is *whether until quite recent times abortion was regarded as wrong when it was known with reasonable certainty that a human life was present, and regarded as wrong because it involved the destruction of a human life*. In answering that question, what is at issue is often not the historical facts, but the emphasis placed on them, and the inferences drawn from them.

In assessing the historical record it is useful to break it into four broad areas: pre-literate and ancient societies; the traditions of Judaism and the Christian Church, up to the 19th century; the treatment of abortion in English common

law and in the American colonies; and finally the changes
which occurred in the 19th century. In each case an attempt
will be made to make clear the various claims being
advanced. After presenting the pro-choice account of each
period, I will review some of the pro-life literature on the
topic to see if it suggests any significant revision of that
account. This paper is not based on research in the
sources, but is a broad review of some of the accounts the
topic, accompanied by an examination of some of the
historical events discussed in that literature, in an attempt
to appraise the validity of the assertions being made.
There is a need for a comprehensive treatment of the
history of abortion laws, attitudes and practices, but this
account is not it. To reiterate, this paper simply asks one
question: can the present day pro-life movement plausibly
assert a valid claim to be the continuation of a long and
respected tradition, which for over one and a half millennia
was the predominant one in the Western world?

To its enemies the right-to-life movement does not
represent a defense of traditional values but is rather, in
Michael A. Cavanaugh's phrase, "a non traditional
traditionalism." Accepting the pro-choice account of the
historical record at face value Cavanaugh argues that

> The contemporary position with the best traditional pedigree is not
> unqualified opposition to abortion. Rather it is the liberty to elect
> abortion. Traditionally abortion was medically available, legally
> permissible, and carried on below the threshold of moral awareness.[3]

To begin, it is useful to examine the frequently made
claim that abortion has been practiced by all cultures, and
that by implication it is an acceptable institution with little
stigma attaching to it. Consultation of the work of George
Devereux, who reviewed attitudes to abortion in a wide
range of pre-literate cultures, leads to a somewhat different
conclusion. While some societies feel no repugnance,
others condemn it; thus, he reports, a Cherokee "had

trouble 'understanding' what the anthropologist meant by abortion. When he finally 'understood,' he was horrified, exclaiming that one might as well cut off the head of a five-year-old child, and that it was outright murder. After this conversation his regard for whites appears to have decreased."[4] Abortion may indeed be widely practiced, but it is also frequently disapproved of, and often for reasons clearly consistent with the views of the pro-life movement.

In the pagan culture of the ancient Mediterranean world abortion was well known, and medical texts from the period describe methods of performing it.[5] Both Plato and Aristotle saw abortion as an appropriate instrument for population control and contemplated compulsory abortion in certain cases for the good of the state.[6] Aristotle's influential work in biology transmitted the view that has often been invoked in the subsequent history of the controversy over abortion, that after conception there was a succession of souls: first the "nutritive" or "vegetative" soul, then the "sensitive" soul, and then the "rational" soul. This final stage, when true human life was present, occurred when distinct organs were formed: for males this was at 40 days; for females at 90 days. This final stage corresponded, he claimed, with the first movements of the fetus.[7] These limits were to be incorporated into some of the subsequent penal treatment of abortion as a way to determine the severity of sentences.

But there is also some evidence of anti-abortion sentiment in ancient society, most notably in the Hippocratic Oath (*circa* 400 B.C.) with its promise "I will not give to a woman a pessary to cause abortion." The degree to which this oath actually regulated conduct is, however, obscure.[8] A society which allowed the exposure of some newborn infants had little inclination to reject abortion. One Greek philosophical school worth mentioning is that of the Stoics. While a first century Stoic text by Musonius Rufus opposes abortion, it most likely does so because its widespread practice would be detrimental to the family and to the state, not because of a belief in the inherent value of fetal life: the Stoics did not believe that the child was human until it had drawn its first breath.[9]

Abortion was practiced in ancient Rome, but disapproved of when it was performed without the permission of the father, the *paterfamilias*, and when it endangered the life of the mother. There were some countervailing trends: Connery sees a growing tendency "to attribute more and more rights to the fetus"[10] and by the second century legislation against abortion first appeared. Yet the Romans never considered the fetus a human person.[11]

Pro-choice accounts of the history of attitudes to abortion tends to minimize Jewish opposition to the practice by stressing the lack of specific reference to it in Scripture other than the somewhat ambiguous mention in Exodus 21: 22-23. In that passage there is discussion of an abortion caused by an accidental blow to a woman in the course of a struggle between two men. In the Hebrew text a fine is assessed if the fetus dies; if the woman dies the penalty is death. In the Septuagint a key word *'ason* is translated as "form," not "harm," thus introducing the notion that the degree of penalty was dependent on the state of development of the fetus: a fine if it was "unformed", death if it was "formed." While Scripture provides little direct clue to attitudes to abortion, its general emphasis on the beauty and value of life as a gift from the Creator, and its celebration of large families certainly indicates an anti-abortion orientation.

The Talmud deals with the issue more clearly. The fetus was not considered "a separate entity but part of the mother until it is born."[12] This does not mean, however, that the fetus was held to have no value, but that it had less value than the mother. Hence, therapeutic abortion was allowed, but there is no reason to believe that there was any acceptance of abortion as a right or as a frequently practiced operation. The fact the Talmud in one instance gives permission for a therapeutic abortion, specifying that "her life takes precedence over its life," seems to indicate that ordinarily abortion was forbidden,[13] for if abortion was unrestricted, it would hardly be necessary to specifically approve of it in such compelling circumstances. The Septuagint translation, with its echoes of the Aristotelian view of human development, became the basis of the Alexandrian school of Jewish thought on the subject: after "formation" the fetus was treated as a full human being. It is clear in this tradition that abortion, at least the abortion a "formed" fetus, was not only wrong but a form of homicide. Thus Philo, a first century Jewish philosopher argued that the accidental aborting of a formed fetus was akin to the destruction of a completed sculpture which had not yet left the artist's workshop. It should be stressed that this tradition does not regard the unformed fetus as of no value - its destruction, though not a homicide, is still an offense against life, for, in Connery's words, it prevents "nature from bringing into existence a human life."[14] The Hebrew text, which stressed the "harm" done to the mother, was used in the Palestinian Jewish approach to the topic, which did not see the fetus as a person but as part of the mother. Some saw conception as the time of ensoulment, others saw "formation" and others believed that this took place at birth. It should be stressed, however, that while several schools of thought on abortion and the nature of the fetus developed in Jewish thought, there is no sign that abortion was envisioned for anything other than very serious reasons, most notably threats to the life of the mother.[15] In the words of a distinguished contemporary Jewish scholar,

The destruction of an unborn child, let alone of an embryo in the earliest stages of gestation, does not constitute murder, since the unqualified entitlement to life — equal to the claim to inviolability of any other human being — sets in only at birth. Nevertheless, the germinating product of conception enjoys a very sacred title to life which may be set aside by deliberate destruction or abortion only in the most exceptional cases of medical urgency, notably to save the life of the mother if this would otherwise be at risk.[16]

While the pro-life movement does not find a position identical to its own in this part of the Jewish tradition, it can discern here an appreciation of the fetus's "sacred title to life" and an aversion to abortion for anything other than a threat to the mother's life. It is certainly the case that the pro-choice opinion has little support in this tradition, while the pro-life position can see in it a kindred viewpoint.

How is the pro-choice case argued with respect to the history of Christianity? Dallas Blanchard's recent pro-choice account, written for popular consumption, *The Anti-Abortion Movement and the Rise of the Religious Right: From Polite to Fiery Protest*, contains a short history of abortion. He claims that "some" of the "early church elders condemned the practice of abortion" but that "between 450 and 1450, church doctrine allowed abortion only before quickening." Until the 19th century

most theologians believed that ensoulment occurred at the time of quickening. Thus the practices of women and the positions of the church, as well as the later common law, usually coincided.... Between 1450 and 1750 church teaching generally held to the allowance of abortion before quickening and also allowed it after to save the woman's life.... Pope Gregory XIII, who led the church from 1572 to 1585 allowed it in the first 40 days of pregnancy and for single women under extenuating circumstances.[17]

Remarkably Blanchard cites as his source for these statements the works of John Noonan, the very scholar who proclaimed opposition to abortion an "almost absolute value" in history and who makes no statements even remotely resembling those for which he is cited as an authority.[18] Something like this account can be found in a number of popular writings.

A more moderate statement of similar views is given in Kristin Luker's widely used *Abortion and the Politics of Motherhood*, which argues that church councils outlined penalties only for women who committed abortion after a sexual crime and that early Christian thought was divided as to whether early abortion was murder. She asserts that "different sources of church teachings and laws simply did not agree on the penalties for abortion or whether early abortion is wrong."[19] Angus McLaren, a prominent historian of contraception and abortion, stresses another theme. Christian opposition to abortion did not arise from a concern for fetal life: "Catholic historians such as John Noonan, who defend contraception but oppose abortion, have argued that early Christians, like their 20th century counterparts, condemned abortion because it entailed the killing of a live fetus. But this was not quite the case. Early abortion and contraception were regarded by some early Christians not as different but as very much the same thing — attempts to enjoy sexual pleasure without bearing children."[20] This position is echoed by Daniel Dombrowski in his analysis of Augustine's reasons for opposition to abortion. Dombrowski suggests that such interpreters as Noonan, Connery and Gorman are in error in ascribing to Augustine any concern for the protection of human life in his rejection of early abortion. Rather Augustine opposed these abortions because of his rejection of any sexual activity which was not procreative.[21] Another direct attack on Noonan's position is found in Dunstan's writings, particularly "The Human Embryo in the Western Moral Tradition." He writes that "the claim to absolute protection for the human embryo 'from the beginning' is a novelty in the Western, Christian and specifically Roman Catholic moral traditions. It is virtually a creation of the late 19th century, a little over a century ago; and that is a novelty as traditions go."[22] Dunstan bases this claim on a review of the long-standing distinction between "formed" and "unformed" fetuses and the differential penalties which attached to the destruction of the being in the woman's womb depending on its state of development.

What can be said in response to these claims? In reviewing Christian attitudes to abortion, we should note that there is no explicit discussion of the subject in the New Testament: the reference in Galatians 3:1-6 to *pharmakeia* is possibly to abortifacient drugs, among others, but it is not very explicit.

Proof of Christian repugnance to abortion is found very early, however. The *Didache*, from the second century (and possibly earlier) explicitly condemns abortion: "You shall not kill the fetus by abortion or destroy the infant already born." A nearly identical condemnation is found in the *Epistle of Pseudo-Barnabas*. Connery suggests that the reason why abortion is directly condemned in the early Christian writings, but not in Jewish writings, is that the Christian documents "were addressed to gentiles, people coming from a culture where both abortion and infanticide were practiced with frequency.... For the most part the New Testament was addressed to a Jewish audience who did not have this practice or tradition."[23]

That abortion was condemned as an attack on life, and not only as an ancillary to sexual sins is clear from the *Plea for Christians* by Athenagoras in the second century. He defends Christians from the pagan claim that they were cannibals (a claim based on a false understanding of the Eucharist) by pointing out that Christians are opposed to all killing - including infanticide and abortion.

Other texts from this era could be cited, but a final example will be taken from Tertullian, who also defended Christians from the charge of child sacrifice, by pointing out that the Romans practiced infanticide — which Christians condemned, along with abortion. He sees abortion as an anticipated homicide.[24] Though in another work he indicated that the fetus is not a man until it is formed (he appealed here to the Septuagint distinction), there is no reason to believe that he approves of abortion before the fetus is "formed."[25] What is reflected here is rather an ignorance of biological processes and the resulting uncertainty about when abortion becomes homicide rather than another kind of sin against life.

One such controversial passage from Tertullian has been read as approving therapeutic abortion where a difficult birth imperils the woman's life. In fact the main point of the passage is to prove that the fetus is alive — contrary to the Stoic claim that birth is the crucial dividing line — since otherwise it would not be necessary to kill the child. Whether he really believes the abortion "necessary" in the sense of justified is dubious in view of the negative phrases he uses in conjunction with it.[26]

The first church legislation dealing with abortion comes from the Council of Elvira in 305. In canons 63 and 68 women who have abortions to conceal adultery are subject to severe penance. Some pro-choice authors have interpreted this as a sign that what is really being condemned is the sexual sin, and that abortion was abhorred because of it, not because it represented an attack on human life. A separate canon dealt with adultery alone, and it prescribed a far less severe sentence; thus it would be reasonable to conclude that the attack on life simply compounded the offense.

The Council of Ancyra in 314 modified the severe penalties of Elvira: it seems most likely that this was a pastoral judgment related to recognition of the pressures on a pregnant woman, not the result of a more tolerant view of abortion.

The writings of Basil the Great later in the fourth century contain a condemnation of abortion which equated it with homicide. Significantly, he rejects the distinction between the formed and unformed fetus.[27] For other writers, however, this distinction becomes an important one, and yet no clear agreement about the time of "animation" emerged. Jerome, although a consistent and clear opponent of abortion, is unclear about the time of animation. The issues here are complex and involve a tangled debate about the nature of the soul and its relation to the body.[28]

Augustine's writings on abortion are numerous and influential. The section of his *Marriage and Concupiscence* known to posterity as *Aliquando* condemns those married who "procure poisons of sterility, and if they do not work, they extinguish the fetus in some way in the womb, preferring that their offspring die before it lives, or if it is already alive in the womb, to kill it before it was born."[29] Here he distinguishes contraception, the killing of the unanimated fetus, and abortion of the animated fetus. This distinction between two stages of fetal life with reference to abortion became commonly (though not universally) made. But it should be noted that abortions at both stages are condemned.

As mentioned earlier Dombrowski disagrees with the interpretations of Augustine offered by Noonan, Connery and Gorman. He stresses the distinction made by Augustine between the formed and unformed fetus, and the clear implication at a number of points in his writing that the unformed fetus is not a human being. He suggests that the real source of Augustine's condemnation of early abortion, as of contraception, is a condemnation of any divorce between sex and procreation, a condemnation which he alleges is rooted in Augustine's negative view of sex for pleasure. Dombrowski makes a strong case that Augustine does not view early abortion as homicide, the killing of a human being,[30] but it is less clear that Augustine's sole basis for condemning of it is his view of sex. Dombrowski has set up an arbitrarily forced dichotomy by holding that this condemnation can only be the result of either a belief in the humanity of the fetus, or a hatred of sexual pleasure. Are other alternatives possible? A closer look at Augustine's work, in the light of Dombrowski's argument seems appropriate.

Augustine was frequently concerned by the problem of the formed/unformed, animated/unanimated fetus. For example:

> If the embryo is still unformed, but yet in some way ensouled while unformed... the law does not provide that the act pertains to homicide, because still there cannot be said to be a live soul in a body that lacks sensation, if it is in flesh not yet formed and thus not yet endowed with senses.[31]

It should be mentioned here that while the terms "formed" and "unformed" and "animated" and "unanimated" and later "quickened" and "unquickened" eventually came to be seen as equivalent pairs, there was considerable controversy about this point and Augustine's attempts to grapple with the subject illustrate its complexity.[32]

The distinction between "formed" and "unformed" fetuses continued to be made in later centuries. With the development of the tradition of private penance, various penitential books of instruction for confessors appeared which recommended different penalties for the two sins. Commonly a period of one year of penance for the abortion of an unformed fetus was assessed, while three years was given for abortion at later stages of development.

An important tenth century development was the collection *Libri Synodates* by Regino of Prum. In canon 89 of Book II, known by its initial words, *Si aliquis*, anyone who deliberately causes sterility is held to be a murderer. This canon would play a crucial role in later centuries, for it suggested that all abortions be treated as homicides, regardless of the stage of development.

In response to a question regarding the status of a monk who had accidentally caused an abortion (thereby, under *Si aliquis*, being guilty of homicide and subject to loss of his ministry) Innocent III issued the decree *Sicut ex* that if the fetus had been unformed he would not face loss of ministry. Since the earlier canon *Si aliquis* continued in force, a contradiction or at least confusion existed which engaged attention in subsequent centuries. Later authors inclined to accept the view that while all abortions were in some sense homicide, not all led to clerical irregularity.

The later Middle Ages saw two important developments: the rediscovery of Aristotle's biology, with its claim that males and females were animated at different gestational ages; and the origin of a discussion about therapeutic abortion. Some theologians held that the abortion of an unanimated fetus was licit in order to save the mother's life; abortion of the formed fetus continued, for these writers, to be homicide. In the case of doubt as to the fetus' state, the abortion should not be done. In later centuries the debate over therapeutic abortion widened; it is impossible in the space available here to give an adequate account of it. The fullest and best known development of these theories was by the 16th century Jesuit, Tomas Sanchez. Over time the distinction was drawn more clearly between means tending directly to procure an abortion and those treatments which had an unintended abortifacient effect. Noonan notes with respect to this debate that, "the balance struck by the casuists and now set out by St. Alfonso treated the embryo's life as less than absolute, but only the value of the mother's life was given greater weight."[33]

These speculations by moralists, however, ought not to be confused with Church law. The tradition of *Si aliquis* continued in force, although penalties varied depending on whether or not 40 days had been reached in gestational age; penalties were also lighter than for other homicides, not because the crime was objectively less, but because extenuating circumstances often existed.

A more severe view was taken by Pope Sixtus V in his 1558 bull *Effraenatam* which applied the same penalties —

including excommunication — for abortion at any stage of development. This bull was revoked in 1591; however, the penalty of excommunication continued to be attached to the abortion of the ensouled fetus.

Up to this point we have considered the treatment of abortion in the Roman Catholic Church. What of the Protestant tradition? A study by Germain Grisez notes that there is little in the writings of the early reformers bearing on it, although Calvin does argue that just as it is worse to kill a man in his own house, "it ought to be regarded as more atrocious to kill a fetus who has never seen the light of day, in the womb."[34] Other examples are cited by Grisez. In general the Reformation spelled no break with the unchanging Christian opposition to abortion. Grisez detects in Lutheranism some tendency to "mitigate" traditional views, while Calvinism maintained traditional beliefs with full force. Nonetheless, Grisez also points to Lutheran theologians who of the 17th century took a more restrictive view of therapeutic abortion than some of their Catholic contemporaries.[35] In more modern times, the opposition to abortion expressed by Karl Barth and Dietrich Bonhoeffer is worth noting.[36]

In the light of the foregoing account it is possible to reply to the pro-choice view of the treatment of abortion by the Church. First of all, there is absolutely no basis for the frequently made statement that abortion was ever allowed in the period prior to what was thought of as animation or formation. Blanchard's statement, quoted above, that abortion was allowed by the church in the first 40 days, is utterly without foundation. How he believed that Noonan's work led to such conclusions is difficult to imagine. Penalties may have varied for early abortion, but there is no reason to suppose that it was permitted. Nor is there reason to support Luker's claim that there was no agreement on whether early abortion was wrong. Given the early Church's hostility to contraception, it is difficult to imagine that the abortion of the fetus in its early stages would normally be regarded as acceptable. This is clear from McLaren's account, mentioned above, which observes that while abortion was regarded by some as acceptable to save the mother's life, in general it, like contraception, was regarded with profound hostility. Dombrowski concedes that "John Noonan has correctly noted that condemnation of abortion has been "an almost absolute value in history," specifically in the history of Catholicism."[37] Two points are clear. First, abortion at any stage of development was not accepted. The sources to prove this point are legion and the works of John Noonan, John Connery, Michael Gorman and Gerald Bonner[38] all testify to this. Connery concludes that:

Whatever one would want to hold about the time of animation, or when the fetus became a human being in the strict sense of the term, abortion from the time of conception was considered wrong, and the time of animation was never looked on as a moral dividing line between permissible and immoral abortion.[39]

Second, abortion after quickening or after the fetus was "formed" was commonly denounced as homicide. Thus St. Jerome explained that "seeds are gradually formed in the uterus, and it is not reputed homicide until the scattered elements receive their appearance and members."[40]

The pro-life claim to represent a long-standing tradition appears imperiled, however, by the interlinked assertions that while the abortion of early term fetuses was condemned, it was not regarded as homicide because it was not believed that animation had occurred and that the condemnation of abortion at this stage represented not a regard for human life but repressive sexual attitudes. While the first assertion is true for the majority of the Church Fathers, the second needs to be qualified. That is, while it is the case that the condemnation of early abortion was heavily colored by a loathing of sexual sin, it is true that it was also regarded as an attack on life, even if not necessarily homicide. The presence of a concern about sexual sin does not preclude the simultaneous existence of a concern for life in the condemnation of abortion by many of the Church Fathers.[41] Even if we were to assume that both of the pro-choice claims are unreservedly true, would it follow that there is not a tradition which rejects the killing of all innocent human life? We should review the history of the tradition that a distinction can be made between early and later fetuses.

The principal sources of the distinction are, of course, the biology of Aristotle and the Scriptural treatment in Exodus. The writings of the early Church reflect these distinctions, as Dunstan and others have stressed, and clearly for many (but not for all) the abortion of an "unformed" fetus was not homicide. St. Basil declared that "A woman who deliberately destroys a fetus is answerable for murder. And any fine distinction as to its being completely formed or unformed is not admissible among us."[42]

The distinction between "formed" and "unformed" fetuses continued to be made in later centuries and is at the core of the pro-choice account of the history of abortion. What exactly does it prove? Dunstan seems clear about its significance: "the claim for absolute protection for the human embryo 'from the beginning' is a novelty in the Western, Christian and specifically Roman Catholic moral traditions." Later he asserts that

The aim of this chapter has been, not to claim contemporary relevance for either an outmoded embryology or an outmoded philosophical speculation on the soul and the time of its 'entering' (if it does) the body; nor yet to ventilate again the liceity of abortion. It has been to recall a moral tradition *expressed in terms* of these three things, persisting to the end of the 19th century, and for those cognizant of the arcane casuistry of medical practice beyond that date into this day. The tradition attempted to grade the protection accorded to the nascent human being according to the stages of its development.[43]

To assess this claim we must consider more closely the reasons offered in the ancient world for differentiating between the formed and unformed fetus. On examination it is clear that they reflect a profound — and fully understandable — ignorance of the nature of fetal development. Consider, for example, Aristotle's belief that movement in males first occurred at 40 days, and at 90 days in the case of females. Obviously this is wrong, not merely at a simple level — males and females do not differ in the fashion Aristotle describes, and fetal movement, we now know, occurs far earlier — but in a far deeper way. The role of DNA, the real nature of sperm and egg, the self directing character of the fetus, which secretes hormones to stop the mother's periods, were all either unknown or only partially understood by Aristotle and other ancient thinkers. This is hardly to their discredit, since they were limited to the observation of external phenomena — the physical appearance of aborted fetuses, the mother's sensation of movement — but it is rather the case that they could not adequately perceive the inner dynamics of fetal life. Of necessity their appreciation of when "life" or the "soul" could be posited was radically limited. To attribute *moral* significance to this ignorance is to allow contemporary beliefs to dictate our historical sense.

Dunstan's argument that the protection of human life "from the beginning" is a novelty is simply not supported by his own evidence. His work has made it clear that it was precisely because human life was not seen as beginning at conception that less protection was afforded to early fetal life. The profound limitations of the biological knowledge available shaped the decisions made, and hence Dunstan's caveat that he does "not claim contemporary relevance for an outmoded embryology" is misleading. When the Church fathers and later Christian writers knew that human life was present they afforded it full protection; when they had reason to doubt that it was they imposed lesser penalties. To the question *whether there is the sanction of tradition for a movement which seeks full protection for human life from the earliest period where we have good grounds to believe that it exists* the answer is clearly yes. The modern pro-life movement, if somehow brought to the attention of the early Church fathers might seem odd to them on a number of counts — not least in its unconscious acceptance of a "rights" orientation — but it would surely appear congruent with their approach and, in the light of scientific discoveries, a logical development of it.

We should bear in mind the question we are asking, which is surely not *whether the exact set of beliefs of the right to life movement of the late 20th century have existed unchanged from the earliest days of the Church to the present*. Rather, as stated at the start of this essay, we want to see *if until quite recent times abortion was regarded as wrong when it was known with reasonable certainty that a human life was present, and regarded as wrong because it involved the destruction of a human life*. That a concern about sexual sin was mixed with a concern to protect life or that less protection was afforded life in stages when its existence as human life was arguable does not negate the existence of a pro-life tradition. We are, after all, concerned to prove the existence of that tradition, not to prove the unchanging character of biological knowledge.

Turning to the question of English common law and the status of abortion in the Anglo-American world prior to the 19th century, we have a handy compendium of the views of pro-choice scholars: the *amicus* brief submitted in *Casey v. Planned Parenthood* by 250 historians:

As this Court demonstrated in *Roe v. Wade*, abortion was not illegal at common law. Through the 19th century, American common law decisions uniformly reaffirmed that women committed no offense in seeking abortion. Both common law and popular American understanding drew distinctions depending upon whether the fetus was "quick", i.e., whether the woman perceived signs of independent life. There was some dispute whether a common law misdemeanor occurred when a third party destroyed a fetus, after quickening, without the woman's consent. But early common law recognition of this crime against a pregnant woman did not diminish the woman's liberty to end a pregnancy herself in its early stages.... Recent studies of the work of midwives in the 1700[s] report cases in which the midwives appeared to have provided women abortifacient compounds. Such treatments do not appear to have been regarded as extraordinary or illicit by those administering them.[44]

The principal secondary sources quoted in support of these statements are James Mohr's *Abortion in America*,[45] Carol Smith-Rosenberg's *Disorderly Conduct*,[46] Cyril Means's "The Phoenix of Abortional Freedom,"[47] and Angus McLaren's *Reproductive Rituals*.[48] There is no reference to the large group of studies by pro-life scholars which contest these points. Particularly notable is the absence of any reference to the works of legal scholars such as John Keown[49], Robert Byrn[50], Clarke Forsythe[51] and others.[52] Particularly notable is the lack of reference to the work of Joseph Dellapenna. Dellapenna, like the pro-choice historians, had presented an *amicus* brief in *Casey*,[53] and had earlier presented one in *Webster v. Reproductive Health Services*.[54]

In these and other *amicus* briefs Dellapenna has demonstrated that, contrary to Means and others, a substantial body of evidence exists to show that there was no common law "liberty" to commit abortion:

Common law indictments and appeals of felony for abortion are recorded as early as 1200. While the terse records often do not indicate the outcome of the proceedings, the many clear records of punishment and judgments of "not guilty" (rather than dismissal) prove that the indictments and appeals were valid under common law. Means was simply wrong to assert that only two cases dealt with abortion before 1600 and that the courts in both cases doubted whether abortion was a crime....[55]

It should be noted that even scholars sympathetic to a pro-
choice view dismiss Means's claim to an unlimited
common law "right" to abortion.[56]

With regard to the assertion that abortion was a right
prior to "quickening," we should consider the argument of
Robert Byrn that

"quickening" was utilized in the later common law as a practical
evidentiary test to determine whether the abortion had been an assault
upon a live human being in the womb and whether the abortional act
had caused the child's death; this evidentiary test was never intended
as a judgment that before quickening the child was not a live human
being; and... at all times, the common law disapproved of abortion as
malum in se and sought to protect the child in the womb from the
moment his living biological existence could be proved.[57]

The difficulty faced by the court in proving that the
aborted child had been indeed "quick" made prosecution
complicated. For abortion to be a crime it was necessary
to prove that what was killed had indeed been alive: given
the primitive biological knowledge of the time, this was
difficult to do. Nonetheless abortion continued to be a
crime. In the 17th century in the case of *R. v. Sims* it was
declared that if the child was born alive and subsequently
died from the abortion procedure, then the crime was
murder; if it was still-born, then murder could not be
proved because it was not clear that the child had been
alive at the time of the abortion. Subsequently Sir Edmund
Coke (Attorney General at the time of the *Sims* case) in his
enormously influential legal writings maintained that if the
child was delivered dead "this is a great misprision
[misdemeanor] and no murder but if the child be born
alive, and dieth of the Potion, battery, or other cause, this
is murder, for in law it is accounted a reasonable creature,
in rerum natura, when it is born alive."[58]

Does Coke's view mean that the unborn child was not
accounted as a person *in rerum natura* before birth? No,

Byrn argues, for he was "referring only to the law of homicide where the exigencies of proof prevented labelling the intra-uterine killing a murder. For other purposes, such as inheritance, the unborn child was recognized as a person *in rerum natura* in the womb."[59]

Moreover, in 1670 Chief Justice Hale held that if a woman died as the result of an attempted abortion at *any* stage in her pregnancy, the person performing the abortion was accounted guilty of a murder. Dellapenna suggests that this was either "akin to felony murder, with the *mens rea* against the child linked to the *actus reus* of killing the mother to support the charge of murder." Alternatively it could be because "the act was one of extreme recklessness, endangering the mother's life, and, therefore, murder."[60] Either way, this hardly equates with the pro-choice claim that abortion was an accepted practice. Clarke Forsythe puts the issue in somewhat different terms:

During the period of the formation of the common law, quickening was the most important point in pregnancy in both law and medicine. It was assumed that the fetus first became alive at quickening. At common law, the primitive state of medical knowledge made quickening legally significant, "since quickening was determinable at least by the mother, in a time when little else about the fetus was readily understood." Later, in the 19th century, physicians came to understand that the fetus was alive at conception. Nevertheless, prior to the 20th century, quickening remained the first reliable proof that the mother was pregnant.[61]

We have evidence that not only was abortion legally disapproved, but it was regarded with disapproval by much of society. This is not to say that it was not practiced, but only that a strong tradition of abhorrence of it is also part of the historical record. Even pro-choice historians cite numerous hostile references to abortion, and although they assert that abortion prior to quickening was accepted by many women as moral, the fact remains that once it was known that a living fetus was involved, there was frequent condemnation of the practice and even at the earlier stages it had a disreputable character.[62]

In this context it is instructive that midwives in England took oaths not to help with abortions and that the Common Council of New York City in 1716 adopted an ordinance forbidding midwives from performing them: "You [midwives] Shall not Give any Counsel or Administer any Herb Medicine or Potion, or any other thing to any Woman being with Child whereby She Should Destroy or Miscarry of that she goeth withal before her time."[63]

Another area which bears examination is the change which took place in both secular and Church legislation in the 19th century with respect to abortion. This is a critical period for the pro-choice argument: it is necessary for it to portray the significant tightening of abortion restrictions in this era, and the abolition of the "quickening" distinction as an aberration, as a deviation from the "true" tradition of the West. To do this it is necessary to argue that the change took place not because of increased scientific knowledge, which rendered the old distinction absurd, but because of more sinister and discreditable reasons. For a summary of the pro-choice view we can turn to Blanchard, who asserts there were four motives for the introduction of statutory bans on abortion in 19th century America: "the drive for medical professionalization, a call for moralism, concern for women's health and a mix of social forces stemming from industrialization and mass immigration."[64] As he puts it, "thus a coalition of medical professionals, moralists, xenophobics, anti-Catholics and anti-semites managed to get the various state legislatures to enact laws restricting abortion."[65] Note that there is no mention of a concern for the value of fetal life: by implication there is no pro-life tradition, only a variety of selfish or discreditable motives. This analysis appears as well in the historians' *Casey* brief, although somewhat more moderately phrased.

That brief's treatment of the period became the focus of attacks on its credibility, most notably in an article in *First Things* entitled "Academic Integrity Betrayed."[66] Illuminating as well was a roundtable discussion reprinted in *The Public Historian*, in which a number of those involved in preparing the historians' brief spoke candidly about some of the issues involved. James C. Mohr admitted that he did not "ultimately consider the brief to be history, as I understand that craft. It was instead legal argument based on historical evidence. Ultimately it was a political document."[67]

Strikingly the negative view of the 19th century American abortion reformers ignores what is actually in the source most frequently cited by pro-choice historians, James Mohr's *Abortion in America*. That work makes it clear that moral concern for the life of the fetus was of central importance. Even when suggesting that professional self-interest helped drive the anti-abortion crusade by 19th century physicians, he acknowledged the reality of their moral concern:

Compelling personal factors certainly added to the substantial professional motives for an anti-abortion crusade on the part of America's regular physicians. The first was a no doubt sincere belief on the part of most regular physicians that abortion was morally wrong. The fact that this belief coincided nicely with their professional self-interest is no reason to accuse physicians of hypocrisy on the issue; instead the convergence probably helps to explain the intensity of their commitment to the cause. As was pointed out in an earlier context, 19th century physicians knew categorically that quickening had no special significance as a stage in gestation.[68]

This is made even clearer in Marvin Olasky's very fine and little recognized work, *Abortion Rites: A Social History of Abortion in America*. He notes the real concern for human life manifested by the physicians who led the anti-abortion crusade and suggests that for many of them the slaughter they had witnessed during the Civil War had sensitized them to any attack on life.[69]

Two other things stand out in looking at the 19th century's attitude to abortion. One is the complete lack of any organized opposition to the new anti-abortion legislation. As Michael Grossberg has observed, "the public advocacy of contraception by sexual radicals and reformers.... had no pro-abortion counterparts."[70] If abortion was indeed a cherished common law "liberty," it is hard to imagine why legislature after legislature passed laws abolishing the "quickening" distinction and proscribing abortion. The most reasonable explanation is surely that as the scientific case became clearer that fetal development was continuous after conception, the public extended to abortion in early pregnancy the same disapproval with which late-term abortion had always been regarded.

Another notable circumstance is the opposition to abortion manifested by early advocates of women's rights. As Mohr observes, "Virtually all feminists, even those around Victoria Woodhull, viewed the prevalence of abortion in the United States as understandable, under the circumstances, but looked forward to its elimination rather than its wholesale adoption by all women."[71] If abortion restriction really was a plot by the patriarchy to oppress women, then why was it so fervently advocated by feminists?

Angus McLaren has greatly extended the reach of the "discreditable motives" argument, first to Britain and then to the Pope. In the case of Britain, McLaren asserts that the attacks made by doctors on the quickening doctrine reflected not so much the advance of scientific knowledge as a concern "to assert that only medical men could authoritatively discuss issues relating to physiology." While McLaren's assertion about motives is debatable, it is unquestionably true, as even he admits, that "the notion that the mother's awareness of fetal movements signified some clear stage of development was by the 19th century clearly no longer scientifically tenable...."[72] The mixed motives of the medical profession in advocating abortion restriction were earlier noted by John Keown, but Keown rightly insists on the reality of the moral concerns of doctors, particularly in the light of new scientific knowledge about fetal development.[73] The existence of mixed motives does not negate the existence of a pro-life tradition: a concern to protect human life, from the earliest time it was known to exist, was a part of Victorian England, as it was in America at the same time.

More daring is McLaren's suggestion that changes in the Roman Catholic Church also reflected base motives. The argument, advanced by Noonan and others that the Papacy moved to drop references to the "ensouled fetus" in its 1869 legislation on abortion because of the advance of scientific knowledge is rejected by McLaren. He insists that

the argument that the Church was concerned with scientific findings does not tally with the traditional view of Pius IX — the reactionary propounded of the Syllabus of Errors, the declarer of Papal Infallibility, and the institutor of the Dogma of the Immaculate Conception.[74]

This is a curious argument, which relies for its force on crude stereotyping: apparently anyone who believes in the Immaculate Conception is incapable of understanding science. The real core of his argument, however, is in the suggestion that the Church was responding to the increased power claimed by doctors over pregnancy:

The Church was more alarmed than relieved by the reports of doctors' increased ability to not only observe but to intervene in the process of reproduction. Pius, in dropping the reference to the 'ensouled fetus' and thereby condemning all abortions, was clearly launching the Church in a campaign against medical intervention in childbirth. Doctors might pride themselves on having led an attack against criminal abortions but they now found themselves in turn attacked by Catholics for their provision of therapeutic abortions.[75]

The argument advanced by McLaren is most unconvincing: it is in fact pure speculation presented with the utmost self-confidence. Even if the Church was spurred into action by concern over the actions of doctors in the 19th century — something which he does not prove — there is no case made that the growth of scientific knowledge was an irrelevancy. The changes in Church law represented not the abandonment but the development of a tradition: the truly reactionary position would have been to insist, in the face of increased knowledge, on the maintenance of distinctions regarding fetal life which arose from ignorance.

More persuasive is the view advanced by Noonan and Connery, that from the 17th century on several streams of thought contributed to wiping out the distinction between formed and unformed fetuses. One was the growing medical opinion that ensoulment occurred at conception, or very shortly thereafter. What was under attack here was the Aristotelian biology which had long been so influential. Another influence was the growing attention paid to the Immaculate Conception of Mary, and a concomitant tendency to see life as beginning with conception. The logical result was the 1869 extension of excommunication to all cases of abortion, not just for those where the fetus was older than 40 days. The tightening continued with the new Code of Canon Law in 1917, which made clear that all those involved in abortion - doctors and mothers - were excommunicated. During the same period the therapeutic abortion exceptions taught by some theologians were declared invalid by the Vatican. In 1930 the encyclical *Casti connubii* made crystal clear the utterly unacceptable character of abortion under any circumstances. This was reaffirmed by the Second Vatican Council.

The changes in abortion attitudes in English law, the corresponding tightening of American abortion laws, as well as the more restrictive Papal legislation, all must be set in the context of growing scientific knowledge about the nature of life before birth. The Aristotelian biology had fallen into discredit and scientists inclined more and more to the view that pregnancy was a biologically continuous process. The existence of the ovum was scientifically demonstrated in 1827, completing the triumph of the "ovists" - those who believed that human beings developed from eggs which were in some fashion activated by sperm. The rival theorists, the "animaliculists," believed that life developed from the sperm. As Carl Degler has put it, "what is spoken today as the moment of conception, the time when egg and sperm unite, had no specific meaning, or even conceptualization for people at the opening of the 19th century. About all that physicians and lay people alike knew was that at some point after sexual intercourse the male sperm (or the egg) began to develop into a recognizably potential human being." He notes that:

With the scientific establishment of the existence of the ovum and the idea of conception as the moment at which sperm united with egg to begin the process of growth that would eventuate in a baby, the whole matter took on a different aspect. Since the process from conception to birth was now viewed as continuous, whatever sanctity had been attached to the life of the fetus after quickening now had to be extended to the full life of the fetus before quickening began, that is, from the moment of conception.[76]

To conclude, it is clear that the pro-life movement has deep roots in the past, reaching back several millennia at least. There indeed existed a tradition which graded the protection accorded a fetus according to its stage of development, but that tradition rested on a view of fetal life no longer supportable in the light of the medical discoveries made by the early 19th century. The changes in the laws of Church and state in the 19th century represent a development, not a repudiation of that tradition. To deny this is of necessity to ignore the statements made by those effecting the change and to give credence instead to theories which attempt to place the full weight for these changes on discreditable motives. Such motives no doubt existed, but to make them the whole of the story is bad history. The pro-life movement should not look upon the years before the 1960ˢ as some sort of pro-life golden age: it was not. But it can see its concerns as part of a long and honored tradition.

NOTES

1. Joyce Appleby, Lynn Hunt and Margaret Jacob, *Telling the Truth About History* (New York: W. W. Norton 1994) 195.

2. John Noonan, "An Almost Absolute Value in History" in John Noonan, ed., *The Morality of Abortion: Legal and Historical Perspectives* (Cambridge: Harvard Univ. Press 1970) 1-59.

3. Michael A. Cavanaugh, "Secularization and the Politics of Traditionalism: The Case of the Right-to-Life Movement" in *Sociological Forum* 1/2 (1986) 251-283 at 260.

4. George Devereux, *A Study of Abortion in Primitive Societies* (New York: International Univ. Press 1976; 1ˢᵗ ed. 1955) 53. See also his "A Typological Study of Abortion in 350 Primitive, Ancient and Pre-Industrial Societies" in Harold Rosen, ed., *Abortion in America* (Boston: Beacon 1967).

5. Noonan 3-4.

6. Noonan 5. See also John M. Riddle, *Contraception and Abortion from the Ancient World to the Renaissance* (Cambridge: Harvard Univ. Press 1972) 18.

7. Aristotle, *Generation of Animals* II, 3 and *History of Animals* VII, 3 in Jonathan Barnes, ed., *The Complete Works of Aristotle*, Vol. I (Princeton: Princeton Univ. Press 1984) 1142-1144 and 913-914. Aristotle's theories are discussed in John Connery, S.J., *Abortion: The Development of the Roman Catholic Perspective* (Chicago: Loyola Univ. Press 1977) 17-18. Also see D. M. Balme, "*Anthropos anthropon genna*, Human is Generated by Human" in G. R. Dunstan,

ed., *The Human Embryo: Aristotle and the Arabic and European Traditions* (Exeter: Univ. of Exeter Press 1990) 20-31. Balme (p.30) writes that "Aristotle envisages conception as taking place slowly, over some days. But when then semen has, as he expresses it, 'set' the menstrual blood as rennet sets milk, the female's residue has acquired the necessary source of movement and has become a fetus.... It now possesses in potentiality all the soul faculties including nous." Also informative is Helen King's, "Making a Man: Becoming Human in Early Greek Medicine" in Dunstan 10-19.

8. A very restrictive reading of the oath is given by Riddle (pp. 7-10).

9. Michael J. Gorman, *Abortion and the Early Church: Christian, Jewish and Pagan Attitudes in the Greco-Roman World* (Downers Grove: Intervarsity Press 1982) 29-30; Riddle 21.

10. Connery 23.

11. Connery 22.

12. Connery 16.

13. Connery 15.

14. Connery 19. As Gorman says in *Abortion and the Early Church* (37), "While the translators of the Septuagint and the philosopher Philo distinguished the nonhuman from the human fetus, ... this legal concern should not be seen as the primary aim of these writers or of Alexandrian Judaism generally. Rather, their fundamental concern is the serious immorality of killing any unborn, especially when the killing is deliberately executed."

15. For fuller discussions of this complex topic see Gorman and Connery. Particularly useful is David M. Feldman, *Marital Relations, Birth Control and Abortion in Jewish Law* (New York: Schocken Books 1974). Especially significant is Feldman's statement (284) that non-therapeutic abortions are "very likely not even contemplated in the Mishnaic law." The claim by Riddle (20) that the passage in Exodus "seems to support abortion implicitly" does not seem tenable.

16. Sir Immanuel Jakobovits, "The Status of the Embryo in the Jewish Tradition" in G. R. Dunstan and Mary J. Seller, *The Status of the*

Human Embryo: Perspectives From Moral Tradition (London: King Edward's Hospital Fund for London 1988, printed and distributed by Oxford Univ. Press) 62-73 at 70. He expresses the same view in "Jewish Views on Abortion" in *Human Life Review* 1/1 (Winter 1975) 76: "While the destruction of an unborn child is never regarded as a capital act of murder (unless and until the head or the greater part of the child has emerged from the birth canal), it does constitute a heinous offense except when indicated by the most urgent medical considerations."

17. Dallas Blanchard, *The Anti-Abortion Movement and the Rise of the Religious Right: From Polite to Fiery Protest* (New York: Twayne Publishers 1994) 11.

18. Blanchard has almost certainly been confused by Noonan's discussion of the relative penalties attached to abortion at different stages and the fact that the abortion of the pre-quickened fetus was frequently not considered homicide. Whatever the penalties, abortion was always a sin and hardly "allowed" by the Church at any time.

19. Kristin Luker, *Abortion and the Politics of Motherhood* (Berkeley: Univ. of California Press 1984) 13.

20. Angus McLaren, *A History of Contraception* (Oxford: Basil Blackwell 1990) 82.

21. Daniel A. Dombrowski, "Augustine, Abortion and *Libido Crudelis*" in *Journal of the History of Ideas* 39/1 (Jan-Mar 1988) 151-154.

22. In Dunstan and Seller 39-57 at 40.

23. Connery 36-37.

24. Connery 39-40.

25. Connery 40-41, Gorman 57-58.

26. Connery 41-42. See also Noonan 13.

27. Connery 49, Gorman 66-67.

28. Connery 53-54.

29. Noonan 16, Connery 55-59, Gorman 70-72.

30. Dombrowski.

31. Quoted in Riddle 21.

32. For a discussion of this issue for several early writers, see Connery, ch. 4.

33. Noonan 32.

34. Quoted in Germain Grisez, *Abortion: the Myths, the Realities and the Arguments* (New York: Corpus Books 1970) 157-58; the other information in this paragraph also comes from Grisez 156-65.

35. Grisez 161.

36. Grisez 297-98.

37. Dombrowski 151.

38. See notes 2, 7, 9 above. Gerald Bonner, "The Teaching of the Early Church as regards Abortion" in Joseph W. Koterski, S.J., ed., *Life and Learning IV* (Washington, D.C.: Univ. Faculty For Life 1995) 230-252.

39. Connery 304.

40. Quoted in Noonan 15. Augustine's similar view is cited on the same page.

41. See Connery 54.

42. Quoted in Dunstan 44.

43. Dunstan 40, 55.

44. "Brief of 250 American Historians as *Amici Curiae* in Support of the Petitioners," reprinted in Leon Friedman, *The Supreme Court Confronts Abortion: The Briefs, Arguments and Decision in Planned*

Parenthood v. Casey (New York: The Noonday Press, Farrar, Strauss and Giroux 1993) 136-163.

45. James C. Mohr, *The Origins and Evolution of National Policy, 1800-1900* (New York, Oxford Univ. Press 1978).

46. Carroll Smith-Rosenberg, "The Abortion Movement and the AMA, 1850-1880" in *Disorderly Conduct: Visions of Gender in Victorian America* (New York: Oxford Univ. Press 1985) 217-244.

47. Cyril B. Means, "The Phoenix of Abortional Freedom: Is a Penumbral or 9th Amendment Right About to Arise from the 19th Century Legislative Ashes of a 14th Century Common Law Liberty?" in *New York Law Forum* 17 (1971) 335.

48. McLaren (note 20 above).

49. John Keown, *Abortion, Doctors and the Law: Some Aspects of the Legal Regulation of Abortion in England from 1803 to 1982* (Cambridge: Cambridge Univ. Press 1988).

50. Robert M. Byrn, "An American Tragedy: The Supreme Court on Abortion" in *Fordham Law Review* 41 (1973) 807.

51. Clarke D. Forsythe, "Homicide of the Unborn Child: The Born Alive Rule and Other Legal Anachronisms" in *Valparaiso Law Review* 21/3 (Spring 1987) 563-629.

52. For example, Robert Destro, "Abortion and the Constitution: The Need for a Pro-Life Protective Amendment"in *California Law Review* 63 (1975) 1250; James Witherspoon "Re-examining Roe: Nineteenth-Century Abortion Statutes and the Fourteenth Amendment" in *St. Mary's Law Journal* 17 (1985) 29; John D. Gorby, "The 'Right' to an Abortion: The Scope of Fourteenth Amendment 'Personhood' and the Supreme Court's Birth Requirement" in *Southern Illinois University Law Journal* 1 (1979) 1-36.

53. Brief of the American Academy of Medical Ethics as *Amicus Curiae* in Support of the Respondents and Cross Petitioners Robert P. Casey *et al.* (April 6, 1992).

54. Brief of the Association for Public Justice and the Value of Life Committee, Inc. (Feb. 23, 1989). This brief is reprinted as "The Historical Case Against Abortion" in *Continuity* 13 (Spring/Fall 1989) 59-83. See also Dellapenna's "The History of Abortion: Technology, Morality and Law" in *The University of Pittsburgh Law Review* 40/3 (Spring 1979) 359-428.

55. Dellapenna (see note 53 above) 7-8.

56. Shelley Gavigan "The Criminal Sanction as It Relates to Human Reproduction" in *The Journal of Legal History* 5/1 (May 1984) 20-41.

57. Byrn 815-16.

58. Quoted in Byrn 819-20.

59. Byrn 820.

60. Dellapenna (1979) 387-389.

61. Forsythe 568.

62. McLaren (89-112) makes reference to a number of these.

63. For references to the oaths imposed on English midwives, see Catherine M. Scholten, "On the Importance of the Obstetrick Art: Changing Customs of Childbirth in America, 1760 to 1825" in *William and Mary Quarterly* 34/3 (July 1977)429. Dellapenna reprints the 1716 ordinance adopted by the Common Council of New York as an appendix to his *Casey* brief, p. 37a. See also Dennis J. Horan and Thomas J. Marzen, "Abortion and Midwifery: A Footnote in Legal History" in Thomas W. Hilgers, Dennis J. Moran and David Mall, eds., *New Perspectives on Human Abortion* (Frederick, Md.: Univ. Press of America 1981) 199-204.

64. Blanchard 12.

65. Blanchard 15.

66. Gerald V. Bradley, "Academic Integrity Betrayed" in *First Things* 5 (Aug./Sept. 1990) 10-12. Significantly, one of the most notable signatories of the 1988 brief, James Mohr, did not sign the 1992 brief.

67. James B. Mohr, "Historically Based Legal Briefs: Observations of a Participant in the *Webster* Process" in *The Public Historian* 12/3 (Summer 1990) 25.

68. Mohr 164-165.

69. Marvin Olasky, *Abortion Rites: A Social History of Abortion in America* (Wheaton: Crossway Books 1992) 119-22.

70. Michael Grossberg, *Governing the Hearth: Law and Family in Nineteenth-Century America* (Chapel Hill: Univ. of North Carolina Press 1985) 169.

71. Mohr 111-12.

72. Angus McLaren, "Policing Pregnancies: Changes in Nineteenth-Century Criminal and Canon Law" in Dunstan 193.

73. Keown 38-48.

74. McLaren in Dunstan 196.

75. McLaren in Dunstan 196.

76. Carl Degler, *At Odds: Women and the Family in America from the Revolution to the Present* (New York: Oxford Univ. Press 1980) 240-41.

MAX SCHELER'S PRINCIPLE OF MORAL SOLIDARITY AND ITS IMPLICATIONS FOR THE PRO-LIFE MOVEMENT

John F. Crosby

When he addressed us at the UFL conference two years ago, Richard John Neuhaus made the following statement: "The great question, it seems to me, in the abortion debate — I've argued this for years — is not "When does life begin?" When life begins is not a moral question. It is self-evident to all sane people on grounds of undeniable empirical scientific evidence. But the great question is who belongs to the community for which we accept common responsibility..."[1] This caught my attention, for it was very challenging to me; I had always opened in abortion discussions with the personhood of the embryo, and here was Fr. Neuhaus saying that the real center of gravity in the debate lies elsewhere, it lies in a certain question of co-responsibility. In one point I disagreed with Fr. Neuhaus and still do disagree; in addition to the question when life begins in utero, which really is an empirical question, there is also the question when each human being as person begins to exist, which is not an empirical but a philosophical question. Nor is the answer to the question so obvious to all sane people as to render all discussion of it superfluous. Nor is it unimportant for our stance on abortion to be able to explain the personhood which the human embryo has from conception on. And yet I thought at the time, and I still think, that Fr. Neuhaus was right to object to a too exclusive preoccupation with the question of the status of the human embryo, and was right to warn against an unbalanced individualism which can prevent many people from understanding our pro-life commitment to pre-born human beings.

In what follows I will take for granted the personhood of the human embryo, and will try to explain to my own satisfaction, and hopefully to yours as well, some of the truths at which Fr. Neuhaus was hinting. And I will try to do this with the help of the great German philosopher, Max Scheler (1874-1928). Some of you may know of Scheler as the philosopher who, in the earliest days of the phenomenological movement (at the beginning of this century), brought the methods of phenomenology for the first time into contact with Christian thought. Except for the tragic last years of his life, Scheler did all of his so seminal work in philosophy as a convinced Catholic Christian. Of particular interest to us is his extensive work in philosophical sociology, such as his great study, *On the Nature of Sympathy*, or the sections on community in his *Formalism in Ethics*. By the way, you may also know of Scheler as the phenomenologist who influenced so profoundly the young Karol Wojtyla, who says at the beginning of *The Acting Person* that he owes the ideas of his book not only to St. Thomas Aquinas, but also to phenomenology in the interpretation of Max Scheler.

In 1917 Scheler wrote a study entitled "The Cultural Reconstruction of Europe," in which we read, probably to our great surprise:

A cultural reconstruction is only possible if an increasingly large proportion of the European peoples learns to look upon this cataclysm [World War I] as resulting from *a common guilt* of European peoples mutually influencing each other.... First, therefore, must come the recognition that in the final analysis there is only *one* answer to the question, Who or what nation is responsible for this war? The answer is You, the asker of the question — by what you have done or left undone.[2]

This way of extending the guilt and responsibility for a war strikes us at first as an exaggeration beyond all measure. But let us set aside for a moment the obvious objections which leap to mind, and let us let Scheler challenge a certain individualism that we all tend to hold. In the following we find him distinguishing between the guilt which concerns him in this essay and the guilt which will concern the politicians at the peace conference after the war: "I do not say that once and for all the politician or historian must refrain from asking where the *political*, historical guilt for the definite occurrence lies, guilt for the outbreak of August, 1914."[3]

In other words, as we might say by way of rendering Scheler's thought more concrete, Serbia had a responsibility for the outbreak of the war that, for example, Belgium did not have; on this level of guilt, Serbia was guilty and Belgium was innocent. But on the deeper level of guilt of which Scheler speaks, we cannot localize the guilt so easily; the guilt is more diffused, and almost everyone has some share in it. Scheler proceeds to explain this deeper guilt as a guilt, not for starting the war, but for creating the moral milieu in which the war was possible at all:

What forms the object of common guilt is not that the War did take place, still less the how and when of its beginning, but that it *could* take place, that *such* an event was possible in this European quarter of the human globe, that it was an event of such a nature as we know it to be. The object of common guilt is its possibility, then, and its quality, not its actual occurrence and real beginning. As you must be aware, within the individual the object of any deeper guilt-feeling is likewise not 'that I did it' but that I *could* so behave, was *such* a person as could do it. Only this common act of insight into the *reciprocity* of the shared responsibilities of every belligerent nation and all its subdivisions down to the family and individual can produce the psychological atmosphere from which European culture can arise renewed.[4]

Scheler means that everyone who in the years before the war did any moral wrong, contributed to the formation of the interpersonal situation in Europe in which a world war was possible. The wrong that each committed did not stay with the wrongdoer but was able to spread throughout the European community, enhancing the possibility of a world war. Many of you will recognize this idea of Scheler as an idea that stands at the center of Dostoevsky's great work, *The Brothers Karamazov.*

In one place Scheler makes an attempt to understand more exactly that transmission of good and bad by which we become co-responsible for so many others.[5] He tries to think through what is involved in me failing to show love to another to whom I should have shown love, and sees typified in this at least one mode of acquiring co-responsibility for others. He says that the other, whom I should have loved, would have been "called" to love me in return if I had loved him, since all love, by its inner logic as love, calls for some requital. My failure to love the other leaves him with one less reason for loving, for it deprives him of the call to requite my love. But in having one less reason for loving, the other grows that much less in the power to love, for the power to love grows by performing acts of love, as Aristotle recognized in his theory of moral virtue. When the other turns to all those who are his others, he turns to them with less power to love than he would have had if I had loved as I should have loved; in this way my failure takes its toll on all of his relations to others, thus making itself felt far beyond anything that I can track, just as the stone falling in the water sends its ripples across the lake and out of the sight of the one who dropped the stone. On the other hand, if I had loved as I should have loved, then I would have been co-responsible for the growth in the power of another to love, and thus co-responsible for the greater love that he would have shown throughout his life in all of his relations with others.

It should be clear that Scheler's *Gemeinschuld* (common guilt) has nothing depersonalizing about it, and that it is in no way meant as a substitute for individual guilt and individual responsibility. Common guilt has its origin in individual persons who are co-responsible for their community, and it is nothing apart from such individual persons. We can say that Scheler, far from denying individual responsibility, extends the range of it, so that it includes not only responsibility for oneself but also co-responsibility for others. It is true that, according to the logic of Schelerian co-responsibility, I am not the only one who is responsible for myself but that others are co-responsible for me, and that, as a result, my responsibility for myself is somewhat modified. But for Scheler these others never prevent me from also being responsible for myself, nor from being in some way co-responsible for all of them.

It is remarkable how the thought of Scheler, which for him can be understood in a properly philosophical way, can be found in a recent papal teaching. In his 1984 Apostolic Exhortation, *Reconciliatio et paenitentia*, John Paul II says (para. 16):

To speak of *social sin* means in the first place to recognize that, by virtue of a human solidarity which is as mysterious and intangible as it is real and concrete, each individual's sin in some way affects others. This is the other aspect of that solidarity which on the religious level is developed in the profound and magnificent mystery of the *Communion of Saints*, thanks to which it has been possible to say that "every soul that rises above itself, raises up the world." To this *law of ascent* there unfortunately corresponds the *law of descent*. Consequently, one can speak of a *communion of sin*, whereby a soul that lowers itself through sin drags down with itself the Church and, in some way, the whole world. In other words, there is no sin, not even the most intimate and secret one, the most strictly individual one, that exclusively concerns the person committing it. With greater or lesser violence, with greater or lesser harm, every sin has repercussions on the entire ecclesial body and the whole human body.

There are several consequences which follow from these ideas of Scheler for our pro-life commitment. The most important of them concerns our understanding of the wrongness of abortion. But before discussing that one, let us also consider this one. The responsibility for abortions is not limited to the women who have them or to the doctors who provide them or to the politicians and judges who legalize them. Scheler challenges even those actively committed to resisting abortion to consider that their own moral failings have contributed to the moral milieu in which easy abortion is taken for granted. If Scheler were still alive and we were to ask him about the guilt for the "culture of death" in which live, we can be sure that he would answer, not only by accusing Justice Blackmun, or President Clinton, but also by saying, "You who ask the question — you are in a way guilty, too. You of the pro-life movement, beware of the idea that the crimes of abortion are taking place completely apart from you. It is not enough to establish the fact that you did not commit the crimes, and in fact did not even instigate them, and have even officially disapproved of them. If you lived more just lives, it would be that much less possible for such a 'culture of death' to have taken root. Even you are to some extent implicated in the immeasurable reciprocity of guilt for our culture of death."

I should add right away that Scheler would, I am certain, have been quick to reject the quietistic consequences that one sometimes tries to draw from his idea of co-responsibility. He would not say that it is hypocritical for us to condemn and to fight against the providers of abortion. He would not try to level all moral differences between those who support and those who condemn abortion, just as he did not try to abolish, as we saw, the difference between the guilty and the innocent states involved in the First World War. He would not do this, because he never intended that his *Gemeinschuld* should substitute for the other levels of guilt where guilt is really more localisable. And yet it is true that those of us who fight abortion will be preserved from a certain pharisaism by remaining mindful that at the deepest level of guilt even we may have some co-responsibility for the culture of death.

But, as I say, this is not yet the most important implication of Scheler's social philosophy for our pro-life commitment. His thought on solidarity and co-responsibility also helps us to overcome a certain individualism that prevents many people from understanding the wrongness of abortion.

We have to realize that the reciprocity of moral influence which Scheler explores is for him not just a matter of empirical fact. Scheler does not think that we human beings could just as well have nothing to do with each other, exercising no influence on each other, and that it is only our factual social condition which occasions the vast mutual influence which we know from experience. No, he thinks that this mutual influence expresses something deeper in man, something metaphysical; the very essence of man as person is working itself out when persons influence each other beyond any possibility of keeping track of the influence. But to understand this we have to go to a more fundamental level of Scheler's thought and say a word about his understanding of the human person.

One finds in Scheler many deep insights into the individual person and the individual responsibility of individual persons; for all of his talk about *Gemeinschuld*, he never dreams of letting the individual get lost in some all-encompassing collectivity. In another lecture from 1917, "Christian Love and the Twentieth Century," he says that the recognition of "the infinite worth of the *individual* soul" is "the *magna carta* of Europe." In the same place he "categorically denies that the individual person is a mere 'modus' of some generality — the State, say, or society, or 'world-reason' or an impersonal... historical process."[6]

Scheler affirms that each individual person has so strong a being-of-its-own that no possible whole could ever encompass him as a mere part of itself. The individual person is a whole of his own. This is why Scheler in this passage speaks of the individual person as a subject of rights. He says that

the separate individual... has an original sphere of action and natural right which is all his own, is independent of the State and its legislation; therein he enjoys the exercise of those 'natural rights' which are innate in the essence of personality....[7]

On the basis of his deep understanding for the individual person Scheler can make telling criticisms of certain forms of social life. Thus, for example, he objects as follows to the ideal of political community that we find in so many ancient Greek thinkers:

they were ignorant of the independent, Stateless, God-created, spiritual and immortal soul, superior in its inmost being to any possible State, possessing an inner world of religion and morality.... Man they confined, to the very roots of his being, in the State, which meant in effect a restriction to things of this earth.[8]

With this personalism Scheler affirms something all-important for our pro-life philosophy; he affirms the basis of the "right to life" which we are always defending. But in this paper I want instead to draw your attention to something else in his understanding of the human person. In the same essay he says that

it is inherent in the *eternal, ideal nature* of a rational person that all its existence and activity as a spirit is from the very beginning just as much a conscious co-responsible, communal reality as a self-conscious, self-responsible, individual reality. The being of a man is just as originally a matter of being, living and acting 'one with another' as it is a matter of existing for oneself.[9]

Just as the distinct selfhood of each person is essential to each person, and not a result of accidental circumstances of our present form of life, so also our existing towards others, our existing with them, our co-responsibility for them. This relation to the other also belongs to the very essence of our personhood; it serves to define our identity as persons.

In another place he expresses the same idea, stressing the co-responsibility which belongs to us as persons:

each individual is not responsible solely for his own character and conduct, responsible through his conscience before his Lord and creator, but each individual... is, in its capacity as "member" of communities, also responsible to God — as fundamentally as for self — for all that bears spiritually and morally upon the condition and the activity of its communities.[10]

It is on this basis that Scheler rejects any and every social philosophy that sees the highpoint of social life in *Gesellschaft,* or society, which for Scheler means that form of living together in which all bonds with others, and all responsibilities for others, arise only through persons explicitly assuming responsibility for others. He rejects the idea that the individual person arbitrarily posits the social relations in which he lives, and that before he acts to posit them he simply stands next to other persons, lacking any bond with them. What he affirms, by contrast, is the idea that persons are bound to each other, and are thus co-responsible for each other, as a result of their very being as persons and in advance of any conscious acting (of course, he does not deny that there is *also* such a thing as an obligation that is freely assumed). Perhaps we can even say that for Scheler individual persons are from the very beginning comprehended in a fundamental human community; they do not create it, but awaken to it; their social existence unfolds within this community, and finds in it a basic norm.

It is clear that Scheler's stress on the individual person, which we were just examining, has nothing to do with the individualism proper to *Gesellschaft*; on the contrary, his personalism is something altogether different as a result of being organically completed by his teaching on co-responsibility.

We are now in a position to understand better Scheler's thought on the so-called common guilt and common responsibility in which we all share. It is because we are by our very natures as persons established one with another in a fundamental human solidarity and so have to do with each other even before assuming any particular responsibility — it is because of this that we dwell in an interpersonal space in which "there is no moral gesture so trivial that does not radiate, like the splashing stone, an infinity of ripples — circles soon lost to the naked eye."[11] From the point of view of *Gesellschaft* the moral condition of each individual remains shut up in the individual until he turns to someone who consciously receives his act. But from the point of view of what Scheler calls "the principle of moral and religious reciprocity or *moral solidarity*,"[12] the moral substance of the individual person essentially tends to fill the already existing interpersonal space and so to affect for better or worse the spiritual atmosphere in which the others breath. In this way each individual person becomes co-responsible for the moral state of more of his fellow human beings than he can possibly count. Thus it is the very essence of the human person, and not just changeable factual circumstances of our social life, which underlies the immeasurable co-responsibility in which we stand.

And now we are in a position to see what follows from Scheler's teaching for our understanding of the wrongness of abortion. As Fr. Neuhaus reminded us two years ago, it is not enough to appeal to the right to life of the unborn. Important as it is, indispensable as it is, to affirm that in every abortion a right is violated, this has to be completed by another affirmation. If our stance in this central moral question of our time is not to suffer a certain individualistic distortion, then we must also appeal to the moral solidarity of all men, to the fundamental responsibility for one another in which we are established. *Then it becomes evident that abortion is not only the violation of a right, but also the betrayal of a brother or a sister. It not only violates the rights of the aborted person, but also the fundamental solidarity in which we stand with him or her.*

Many of you know the article of Judith Thomson that appeared in a philosophy journal some years ago entitled, "A Defense of Abortion." It was very widely read and exercised no little influence. For the sake of her argument she assumed that the human embryo which is aborted is a person. She argued as follows. It is indeed very generous if a woman lets the child live which she has conceived, but the burdens of pregnancy are such that she usually has no obligation to keep it; in most cases the mother who keeps it is a Good Samaritan who goes beyond the call of duty. Abortion is justified from this point of view, not on the grounds that the embryo is not a *human* being, but rather on the grounds that it is not a *fellow* human being. Thomson seems to think that such "fellowship" as we have with others exists only a result of our consciously creating it. Indeed, she writes, exactly in the spirit of Scheler's *Gesellschaft*, "Surely we do not have any such 'special responsibility' for a person unless we have assumed it, explicitly or implicitly."[13] This point of view is challenged precisely by Scheler's principle of solidarity and of the co-responsibility for others in which we are established *even before we do anything in their regard.*

Perhaps we could even take a step beyond Scheler and say that there are also other levels of responsibility for others which lie beyond the level based on our common humanity. The child that the woman carries is not only a fellow human being to her, but is entrusted to her in a more particular way, being flesh of her flesh. If she aborts her child she betrays this maternal trust, in addition to violating a right. People like Judith Thomson will say that the relation of mother to child is at first a merely "biological" relation, and that only some "assumption" of responsibility by the mother lets an authentic interpersonal relation arise between them. This is exactly the point which we ought to contest. There are in reality all kinds of ways in which we are made responsible for one another "by nature," prior to all the responsibility that we freely contract. The mother-child relation is "by nature" a morally charged relation. It is a false body-soul dualism to declare the relation "merely biological"; from the beginning it involves body and soul, and is thus morally binds the mother to her child even before she assumes any responsibility towards the child. Once we have understood with Scheler the basic human solidarity in which we are established with all human beings, we can proceed to understand some of these more particular forms of solidarity in which we are established with certain others. In coming to understand better these various levels of solidarity, we will overcome that individualism which is one main impediment to understanding the pro-life position.

CONCLUSION

We all know the magnificent final chorus of the Ninth Symphony of Beethoven. The text of Schiller and the music of Beethoven celebrate a fundamental solidarity of all men, which is a source of profound joy for them. Dostoevsky has explored this solidarity in *The Brothers Karamazov*. Now Max Scheler has explored it philosophically in his elaboration of "the principle of moral and religious solidarity," which has a central place in his philosophy of the human person. It has lost none of its timeliness since Scheler formulated it at the time of the First World War, and in fact it has much to say to us in the pro-life movement as we try to deepen and develop the philosophical basis of our commitment.

NOTES

1. Richard John Neuhaus, "The Divided Soul of Liberalism" in *Life and Learning: Proceedings of the Third University Faculty for Life Conference,* ed. Joseph W. Koterski, S.J. (Washington, D.C.: University Faculty for Life, 1993) 7.

2. Max Scheler, "The Cultural Reconstruction of Europe" in *On the Eternal in Man,* tr. Noble (Hamden, Conn., 1972) 416-417. I do not think that the translator was well advised to translate *Gemeinschuld* as "collective guilt"; here and elsewhere I have amended his translation to read "common guilt."

3. Ibid.

4. Ibid.

5. See his *Formalismus in der Ethik und die materiale Wertethik* (Bern, 1966) 523-26. He recapitulates this analysis in "Christian Love in the Twentieth Century," 377-78.

6. Ibid. 384.

7. Ibid.

8. Ibid., 383. We need not concern ourselves with the question whether it is really possible to speak so generally of the "ancient Greek ideal of community," or whether one should restrict such characterizations to, say, the Aristotelian philosophy of the polis. What is important for us is that Scheler refuses to let the individual person be absorbed into the political community.

9. Ibid., 373. I have amended the translation in several places.

10. Ibid., 376. The polarity which Scheler recognizes in the human person — existing in oneself and existing towards others — was also affirmed by Vatican II in *Gaudium et spes* 24: "...man, who is the only creature on earth that God has willed for its own sake, can fully discover his true self only in a sincere giving of himself."

11. Ibid., 377.

12. Ibid., 377 (lightly amended by me).

13. Judith Jarvis Thomson, "A Defense of Abortion," originally in *Philosophy and Public Affairs* 1/1 (1971) 47-56; reprinted in *Ethics for Modern Life*, eds. Abelson and Friquegnon (New York: St. Martin's Press, 1987) 137.

About Our Contributors

Francis J. Beckwith (Ph.D., Fordham) teaches philosophy at the Univ. of Nevada, Las Vegas and is the author and editor of several books, including *Do the Right Thing: A Philosophical Dialogue on the Moral and Social Issues of Our Time* (1996), *The Abortion Controversy: A Reader* (1994), and *Politically Correct Death: Answering the Arguments for Abortion Rights* (1993).

Dr. Nigel M. de S. Cameron is Vice-President for Academic Planning and Professor of Theology and Culture at Trinity International University, Deerfield Illinois.

Keith Cassidy is a member of the History Department at the University of Guelph, Ontario. He is at work on a full-length study of the Right-to-Life Movement.

Teresa Stanton Collett, Esq. teaches at the South Texas College of Law in Houston, Texas, and has been a visiting professor at the Univ. of Notre Dame Law School.

William F. Colliton, Jr., M.D., received his medical education at Georgetown University and for over thirty years has had a private practice in obstetrics and gynecology. He is a Diplomate of the American Board of Obstetrics and Gynecology and a Clinical Professor at the George Washington University Medical Center.

John J. Conley, S.J. (Ph.D., Louvain) teaches philosophy at Fordham University. He has published many articles in ethics and is the director of the M.A. in Philosophical Resources at Fordham.

John Crosby (Ph.D., Univ. of Salzburg, 1970) has taught at the Univ. of Dallas, the Int'l. Academy of Philosophy (Liechtenstein), and is now professor of philosophy at Franciscan Univ. of Steubenville.

Eugene F. Diamond, M.D. is professor of pediatrics at Loyola Univ., Stritch School of Medicine. He has been President of the Catholic Physician's Guild and written five books, including *The Large Family: A Blessing and A Challenge* (1995).

Clarke D. Forsythe, Esq. is the President and Executive Director of Americans United for Life, Chicago, Illinois.

Michael J. Gorman is Dean of the Ecumenical Institute & Associate Professor of New Testament & Early Church History, St. Mary's Seminary & University, Baltimore, MD.

Jeff Koloze (M.A. in English, Cleveland State Univ.) is a part-time lecturer in English at Cuyahoga Community College. His dissertation will analyze three right-to-life issues in American fiction.

Joseph W. Koterski, S.J. (Ph.D., St. Louis Univ.) teaches philosophy at Fordham Univ. and is the Editor-in-Chief of the *International Philosophical Quarterly*.

Christine R. Kovach, Ph.D., R.N., teaches research design and gerontology illness management at Marquette University. Her interests are dementia care, special care units, adult day care, and reminiscence therapy.

Monte Harris Liebman, M.D. is a co-founder of the *Pregnancy Aftermath Helpline* and *People for Life of Milwaukee* and is currently the President and counseling instructor for Birthright of Waukesha County, Wisconsin. He has been a practicing psychiatrist and is currently the family day care provider of the Children's Day Child Care Center, Brown Deer, Wisconsin.

Anne M. Maloney (Ph.D., Marquette) is an Associate Professor of Philosophy at the College of Saint Catherine in St. Paul, Minnesota. She is also Vice-President of the Minnesota chapter of Feminists for Life, and a member of the Respect Life Commission for the Archdiocese of Minneapolis and St. Paul.

Judge Joseph W. Moylan received the B.A. in philosophy from Marquette in 1953 and his law degree from Creighton University in 1960. After a dozen years of private law practice he served on the bench of the Juvenile Court in Omaha, Nebr. from 1973 to 1993.

Patricia A. Noonan, M.S., R.N., is a clinical specialist at St. Camillus Health Center and served as one of the case managers for the Hospice Households project.

Robert O'Bannon (Ph.D., Univ. of Florida) is Professor of Health Sciences at Lee College in Cleveland, Tenn. He is an ordained minister in the Church of God and has served as a missionary in the Middle East, Africa, and Europe.

Vincent M. Rue, Ph. D., is Co-Director with his wife, Dr. Susan Stanford-Rue, of the Institute for Pregnancy Loss. He has lectured widely both in the U.S. and internationally. He is a traumatologist, researcher, psychotherapist, and forensic expert.

Susan Stanford-Rue, Ph.D., a professional psychological counselor, is Co-Director (with Dr. Vincent Rue) of the Institute for Abortion Recovery and Research located in Portsmouth, New Hampshire. She is the author of *Will I Cry Tomorrow? Healing Post-Abortion Trauma* (1986, 1990).

Sarah A. Wilson, Ph.D., R.N., is a nurse anthropologist whose research interests are hospice, death and dying, caregivers, and cultural influences on health care. Dr. Wilson is on the faculty of Marquette Univ. and teaches community health, chronic illness, and culture and health to graduate and undergraduate nursing students.

Carl Winderl received a Ph.D. in Creative Writing from New York Univ. and is now Professor of English at Eastern Nazarene College in Wollaston Park, Massachusetts. He has published one book of poems, *Poet at Large*, and nearly one hundred poems in various literary and university magazines.

Christopher Wolfe (Ph.D., Boston College) teaches Constitutional Law at Marquette Univ. and has written *The Rise of Modern Judicial Review* (1986, 1994), *Essays on Faith and Liberal Democracy* (1987), and *Judicial Activism* (1991). In 1989 he founded the American Public Philosophy Institute and currently serves as its President.

UFL Board of Directors*